T0236038

Informatik aktuell

Herausgegeben
im Auftrag der Gesellschaft für Informatik (GI)

Ziel der Reihe ist die möglichst schnelle und weite Verbreitung neuer Forschungs- und Entwicklungsergebnisse, zusammenfassender Übersichtsberichte über den Stand eines Gebietes und von Materialien und Texten zur Weiterbildung. In erster Linie werden Tagungsberichte von Fachtagungen der Gesellschaft für Informatik veröffentlicht, die regelmäßig, oft in Zusammenarbeit mit anderen wissenschaftlichen Gesellschaften, von den Fachausschüssen der Gesellschaft für Informatik veranstaltet werden. Die Auswahl der Vorträge erfolgt im allgemeinen durch international zusammengesetzte Programmkomitees.

Weitere Bände in der Reihe http://www.springer.com/series/2872

Thomas Tolxdorff · Thomas M. Deserno ·
Heinz Handels · Andreas Maier ·
Klaus H. Maier-Hein · Christoph Palm
(Hrsg.)

Bildverarbeitung
für die Medizin 2020

Algorithmen – Systeme – Anwendungen.
Proceedings des Workshops
vom 15. bis 17. März 2020 in Berlin

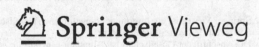

Hrsg.

Thomas Tolxdorff ⓘ
Institut für Medizinische Informatik
Charité – Universitätsmedizin Berlin
Berlin, Deutschland

Heinz Handels ⓘ
Institut für Medizinische Informatik
Universität zu Lübeck
Lübeck, Deutschland

Klaus H. Maier-Hein ⓘ
Medical Image Computing, E230
Deutsches Krebsforschungszentrum (DKFZ)
Heidelberg, Deutschland

Thomas M. Deserno ⓘ
Peter L. Reichertz Institut für Medizinische
Informatik
Technische Universität Braunschweig
Braunschweig, Deutschland

Andreas Maier ⓘ
Lehrstuhl für Mustererkennung
Friedrich-Alexander-Universität
Erlangen, Deutschland

Christoph Palm ⓘ
Fakultät für Informatik und Mathematik
Ostbayerische Technische Hochschule
Regensburg
Regensburg, Deutschland

ISSN 1431-472X
Informatik aktuell
ISBN 978-3-658-29266-9   ISBN 978-3-658-29267-6   (eBook)
https://doi.org/10.1007/978-3-658-29267-6

Die Deutsche Nationalbibliothek verzeichnet diese Publikation in der Deutschen Nationalbibliografie; detaillierte bibliografische Daten sind im Internet über http://dnb.d-nb.de abrufbar.

© Springer Fachmedien Wiesbaden GmbH, ein Teil von Springer Nature 2020
Das Werk einschließlich aller seiner Teile ist urheberrechtlich geschützt. Jede Verwertung, die nicht ausdrücklich vom Urheberrechtsgesetz zugelassen ist, bedarf der vorherigen Zustimmung des Verlags. Das gilt insbesondere für Vervielfältigungen, Bearbeitungen, Übersetzungen, Mikroverfilmungen und die Einspeicherung und Verarbeitung in elektronischen Systemen.
Die Wiedergabe von allgemein beschreibenden Bezeichnungen, Marken, Unternehmensnamen etc. in diesem Werk bedeutet nicht, dass diese frei durch jedermann benutzt werden dürfen. Die Berechtigung zur Benutzung unterliegt, auch ohne gesonderten Hinweis hierzu, den Regeln des Markenrechts. Die Rechte des jeweiligen Zeicheninhabers sind zu beachten.
Der Verlag, die Autoren und die Herausgeber gehen davon aus, dass die Angaben und Informationen in diesem Werk zum Zeitpunkt der Veröffentlichung vollständig und korrekt sind. Weder der Verlag, noch die Autoren oder die Herausgeber übernehmen, ausdrücklich oder implizit, Gewähr für den Inhalt des Werkes, etwaige Fehler oder Äußerungen. Der Verlag bleibt im Hinblick auf geografische Zuordnungen und Gebietsbezeichnungen in veröffentlichten Karten und Institutionsadressen neutral.

Springer Vieweg ist ein Imprint der eingetragenen Gesellschaft Springer Fachmedien Wiesbaden GmbH und ist ein Teil von Springer Nature.
Die Anschrift der Gesellschaft ist: Abraham-Lincoln-Str. 46, 65189 Wiesbaden, Germany

Bildverarbeitung für die Medizin 2020

Veranstalter

IMI   Institut für Medizinische Informatik,
Charité-Universitätsmedizin Berlin

Unterstützende Fachgesellschaften

BVMI	Berufsverband Medizinischer Informatiker
CURAC	Computer- und Roboterassistierte Chirurgie
DAGM	Deutsche Arbeitsgemeinschaft für Mustererkennung
DGBMT	Fachgruppe Medizinische Informatik der Deutschen Gesellschaft für Biomedizinische Technik im Verband Deutscher Elektrotechniker
GI	Gesellschaft für Informatik – Fachbereich Informatik in den Lebenswissenschaften
GMDS	Gesellschaft für Medizinische Informatik, Biometrie und Epidemiologie
IEEE	Joint Chapter Engineering in Medicine and Biology, German Section

Tagungsvorsitz

Prof. Dr. Thomas Tolxdorff
Institut für Medizinische Informatik
Charité-Universitätsmedizin Berlin

Tagungssekretariat

Sabine Sassmann
Institut für Medizinische Informatik
Charité-Universitätsmedizin Berlin
Hindenburgdamm 30
12203 Berlin
Telefon: (030) 450 544 502
Email: medinfo@charite.de
Web: http://bvm-workshop.org

Lokale BVM-Organisation

Prof. Dr. Thomas Tolxdorff, PD Dr. Jürgen Braun, Greta Maltsenko,
Sabine Sassmann, Dr. Thorsten Schaaf, u.v.m.

Verteilte BVM-Organisation

Thomas Deserno, Hendrik Griesche, Sven Neumann, Aaron Wiora und Jamie-Céline Heinzig - Peter L. Reichertz Institut für Medizinische Informatik (PLRI), Technische Universität Braunschweig und Medizinische Hochschule Hannover (Tagungsband)

Heinz Handels und Jan-Hinrich Wrage - Institut für Medizinische Informatik, Universität zu Lübeck (Begutachtung)

Andreas Maier - Lehrstuhl für Mustererkennung, Universität Erlangen (Social Media, Special Issue)

Klaus Maier-Hein, André Klein und Jens Petersen - Abteilung Medizinische Bildverarbeitung, Deutsches Krebsforschungszentrum (DKFZ) Heidelberg (Anmeldung, Mailingliste)

Christoph Palm, Alexander Leis, Leonard Klausmann und Sümeyye R. Yildiran - Regensburg Medical Image Computing (ReMIC), Ostbayerische Technische Hochschule Regensburg (Internetpräsenz, Newsletter, Social Media)

Thomas Tolxdorff und Thorsten Schaaf - Institut für Medizinische Informatik, Charité-Universitätsmedizin Berlin (Internetpräsenz)

BVM-Komitee

Prof. Dr. Thomas M. Deserno, Peter L. Reichertz Institut für Medizinische Informatik (PLRI), Technische Universität Braunschweig und Medizinische Hochschule Hannover

Prof. Dr. Heinz Handels, Institut für Medizinische Informatik, Universität zu Lübeck

Prof. Dr. Andreas Maier, Lehrstuhl für Mustererkennung, Universität Erlangen

PD Dr. Klaus Maier-Hein, Abteilung Medizinische Bildverarbeitung, Deutsches Krebsforschungszentrum Heidelberg

Prof. Dr. Christoph Palm, Regensburg Medical Image Computing (ReMIC), Ostbayerische Technische Hochschule Regensburg

Prof. Dr. Thomas Tolxdorff, Institut für Medizinische Informatik, Charité–Universitätsmedizin Berlin

Programmkomitee

Felix Balzer, Charité-Universitätsmedizin Berlin
Jürgen Braun, Charité-Universitätsmedizin Berlin

Thorsten Buzug, Universität zu Lübeck
Thomas Deserno, TU Braunschweig
Hartmut Dickhaus, Universität Heidelberg
Georg Duda, Charité-Universitätsmedizin Berlin
Jan Ehrhardt, Universität zu Lübeck
Sandy Engelhardt, Hochschule Mannheim
Ralf Floca, DKFZ Heidelberg
Nils Forkert, University of Calgary, Canada
Horst Hahn, Fraunhofer MEVIS, Bremen
Heinz Handels, Universität zu Lübeck
Tobias Heimann, Siemens Erlangen
Mattias Heinrich, Universität zu Lübeck
Alexander Horsch, TU München und Uni Tromsö, Norwegen
Dagmar Kainmüller, MDC Berlin
Ron Kikinis, Harvard Medical School und Fraunhofer MEVIS Bremen
Frederick Klauschen, Charité-Universitätsmedizin Berlin
Dagmar Krefting, Universität Göttingen
Titus Kühne, DHZB Berlin
Andreas Maier, Universität Erlangen
Klaus Maier-Hein, DKFZ Heidelberg
Lena Maier-Hein, DKFZ Heidelberg
Andre Mastmeyer, Hochschule Aalen
Dorit Merhof, RWTH Aachen
Jan Modersitzki, Fraunhofer MEVIS, Lübeck
Heinrich Müller, TU Dortmund
Nassir Navab, TU München
Marco Nolden, DKFZ Heidelberg
Christoph Palm, OTH Regensburg
Fabian Prasser, BIH Berlin
Bernhard Preim, Universität Magdeburg
Petra Ritter, BIH Berlin
Karl Rohr, Universität Heidelberg
Sylvia Saalfeld, Universität Magdeburg
Ingolf Sack, Charité-Universitätsmedizin Berlin
Dennis Säring, Hochschule Wedel
Ingrid Scholl, Hochschule Aachen
Stefanie Speidel, HZDR/NCT Dresden
Thomas Tolxdorff, Charité-Universitätsmedizin Berlin
Klaus Tönnies, Universität Magdeburg
Gudrun Wagenknecht, Forschungszentrum Jülich
René Werner, Universität Hamburg
Thomas Wittenberg, Fraunhofer IIS, Erlangen
Ivo Wolf, Hochschule Mannheim

Sponsoren des Workshops BVM 2020

Die BVM wäre ohne die finanzielle Unterstützung der Industrie und nicht-industrieller Partner in ihrer erfolgreichen Konzeption nicht durchführbar.

Dieses Buchprojekt wurde durch die großzügige Förderung des Berliner Institut für Gesundheitsforschung / Berlin Institute of Health (BIH) ermöglicht, wofür wir uns an dieser Stelle herzlich bedanken möchten.

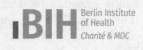

Darüber hinaus freuen wir uns sehr über die langjährige kontinuierliche Unterstützung mancher Firmen sowie auch über das neue Engagement anderer:

Platin-Sponsoren

Agfa HealthCare GmbH
Konrad-Zuse-Platz 1, 53227 Bonn

arxes-tolina GmbH
Piesporter Straße 37, 13088 Berlin

Bechtle AG
Kaiserin-Augusta-Allee 14, 10553 Berlin

Canon Medical Systems GmbH
Hellersbergstraße 4, 41460 Neuss

DEKOM Engineering GmbH
Hoheluft-Chaussee 108, 20253 Hamburg

Dell Technologies GmbH
Raffineriestraße 28, 06112 Halle (Saale)

ID GmbH & Co KGaA
Platz vor dem Neuen Tor 2, 10115 Berlin

Moysies & Partner IT Managementberatung
Adolfstraße 15, 65343 Eltville am Rhein

Philips GmbH
Röntgenstraße 22, 22335 Hamburg

Sectra Medical
Systems GmbH Gustav-Heinemann-Ufer 74c, 50968 Köln

Visage Imaging GmbH
Lepsiusstraße 70, 12163 Berlin

Gold-Sponsoren

Geschäftsbereich IT der Charité-Universitätsmedizin Berlin
Charitéplatz 1, 10117 Berlin

Chili GmbH
Digital Radiology Friedrich-Ebert-Straße 2, 69221 Dossenheim

Siemens Healthineers GmbH
Henkestraße 127, 91052 Erlangen

Silber-Sponsoren

ADR AG
Ludwig-Wagner-Straße 19, 69168 Wiesloch

Ayacandas GmbH
Neuer Zollhof 3, 40221 Düsseldorf

Circle Cardiovascular Imaging Inc.
Am Sandwerder 37, 14109 Berlin

Eizo Europe GmbH
Helmut-Grashoff-Straße 18, 41179 Mönchengladbach

FUJIFILM Europe GmbH
Heesenstrasse 31, 40549 Düsseldorf

Haption GmbH
Dennewartstraße 25, 52068 Aachen

Bronze-Sponsoren

AlgoMedica Europe GmbH
Waldhofer Str. 102, 69123 Heidelberg

GuiG – Gesellschaft für Unternehmensführung im Gesundheitswesen mbH
Rochusweg 8, 41516 Grevenbroich

Medneo GmbH
Hausvogteiplatz 12, 10117 Berlin

Medtron AG
Hauptstraße 255, 66128 Saarbrücken

Springer Vieweg Verlag
Abraham-Lincoln-Straße 46, 65189 Wiesbaden

Preisträger der BVM 2019 in Lübeck

Beste wissenschaftliche Arbeiten

1. **Katharina Breininger**
   (FAU Erlangen-Nürnberg)
   Breininger K, Hanika M, Weule M, Kowarschik M, Pfister M, Maier A:
   3D-Reconstruction of Stiff Wires from a Single Monoplane X-Ray Image.

2. **Lasse Hansen**
   (Institut für Medizinische Informatik, Universität zu Lübeck)
   Hansen L, Siebert M, Diesel J, Heinrich MP:
   Regularized Landmark Detection with CAEs for Human Pose Estimation in the Operating Room.

3. **Nils Gessert**
   (Medical Technology, Hamburg University of Technology)
   Gessert N, Wittig L, Drömann D, Keck T, Schlaefer A, Ellebrecht DB:
   Feasibility of Colon Cancer Detection in Confocal Laser Microscopy Images Using Convolution Neural Networks.

Bester Vortrag

Fabian Isensee
(Department of Medical Image Computing, German Cancer Research Center, Heidelberg)
Isensee F, Petersen J, Klein A, Zimmerer D, Jaeger PF, Kohl S, Wasserthal J, Koehler G, Norajitra T, Wirkert S, Maier-Hein KH:
nnU-Net: Self-adapting Framework for U-Net-Based Medical Image Segmentation.

Bestes Poster

Johannes Maier
(Regensburg Medical Image Computing (ReMIC), OTH Regensburg)
Maier J, Weiherer M, Huber M, Palm C:
Imitating Human Soft Tissue with Dual-Material 3D Printing.

Vorwort

Die Analyse und Verarbeitung medizinischer Bilddaten hat sich nach vielen Jahren rasanter Entwicklung als zentraler Bestandteil diagnostischer und therapeutischer Verfahren fest etabliert. Von Wissenschaft und Industrie kontinuierlich fortentwickelte Methodik und Gerätetechnik sorgen für eine stetig steigende Datenkomplexität. Diese Informationsvielfalt, gepaart mit ständig wachsender Verarbeitungsgeschwindigkeit von Rechnersystemen, verlangt neue Methoden, um die möglich gewordenen Vorteile zum Wohl von Patienten erschließen zu können. Die computergestützte Bildverarbeitung wird mit dem Ziel eingesetzt, Strukturen automatisch zu erkennen und insbesondere pathologische Abweichungen aufzuspüren und zu quantifizieren, um so beispielsweise zur Qualitätsverbesserung in der Diagnostik beizutragen.

Doch die Anforderungen sind hoch, um die Fähigkeiten eines Experten bei der Begutachtung von medizinischem Bildmaterial sinnvoll zu unterstützen. Dennoch gelingt dies durch zielgerichtete Algorithmen in Kombination mit der Leistungsfähigkeit moderner Computer. So wird es möglich, die Methoden der medizinischen Bildverarbeitung zur Unterstützung der Medizin und zum Nutzen der Patienten einzusetzen. Der Workshop Bildverarbeitung für die Medizin (BVM) bietet hier ein Podium zur Präsentation und Diskussion neuer Algorithmen, Systeme und Anwendungen.

Die BVM konnte sich durch erfolgreiche Veranstaltungen in Aachen, Berlin, Erlangen, Freiburg, Hamburg, Heidelberg, Leipzig, Lübeck und München als ein zentrales interdisziplinäres Forum für die Präsentation und Diskussion von Methoden, Systemen und Anwendungen der medizinischen Bildverarbeitung etablieren. Ziel ist die Darstellung aktueller Forschungsergebnisse und die Vertiefung der Gespräche zwischen Wissenschaftlern, Industrie und Anwendern.

Die BVM richtet sich dabei erneut ausdrücklich auch an Nachwuchswissenschaftler, die über ihre Bachelor-, Master-, Promotions- und Habilitationsprojekte berichten werden.

Der diesjährige Workshop findet nunmehr zum fünften Mal in Berlin statt und verbindet in diesem Jahr insbesondere wissenschaftlich hochaktuelle Themen mit dem klinischen Alltag. Neben spannenden Beiträgen der Teilnehmer konnten hierzu zwei hochinteressante eingeladene Vorträge gewonnen werden:

- Prof. Dr. Anja Hennemuth aus dem Institut für kardiovaskuläre Computerassistierte Medizin der Charité–Universitätsmedizin Berlin wird in ihrem eingeladenen Vortrag eine Übersicht über die Bildbasierte Modellierung in der Kardiologischen Medizin geben.
- Prof. Dr. Marcus Makowski aus dem Institut für Radiologie der Charité–Universitätsmedizin Berlin thematisiert die gewebecharakterisierende Bildgebung bei kardiovaskulären und abdominalen Pathologien mit Hilfe der reproduzierbaren Relaxationsparameter T1 und T2 in der quantitativen Kernspintomographie.

Die auf Fachkollegen aus Berlin, Braunschweig, Erlangen, Heidelberg, Lübeck und Regensburg verteilte Organisation hat sich auch diesmal wieder bewährt. Die web-basierte Einreichung und Begutachtung der Tagungsbeiträge wurde dankenswerterweise wieder von den Kollegen in Lübeck durchgeführt und ergab nach anonymisierter Bewertung durch jeweils drei Gutachter die Annahme von 76 Beiträgen: 28 Vorträge, 47 Poster und eine Softwaredemonstration. Die Qualität der eingereichten Arbeiten war insgesamt wieder sehr hoch. Die besten Arbeiten werden auch in diesem Jahr mit wertvollen BVM-Preisen ausgezeichnet. Die schriftlichen Langfassungen erscheinen in diesem Tagungsband, der von den Braunschweiger Kollegen aufbereitet und vom Springer-Verlag herausgegeben wird. Die LaTeX-Vorlage zur BVM wurde erneut verbessert und der gesamte Erstellungsprozess ausschließlich über das Internet abgewickelt, ebenso wie die von den Heidelberger Kollegen organisierte Tagungsanmeldung. Die Internetpräsentation des Workshops wird in Regensburg gepflegt und bietet ausführliche Informationen über das Programm und organisatorische Details rund um die BVM 2020. Sie sind zusammen mit den Inhalten der vergangenen Workshops auch über den Tagungstermin hinaus abrufbar unter der Adresse

https://www.bvm-workshop.org

An dieser Stelle möchten wir allen, die bei den umfangreichen Vorbereitungen zum Gelingen des Workshops beigetragen haben, unseren herzlichen Dank für ihr Engagement bei der Organisation des Workshops aussprechen: den Referenten der Gastvorträge, den Autoren der Beiträge, den Industrierepräsentanten, dem Programmkomitee, den Fachgesellschaften, den Mitgliedern des BVM-Organisationsteams und allen Mitarbeitern des Instituts für Medizinische Informatik der Charité.

Wir wünschen allen Teilnehmerinnen und Teilnehmern des Workshops BVM 2020 interessante Vorträge, nachhaltige Gespräche an den Postern und in der Industrieausstellung sowie spannende neue Kontakte zu Kolleginnen und Kollegen aus dem Bereich der medizinischen Bildverarbeitung.

Januar 2020

Thomas Tolxdorff (Berlin)
Thomas Deserno (Braunschweig)
Andreas Maier (Erlangen)
Heinz Handels (Lübeck)
Klaus Maier-Hein (Heidelberg)
Christoph Palm (Regensburg)

Inhaltsverzeichnis

Die fortlaufende Nummer am linken Seitenrand entspricht den Beitragsnummern, wie sie im endgültigen Programm des Workshops zu finden sind. Dabei steht V für Vortrag, P für Poster und S für Softwaredemonstration.

Postersession 1

Postersession 2

Session 3: Registrierung

Session 4: Bildrekonstruktion und -verbesserung mit KI-Methoden

Session 5: Segmentierung

Session 6: Neuroimaging

Postersession 3

Postersession 4

Software-Demo

Session 7: Trainings- und Planungstools

Inter-Species, Inter-Tissue Domain Adaptation for Mitotic Figure Assessment

Learning New Tricks from Old Dogs

Marc Aubreville[1], Christof A. Bertram[2], Samir Jabari[3], Christian Marzahl[1], Robert Klopfleisch[2], Andreas Maier[1]

[1]Pattern Recognition Lab, Computer Sciences, Friedrich-Alexander-Universität Erlangen-Nürnberg, Erlangen, Germany
[2]Institute of Veterinary Pathology, Freie Universität Berlin, Germany
[3]Institute of Neuropathology, Friedrich-Alexander-Universität Erlangen-Nürnberg, Erlangen, Germany
marc.aubreville@fau.de

Abstract. For histopathological tumor assessment, the count of mitotic figures per area is an important part of prognostication. Algorithmic approaches - such as for mitotic figure identification - have significantly improved in recent times, potentially allowing for computer-augmented or fully automatic screening systems in the future. This trend is further supported by whole slide scanning microscopes becoming available in many pathology labs and could soon become a standard imaging tool. For an application in broader fields of such algorithms, the availability of mitotic figure data sets of sufficient size for the respective tissue type and species is an important precondition, that is, however, rarely met. While algorithmic performance climbed steadily for e.g. human mammary carcinoma, thanks to several challenges held in the field, for many tumor types, data sets are not available. In this work, we assess domain transfer of mitotic figure recognition using domain adversarial training on four data sets, two from dogs and two from humans. We were able to show that domain adversarial training considerably improves accuracy when applying mitotic figure classification learned from the canine on the human data sets (up to +12.8% in accuracy) and is thus a helpful method to transfer knowledge from existing data sets to new tissue types and species.

1 Introduction

Mitotic figures, i.e. cells undergoing cell devision, are an important marker for tumor proliferation and their density is used in many tumor grading schemes for prognostication [1]. Fostered by the availability of datasets, this field has seen significant algorithmic advances in the very recent past. Especially in the field of human mammary carcinoma, one of the most common tumors in women, data

© Springer Fachmedien Wiesbaden GmbH, ein Teil von Springer Nature 2020
T. Tolxdorff et al. (Hrsg.), *Bildverarbeitung für die Medizin 2020*,
Informatik aktuell, https://doi.org/10.1007/978-3-658-29267-6_1

sets like MITOS [2] were able to include a great deal of variance that are typical in pathology. Since mitosis is a multi-phase process, the visual variability of its appearance in microscopy images is high. Besides this, there is a number of other factors that increase variance: staining is a manual or semi-automated process, and such is the preparation of the tissue sections to put on the microscopy slide. Another source of variance is the tissue itself, as especially macroscopic structures are differing considerably between tissue types. On top of that, we can expect differences between humans and other species - however, it could be well debated if, given a significant sources of variability, these would always play a major role.

All these factors cause a domain shift between data sets that is well-known in digital histopathology, and thus machine learning algorithms that have been trained on one data set will rarely directly transfer to another. Two classes of algorithmic adaptations to models are typically used in this regard: First, we can train a model on a large data set in one domain, which will allow to provide the model with a good initialization of its feature space for the next task, which is training the model with a (smaller) set of images in the target domain - typically referred to as *transfer learning*. This, however, requires annotated images in the target domain, which are also not always available to a sufficient amount.

Another approach is domain adaptation, which can also be done unsupervised, i.e. without any annotation and just images available in the target domain. These approaches rely solely on statistical properties of the input distributions, and will only work sufficiently if the derived real labels of the respective known source domain and the (assumed to be unknown) target domain follow the same ruleset. This is especially tricky in the field of mitotic figure detections, where individual thresholds play a significant role and thus the labels are significantly dependent on the expert defining the label.

Recently, Li et al. have shown, that a combination of an object detection network and a refining second stage classifier [3] show superior performance in mitosis detection, which was in line with our own findings [4]. Due to this, it seems interesting to have a first stage identifying mitotic figures, which acts as a coarse classifier and do the fine classification in a secondary stage, where domain adaption is most crucial. Thus, this work focuses on the distinguishing of mitotic figures from similar looking cells (hard negatives), which would be the task of the second stage.

2 Material and methods

In this work, we use four data sets, two from canine histopathology slides and two from human histopathology slides. Our research group recently published a data set of canine cutaneous mast cell tumor (CCMCT, a common tumor in dogs), spanning 32 whole slide images and providing annotation for all mitotic figures on the complete slides [4]. For this work, we have generated additionally a data set of canine mammary carcinoma (CMC) which includes 22 tumors also completely annotated blindly by two expert pathologists and with consensus found

Table 1. Comparison of the data sets used in this study. CMC and HUMMEN are unplublished (CMCT=cutaneous mast cell tumor; MC=mammary carcinoma; MF=mitotic figures; MFL=mitotic figures look-alikes; ME=meningioma)

data set name	species	tumor	cases	MF	MFL	annotations
CCMCT [4]	dog	CMCT	32	44,880	27,965	complete WSI
CMC	dog	MC	22	13,385	26,585	complete WSI
MITOS 2014 [2]	human	MC	11	749	2,884	selected area
HUMMEN	human	ME	3	782	1,721	complete WSI

for all disagreed cells using an open source solution [5]. As for human tissue, we set up a pilot data set of human meningioma (HUMMEN) consisting of three whole slide images from WHO grades I, II and III. All tissue was sampled for routine diagnostics and, where applicable, institutional review board approval and written consent was given (IRB approval number hidden for review). Additionally, we used the publicly available MITOS2014 data set [2], which contains mitotic figure annotations on human mammary tissue. All four data sets have in common that they contain not only true mitotic figure annotations, but also annotations that can easily be misinterpreted by either an algorithm or a human, but were in final consensus of all experts not found to be mitotic figures. These can be considered truly hard negative, and thus the differentiation between this group and the group of mitotic figures is one of the hardest tasks in mitotic figure detection. As Fig. 1 shows, the domain shift between the data sets can be nicely be spotted in a t-SNE representation, while the cell label is not easily distinguishable.

Domain-adversarial training [6] is an unsupervised network adaptation method, recently also employed in the field of histopathology [7]. It aims

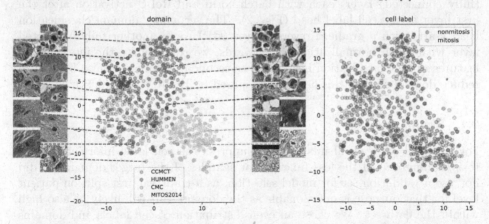

Fig. 1. T-SNE representation of the various domains and classes in our data set, features extracted from a ResNet-18 stem, trained on ImageNet. Human data sets are from mammary carcinoma (MITOS2014) and meningioma (HUMMEN), canine data sets are from cutaneous mast cell tumor (CCMCT) and mammary carcinoma (CMC).

Fig. 2. Domain adversarial training of our network.

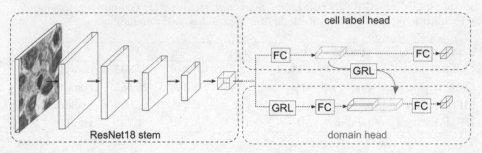

to account for a domain shift in latent space that is known to occur between slides of the same data set, but also, and more severely, between data sets. The core idea is to train a model with a body and two heads, where one head aims to perform classification of the cell class, and the other would aim for the classification of the domain. The latter inherently uses said domain shift to differentiate between data sets, however, it is this domain shift that we want to reduce.

Ganin et al.proposed to use gradient reversal during network training for this task [6]. The gradient reversal layer introduced by them acts as a pure forwarding layer during inference, but inverts the sign of all gradients during back-propagation. We aim to use the method to make the latent space representations for cell classification indistinguishable between source and target domain, and thus improve classification for the target domain in an unsupervised way. Using squared input images of 128px size with the respective cell at it's center, we employed a state-of-the-art network stem (ResNet-18 [8]) for the main feature extraction. After flattening the feature vector, we have two linear (fully connected) layers each with batch-norm and ReLU activation after the first layer as the cell label head (Fig. 2). The secondary domain classification head starts with a gradient reversal layer (GRL) and another fully connected layer with batch normalization. Afterwards, we concatenate the intermediate features of the classification head into the secondary branch, to also be able to reduce domain shift in this layer (as proposed by Kamnitsas et al.[9]).

2.1   Training

For training, we feed all images, and suppress the cell label information (mitosis/nonmitosis) in the loss function for samples of the target domain.We did not use a validation set for model selection, as a train/val/test split on patient level for that purpose is questionable as the domain shift will likely be also high within the data set. We chose an even distribution of cell labels and domains for both, the training and the test set.

We denote the output probability of the cell classification branch and the domain classification branch p_C and p_D, respectively. The true cell class and domain are denoted as y_C and y_D, respectively. We derive the domain classification loss as simple cross-entropy loss

$$L_D(y_D, p_D) = \begin{cases} -log(p_D) & \text{if } y_D = 1 \\ -log(1 - p_D) & \text{otherwise} \end{cases} \qquad (1)$$

With $y_D = 1$ representing the target domain, the cell classification loss is

$$L_C(y_C, p_C, y_D) = \begin{cases} -log(p_D) & \text{if } y_C = 1 \text{ and } y_D = 0 \\ -log(1 - p_D) & \text{if } y_C = 0 \text{ and } y_D = 0 \\ 0 & \text{otherwise} \end{cases} \qquad (2)$$

The total loss is a normalized weighted sum of both, i.e. with uppercase symbols denoting the respective mini batch vectors

$$L = \frac{\gamma}{\sum_i (1 - Y_{D,i})} \sum_i L_C(Y_{C,i}, P_{C,i}, Y_{D,i}) + \sum_i L_D(y_D, p_D) \qquad (3)$$

where γ is a tunable parameter. We trained for 3x30 epochs using super-convergence [10] and Adam as optimizer. For better comparability, we limited the number of cells for the large data sets to 1,600.

3 Results

Domain transfer raised the mean accuracy over 5 runs on the HUMMEN data set by 4.7 percentage points, on the MITOS2014 data set by 12.8 percentage points and in total by 6.5 percentage points (Fig. 3) compared to the baseline (i.e., without domain-adaptation). This improvement can largely be attributed

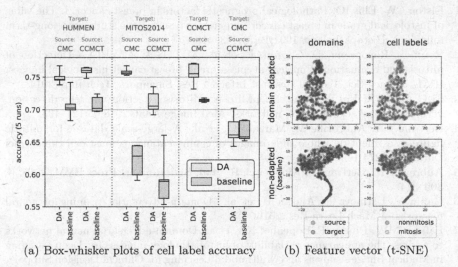

(a) Box-whisker plots of cell label accuracy   (b) Feature vector (t-SNE)

Fig. 3. Results of domain transfer. Plot a) shows accuracy for 5 runs on the different domain transfer tasks, whereas b) shows an example ResNet-18-feature vector with and without domain transfer (CCMCT to MITOS2014 task).

to a reduced domain shift in latent space (Fig. 3(b)). The performance varied both for the domain-adapted and the non-adapted case, and was especially large, where the original domain shift was most severe (MITOS2014 target data set). In this case, we achieved the best results when training on the same tissue type for a different species (CMC).

4   Discussion

Our results indicate that domain adversarial training is a suitable unsupervised learning method to perform mitotic figure domain adaptation between tissue and, equally importantly, also species. This is especially beneficial as publicly available, large datasets can be used for new domains - regardless of tissue/tumor type or species (animal or human). Further, we find a clear dependency on source and target data set, which is not surprising considering the initial latent space distributions. While the results showed clear benefits for the given task, we should point out our method needs access to pre-selected mitotic figures candidates, which we extracted beforehand. This step could, however, be taken over by generalizing model that was trained on a broad range of tissue, which we aim to investigate in future research.

Acknowledgement. CAB gratefully acknowledges financial support received from the Dres. Jutta & Georg Bruns-Stiftung für innovative Veterinärmedizin.

References

1. Elston CW, Ellis IO. Pathological prognostic factors in breast cancer. I. The value of histological grade in breast cancer: experience from a large study with long-term follow-up. Histopathology. 1991;19(5):403–410.
2. Roux, L, Racoceanu, D, Capron, F, et al. MITOS & ATYPIA - Detection of mitosis and evaluation of nuclear atypia score in breast cancer histological images. IPAL, Agency Sci, Technol Res Inst Infocom Res, Singapore, Tech Rep. 2014;.
3. Li C, Wang X, Liu W, et al. DeepMitosis: Mitosis detection via deep detection, verification and segmentation networks. Med Image Anal. 2018;45:121–133.
4. Bertram CA, Aubreville M, Marzahl C, et al. A large-scale dataset for mitotic figure assessment on whole slide images of canine cutaneous mast cell tumor. Sci Data. 2019;274:1–9.
5. Aubreville M, Bertram C, Klopfleisch R, et al. SlideRunner. Procs BVM. 2018; p. 309–314.
6. Ganin Y, Ustinova E, Ajakan H, et al. Domain-adversarial training of neural networks. J Mach Learn Res. 2016;.
7. Lafarge MW, Pluim JP, Eppenhof KA, et al. Domain-adversarial neural networks to address the appearance variability of histopathology images. In: Deep Learning in Medical Image Analysis and Multimodal Learning for Clinical Decision Support. Springer; 2017. p. 83–91.
8. He K, Zhang X, Ren S, et al. Deep residual learning for image recognition. Procs CVPR. 2016; p. 770–778.

9. Kamnitsas K, Baumgartner C, Ledig C, et al. Unsupervised domain adaptation in brain lesion segmentation with adversarial networks. Int Conf on Inf Proc in Med Imaging. 2017; p. 597–609.

10. Smith LN, Topin N. Super-convergence: very fast training of neural networks using large learning rates. In: Pham T, editor. Artificial Intelligence and Machine Learning for Multi-Domain Operations Applications. International Society for Optics and Photonics; 2019. p. 1100612.

Deep Segmentation of Bacteria at Different Stages of the Life Cycle

Roman Spilger[1], Tobias Schwackenhofer[1], Charlotte Kaspar[2,3], Ilka Bischofs[2,3], Karl Rohr[1]

[1]Biomedical Computer Vision Group, BioQuant, IPMB, Heidelberg University
Im Neuenheimer Feld 267, 69120 Heidelberg, Germany
[2]BioQuant, Center for Molecular Biology (ZMBH), Heidelberg University
[3]Max Planck Institute for Terrestrial Microbiology, 35043 Marburg
roman.spilger@bioquant.uni-heidelberg.de

Abstract. Segmentation of bacteria in live cell microscopy image sequences is a crucial task to gain insights into molecular processes. A main challenge is that some bacteria strongly change their appearance during the life cycle as response to fluctuations in environmental conditions. We present a novel deep learning method with shape-based weighting of the loss function to accurately segment bacteria during different stages of the life cycle. We evaluate the performance of the method for live cell microscopy images of Bacillus subtilis bacteria with strong changes during the life cycle.

1 Introduction

To cope with fluctuations in their environmental conditions, many bacteria can switch between a proliferative vegetative state and a metabolically inactive dormant state. For example, Gram-positive bacteria such as Bacillus subtilis form endospores as response to environmental stress, foremost starvation. Endospores are very resistant (e.g., to heat, UV irradiation, and antibiotics) and can stay dormant for many years without nutrients. Once growth-permissive conditions return, the bacterial endospores revert from the dormant state to the vegetative growth mode by spore germination and subsequent outgrowth. Imaging the life cycle of individual bacterial cells under changing environmental conditions is a powerful tool to investigate the mechanisms of these state transitions at the cellular and molecular level. However, a main challenge of analyzing the image data is that the appearance of bacteria changes strongly and asynchronously. In this work, we consider Bacillus subtilis bacteria that change their appearance from rod shape to bright and more circular endospores (see Fig. 1).

In previous work, different approaches for segmentation of bacteria in microscopy images have been introduced. In [1], a seeded watershed algorithm was used, and in [2] a threshold-based approach was applied. Liluashvili et al. [3] described an approach based on linear feature detection and probability maps

© Springer Fachmedien Wiesbaden GmbH, ein Teil von Springer Nature 2020
T. Tolxdorff et al. (Hrsg.), *Bildverarbeitung für die Medizin 2020*,
Informatik aktuell, https://doi.org/10.1007/978-3-658-29267-6_2

with splitting of bacteria at highly curved segments. Stylianidou et al. [4] used thresholding and the watershed transform for bacteria segmentation. Sadanandan et al. [5] employed thresholding with prior Hessian-based enhancement. However, classical approaches often have difficulties with high object density, low image contrast, and strongly changing object appearance. Deep learning methods can improve the performance under challenging conditions. This has been demonstrated for different image analysis tasks, including cell segmentation (e.g., [6, 7, 8]) and bacteria identification (e.g., [9]). In [6], the U-Net was introduced and applied to HeLa cells and glioblastoma-astrocytoma cells. In [7], a feature pyramid network to segment and count round cells in synthetic images was presented. In [8], a convolutional long short term-memory was combined with the U-Net [6] for segmentation of HeLa cells. In [9], a ConvNet was used to distinguish bacteria and non-bacterial objects in microscopy images of larval zebrafish intestines. However, none of the previous work on deep learning considered the segmentation of bacteria in temporal microscopy image sequences with strong changes of the appearance during the life cycle.

In this contribution, we introduce a deep learning method for segmentation of bacteria with strong heterogeneous appearance changes at different stages of the life cycle. We investigated different network architectures and introduce a novel shape-based weighting scheme for the loss function. The method was applied to live cell data of Bacillus subtilis bacteria and yields accurate segmentation results.

2   Methods

2.1   Network architectures

We studied different network architectures: U-Net, Residual U-Net, and Feature Pyramid Network (FPN). Compared to the original U-Net architecture [6] we introduced several modifications. The modified U-Net consists of five down-blocks paired with four up-blocks. A down-block consists of two convolutional layers with a kernel of size 3×3, each followed by a ReLU non-linearity and a batch

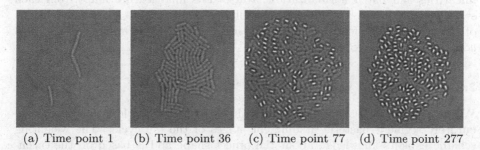

(a) Time point 1   (b) Time point 36   (c) Time point 77   (d) Time point 277

Fig. 1. Example images of Bacillus subtilis bacteria at different stages of the life cycle showing bacteria (time points 1 and 36) and a mixture of bacteria and endospores (time points 77 and 277).

normalization layer. Each down-block, except the last one, is followed by spatial downsampling via a 2×2 average pooling operation. An up-block includes a bilinear interpolation followed by a 1×1 convolution for spatial upsampling. The upsampled input is concatenated with the feature map from the corresponding down-block and passed to two additional 3×3 convolutional layers with ReLU non-linearity and batch normalization. A softmax output layer is used to determine a probability map. Final pixel-wise predictions are obtained by an argmax operation over the computed probability map. The modified U-Net differs in three ways from the original architecture [6]. First, we employ bilinear interpolation followed by a 1×1 convolutional layer, instead of using transpose convolutions for the spatial upsampling operation. This reduces checkerboard artifacts in the output. Second, we include batch normalization layers after the ReLU activations accelerating convergence and improving network accuracy. Third, we use average pooling instead of max-pooling to smooth the feature maps.

We also investigated the modified U-Net described above with short skip connections by incorporating residual blocks [10] (modified Res U-Net). Standard convolutional layers in down- and up-blocks are replaced by two back-to-back residual blocks. Each convolution in the residual blocks is followed by a ReLU non-linearity and a batch normalization layer.

In addition, we studied a feature pyramid network (FPN). While the general architecture with a contracting downsampling path and an expanding upsampling path is very similar to that of the U-Net, the FPN differs greatly in terms of output computation. Down-blocks in the FPN are very similar to the down-block in the residual network, where regular convolutions are replaced by residual blocks. Instead of spatial downsampling with an average pooling layer, we use a convolution with stride 2. In an up-block the feature map from the corresponding down-block is passed through a 1×1 convolution, and summed up element-wise with the (bilinear) upsampled feature map from the previous up-block. An out-block is appended to each up-block to generate the final feature map of the stage and reduce the aliasing effect of upsampling. An out-block comprises two 3×3 convolutions with zero padding, followed by ReLU non-linearities and batch normalization layers. The final feature maps from each stage are upsampled via bilinear interpolation to match the spatial dimensions of the output. The feature maps are stacked and passed through a final 3×3 convolution with zero padding.

2.2   Shape-based weighting of the loss function

We propose a novel shape-based weighting scheme for the loss function to accurately segment bacteria at different stages of the life cycle. The weighting scheme exploits knowledge about the object shape and is based on the eccentricity. The weights are computed as follows. First, regions are identified in the ground truth by connected components labeling. Second, for each region r the best-fitting ellipse is determined, from which the length of the semi-major axis a_r and the length of the semi-minor axis b_r are calculated. Then, the weight w_{ij} at pixel ij based on the eccentricity e_{ij} can be computed by

$$w_{ij} = 1 + w_0 \cdot (1 - e_{ij})^2 \quad , \qquad e_{ij} = \sqrt{1 - \frac{b_r^2}{a_r^2}} \tag{1}$$

where w_0 is an adjustable parameter (we used $w_0 = 10$). Strongly ellipsoidal shapes such as bacteria yield low weights, while more circular shapes such as endospores result in high weights. This weight map enables the network to focus on endospores during training to improve the segmentation of these structures. An example for a computed weight map is shown in Fig. 2.

2.3 Network training

Our dataset consists of 10 temporal microscopy image sequences of Bacillus subtilis each comprising 277 images. Ground truth for all 2770 images was obtained by manual annotation. The dataset is split into 72% for training, 8% for validation, and 20% for testing. We trained the networks using the standard stochastic gradient descent optimizer with a momentum of 0.9 and a batch size of 4. The learning rate is initially set to 0.01 and cosine annealing is used to adjust the learning rate after each batch. We use 128×128 random crops for network training. Standard categorical cross-entropy is employed as loss function.

3   Experimental results

We performed a quantitative evaluation for 554 live cell microscopy images (411×484 pixels). As performance measures, we used the Dice coefficient as well as intersection over union (IoU) which is also known as Jaccard index. We compared FPN, modified Res U-Net, and modified U-Net without and with shape-based weighting of the loss function. Results are provided in Table 1. Bold

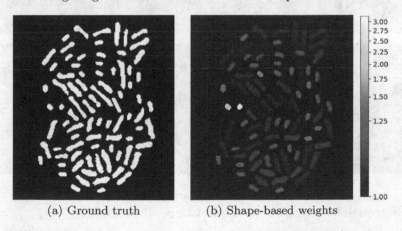

(a) Ground truth   (b) Shape-based weights

Fig. 2. Ground truth segmentation and corresponding weight map.

Table 1. Quantitative results of different network architectures.

	IoU	Dice
U-Net [6]	0.8746	0.9286
FPN	0.9198	0.9569
FPN + weighting	0.9298	0.9625
Modified Res U-Net	0.9352	0.9653
Modified Res U-Net + weighting	0.9387	0.9672
Modified U-Net	0.9385	0.9671
Modified U-Net + weighting	**0.9413**	**0.9687**

indicates the best performance. It can be seen that for all network structures, the proposed weighting scheme improves the result. The best result is obtained by the modified U-Net, which performs much better than the original U-Net [6]. The modified Res U-Net performs slightly worse than the modified U-Net, which indicates that adding skip connections does not improve the result. FPN is worse than the modified U-Net and the modified Res U-Net. The reason is probably that all images in the dataset were acquired with the same magnification and same microscope settings. Therefore, FPN can not take advantage of scale information. Sample segmentation results of the modified U-Net with weighting for different stages of the life cycle (no endospores, mixed, only endospores) are shown in Fig. 3 (time points 39, 69, 100, 157). It can be seen that the images are well segmented.

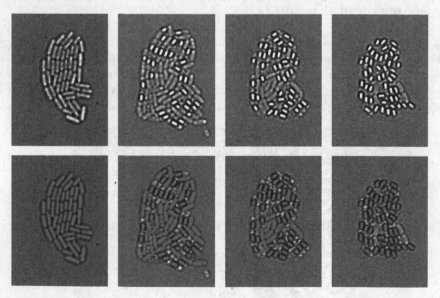

Fig. 3. Example results for different stages of the life cycle (colony growth). True positives (green), false negatives (red), and false positives (purple).

4 Conclusion

We presented a deep learning method combined with a shape-based weighting scheme for the loss function to accurately segment bacteria at different stages of the life cycle. We investigated different network architectures. The method was applied to temporal microscopy image sequences of Bacillus subtilis bacteria with strong changes in appearance. We found that the method yields accurate segmentation results.

Acknowledgement. Support of the DFG within the SFB 1129 and SPP 2202 is gratefully acknowledged. We thank Eva Schentarra for determining ground truth.

References

1. Battenberg E, Bischofs-Pfeifer I. A system for automatic cell segmentation of bacterial microscopy images. Arkin Laboratory for Dynamical Genomics, Lawrence Berkeley National Laboratory; 2006.
2. Chowdhury S, Kandhavelu M, Yli-Harja O, et al. Cell segmentation by multi-resolution analysis and maximum likelihood estimation (MAMLE). BMC Bioinformatics. 2013 Aug;14(10):S8.
3. Liluashvili V, Bergeest JP, Harder N, et al. Automatic single-Cell segmentation and tracking of bacterial cells in fluorescence microscopy images. In: BVM; 2015. p. 239–244.
4. Stylianidou S, Brennan C, Nissen SB, et al. SuperSegger: robust image segmentation, analysis and lineage tracking of bacterial cells. Mol Microbiol. 2016 Aug;102(4):690–700.
5. Sadanandan SK, Baltekin, Magnusson KEG, et al. Segmentation and track-analysis in time-lapse imaging of bacteria. IEEE J Sel Top Signal Process. 2016 Feb;10(1):174–184.
6. Ronneberger O, Fischer P, Brox T. U-Net: convolutional networks for biomedical image segmentation. In: MICCAI; 2015. p. 234–241.
7. Hernández CX, Sultan MM, Pande VS. Using deep learning for segmentation and counting within microscopy data. arXiv. 2018;/1802.10548.
8. Arbelle A, Raviv TR. Microscopy cell segmentation via convolutional LSTM networks. In: IEEE 16th ISBI; 2019. p. 1008–1012.
9. Hay EA, Parthasarathy R. Performance of convolutional neural networks for identification of bacteria in 3D microscopy datasets. PLOS Comput Biol. 2018 12;14(12):1–17.
10. He K, Zhang X, Ren S, et al. Deep residual learning for image recognition. In: IEEE CVPR; 2016. p. 770–778.

Retrospective Color Shading Correction for Endoscopic Images

Maximilian Weiherer[1], Martin Zorn[1], Thomas Wittenberg[2], Christoph Palm[1,3]

[1]Regensburg Medical Image Computing (ReMIC),
Ostbayerische Technische Hochschule Regensburg (OTH Regensburg)
[2]Fraunhofer Institute for Integrated Circuits IIS, Erlangen
[3]Regensburg Center of Biomedical Engineering (RCBE),
OTH Regensburg and Regensburg University
maximilian.weiherer@st.oth-regensburg.de

Abstract. In this paper, we address the problem of retrospective color shading correction. An extension of the established gray-level shading correction algorithm based on signal envelope (SE) estimation to color images is developed using principal color components. Compared to the probably most general shading correction algorithm based on entropy minimization, SE estimation does not need any computationally expensive optimization and thus can be implemented more efficiently. We tested our new shading correction scheme on artificial as well as real endoscopic images and observed promising results. Additionally, an in-depth analysis of the stop criterion used in the SE estimation algorithm is provided leading to the conclusion that a fixed, user-defined threshold is generally not feasible. Thus, we present new ideas how to develop a non-parametric version of the SE estimation algorithm using entropy.

1 Introduction

Endoscopic images often suffer from inhomogeneous illumination due to various imperfections of the image formation process [1]. In endoscopy, inhomogeneous illumination, also referred to as intensity inhomogeneity or shading, manifests itself as an intensity fall off towards the image borders. This effect is commonly known as *vignetting*. To ease further image processing and quantitative analysis shading-free images are desirable. Thus, shading correction is an important pre-processing step to compensate such intensity inhomogeneities, not only for applications dealing with endoscopic images, but also for those operating on images captured by a microscope, computer tomography (CT), ultrasound or magnetic resonance imaging (MRI) [2].

During the last few decades numerous algorithms were developed tackling the problem of retrospective shading correction, which is the process of estimating the best possible corrected image from an observed, shaded image [3]. Commonly used techniques include linear filtering, surface fitting, entropy minimization and

© Springer Fachmedien Wiesbaden GmbH, ein Teil von Springer Nature 2020
T. Tolxdorff et al. (Hrsg.), *Bildverarbeitung für die Medizin 2020*,
Informatik aktuell, https://doi.org/10.1007/978-3-658-29267-6_3

signal envelope (SE) estimation [4, 5]. However, all these methods assume gray-level images. For color images, only few approaches can be found in literature [1]. Basically, these methods try to adapt algorithms designed for gray-level images to color images by

1. converting the RGB image into common color spaces such as YUV or HSV,
2. applying gray-level shading correction to the intensity channels Y or V and finally
3. converting the image back to RGB color space.

A drawback of these approaches is their dependency on perfect separation of intensity and chromaticity. Furthermore, it is assumed that only the intensity of an image is affected by shading. Consequently, Bergen et al. [1] motivated principal component analysis (PCA) in order to construct a suitable color space which perfectly separates the shading effect into one channel.

To date, shading correction methods based on linear filtering, surface fitting and entropy minimization were already extended to color images [1]. In this work, we introduce a novel extension of the retrospective shading correction algorithm based on SE estimation [5] to color images using the PCA-related color space [1]. Additionally, we provide an in-depth analysis of the stop criterion used in the SE estimation algorithm since problems occurred in determining an appropriate user-defined threshold. Finally, new ideas are presented how to develop a non-parametric version of the SE estimation algorithm.

2 Materials and methods

We briefly describe the shading correction algorithm using SE estimation as well as its extension to color images. Finally, our experiments conducted for analysis of the stop criterion will be explained.

2.1 Gray-level shading correction using SE estimation

The algorithm presented by Reyes-Aldasoro [5] assumes that the shaded image N was formed by a linear image formation model, in which an ideal, shading-free image I was corrupted by an additive shading component S_A [4]. Consequently, the corrected image $\hat{I}$ is obtained as the best possible estimate of I, which is

$$\hat{I}(x,y) = N(x,y) - \hat{S}_A(x,y) + C_A \tag{1}$$

where $\hat{S}_A$ is an estimate of the additive shading component S_A and C_A a constant needed to restore a desired gray-level, e.g. the mean intensity of S_A.

In order to calculate $\hat{S}_A$, the algorithm adapts the well-known concept of SE detection used in electronic communications to gray-level images. In this context, the upper (lower) envelope of an image is defined as a smooth surface which outlines the maxima (minima) of the image intensities (Fig. 2(f, g), plotted along a scan line for simplicity). The smooth surface representing the upper (lower) envelope $S_{\max}^k$ ($S_{\min}^k$) is constructed as follows: Firstly, the algorithm blurs N to reduce the effects of noise. Then, $S_{\max}^k$ and $S_{\min}^k$ are calculated using an iterative process in which $S_{\max}^0(x,y) = S_{\min}^0(x,y) := N(x,y)$, initially. In the k-th iteration ($k \geq 1$) of the algorithm, the upper and lower envelope is given by

$$S_{\max/\min}^k(x,y) := \max/\min \left\{ \begin{array}{l} \dfrac{N(x-k,y-k)+N(x+k,y+k)}{2}, \\[2mm] \dfrac{N(x+k,y-k)+N(x-k,y+k)}{2}, \\[2mm] \dfrac{N(x-k,y)+N(x+k,y)}{2}, \\[2mm] \dfrac{N(x,y-k)+N(x,y+k)}{2}, \\[2mm] S_{\max/\min}^{k-1}(x,y) \end{array} \right\} \quad (2)$$

Afterwards, $S_{\max}^k$ and $S_{\min}^k$ are blurred using a kernel size proportional to k. Using an iterative process allows the envelope to adapt to objects of different sizes [5]. To determine a stop criterion, the *smoothness*, quantitatively expressed as magnitude of the gradient $G_{\max}^k$ and $G_{\min}^k$ of upper and lower envelope is calculated

$$G_{\max/\min}^k := \sum_{x,y} \|\nabla S_{\max/\min}^k(x,y)\| \quad (3)$$

where $\nabla S_{\max/\min}^k(x,y)$ denotes the gradient of $S_{\max/\min}^k$ at position (x,y) and $\|\cdot\|$ the euclidean norm. Using $G_{\max}^k$ and $G_{\min}^k$, in each iteration the relative change in smoothness Δ_{smooth} of either upper or lower envelope compared to the previous iteration is obtained as

$$\Delta_{\text{smooth}} = \min \left\{ \left| \frac{G_{\max}^k - G_{\max}^{k-1}}{G_{\max}^{k-1}} \right|, \left| \frac{G_{\min}^k - G_{\min}^{k-1}}{G_{\min}^{k-1}} \right| \right\} \quad (4)$$

The iteration stops when $\Delta_{\text{smooth}} < \delta$ for a user-defined threshold $\delta \in \mathbb{R}^+$. Finally, the smoothest surface, either $S_{\max}^k$ or $S_{\min}^k$ is assigned as additive shading component $\hat{S}_A$ and shading correction is performed using (1). According to [4], C_A is defined as the mean intensity of $\hat{S}_A$.

2.2   Color shading correction using SE estimation

In order to adapt the SE estimation algorithm to color images, we first construct a suitable color space which encodes the shading effect into one channel as suggested in [1]. This is achieved by applying a PCA to a set of pixels in RGB color space sampled from the acquired image $N^{RGB} = \{N^R, N^G, N^B\}$. The result is a transformation matrix $T \in \mathbb{R}^{3 \times 3}$ which aligns the RGB color space with the three principal axes C_1, C_2 and C_3, called *principal color components* (PCC). Thus, the shading effect in an image represented in PCC color space, denoted as $N^{PCC} = \{N^{C_1}, N^{C_2}, N^{C_3}\}$ is separated into the first component N^{C_1}. After calculating T, we follow the typical work-flow for color shading correction as described above:

1. Convert N^{RGB} to PCC color space: $N^{PCC}(x,y) = N^{RGB}(x,y) \cdot T$.
2. Apply gray-level shading correction on N^{C_1} using SE estimation

$$\hat{I}^{C_1}(x,y) = N^{C_1}(x,y) - \hat{S}_A(x,y) + C_A$$

3. Reconvert to RGB color space

$$\hat{I}^{RGB}(x,y) = \hat{I}^{PCC}(x,y) \cdot T^{-1}, \quad \text{where } \hat{I}^{PCC} = \{\hat{I}^{C_1}, N^{C_2}, N^{C_3}\}$$

Note that T is an orthonormal matrix with $T^{-1} = T^T$, where T^T denotes the transpose of T.

2.3   Experiments

Within our experiments, we provide an in-depth analysis of the smoothness-related stop criterion Δ_{smooth} used in the SE estimation algorithm. Aditionally, following Likar et al. [3] who suggested entropy as a global intensity uniformity criterion we evaluate whether or not entropy could serve as a more appropriate stop criterion. Therefore, in each iteration the relative change in entropy Δ_{entropy} of the corrected image $\hat{I}^k$ compared to the previous iteration is defined as

$$\Delta_{\text{entropy}} = \left| \frac{\text{H}(\hat{I}^k) - \text{H}(\hat{I}^{k-1})}{\text{H}(\hat{I}^{k-1})} \right| \tag{5}$$

where $\text{H}(\cdot)$ denotes the well-known Shannon entropy (see, e.g. [3]).

Experiments are based on six test images: three artificial images and three real endoscopic images of the human urinary bladder capured from cystoscopy. Artificial images with known ground truth (which is the true shading-free image) and different amount of shading were generated as described in [1].

For analysis, 100 iterations are performed for each test image and both stop criteria Δ_{smooth} as well as Δ_{entropy} are determined in each iteration. This results in a series of 100 corrected images for each test image. For artificial images the optimally corrected image $\hat{I}_{\text{opt}}$ is given by the minimal *root mean square error* (RMSE) between corrected image $\hat{I}^k$ and true image I. Due to the absence of a ground truth for real endoscopic images, the optimally corrected image could be determined only through visual inspection. Therefore, three individuals were asked to carefully select, from their point of view, the optimally corrected image $\hat{I}_{\text{opt}}$ out of the 100 corrected images. This procedure is repeated for all three endoscopic images.

3   Results

The results of our experiments using artificial and real images are presented separately in the following sections.

3.1   Artificial images

Exemplary, Figures 1(a) and 2(a-c) depict the result for the image corrupted by minor shading. The RMSE-optimally $\hat{I}_{opt}$ is obtained after $k = 11$ iterations ($\bar{k} = 9 \pm 1.63$ on average (Fig. 1(a), gray-shaded area)). The curve of Δ_{smooth} first decreases and then remains nearly constant whereas $\Delta_{entropy}$ falls down to a clearly noticeable minimum, increases and finally decreases again (Fig. 1(a)). Interestingly, both entropy and RMSE show a.very similar curve progression and reach the minimum almost after the same iteration. Thus, a low entropy corresponds to an optimally corrected image, which supports the ideas of Likar et al. [3]. However, the minimum of Δ_{smooth} is located a few iterations later.

Since the minimum of Δ_{smooth} is also greater than 0.01, setting $\delta = 0.01$ as suggested in [5] results in non-termination of the algorithm. However, increasing δ by only 0.5% up to 0.015 leads to $\hat{I}_{opt}$ (Fig. 2(a)). Obviously, for a user it is hardly possible to choose an appropriate value for a delicate parameter like δ.

For visual comparison, Figures 2(b, c) depict the simulated shaded image N and the true image I, respectively.

3.2   Real endoscopic images

An exemplary result for an endoscopic image is shown in Figures 1(b) and 2(d, e). Averaging the corresponding number of iterations and judged by visual observation, $\hat{I}_{opt}$ is obtained after $\bar{k} = 28 \pm 16.63$ iterations (Fig. 1(b), gray-shaded area). Similar to artificial images, Δ_{smooth} first decreases and then remains nearly constant. $\Delta_{entropy}$, however, strongly fluctuates (Fig. 1(b)). Since $\Delta_{entropy}$ reaches a minimum within the range where the optimal or nearly optimal solution is achieved, it further confirms entropy as a global intensity uniformity criterion.

Again, setting $\delta = 0.01$ the algorithm does not terminate within the first 100 iterations. However, already a minor increase of 0.25% up to 0.0125 results in a nearly optimal result (Fig. 2(d)) for the image investigated (Fig. 2(e)). This describes the same effect already observed using artificial images.

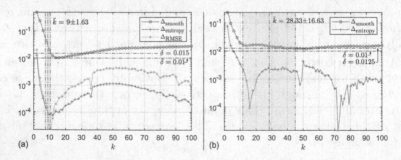

Fig. 1. Results obtained from the analysis of different stop criteria (log-scale) for (a) an artificial image and (b) a real endoscopic image. Instead of absolute RMSE values the relative change in RMSE Δ_{RMSE} is shown. Δ_{RMSE} is calculated analogously to (5).

Fig. 2. Visual results for (a-c) the artificial image and (d, e) the real endoscopic image used for analysis. (a) and (d) $\hat{I}_{opt}$, (b) and (e) N, (c) I. (f) shows intensity profiles of the corrected and (g) shaded C_1-channel of (e) as well as upper and lower envelope.

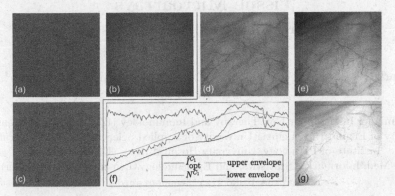

4 Discussion

In summary, no color artifacts were visible when using PCC color space for extending the SE-based shading correction algorithm to color images. Additionally, no computationally expensive optimization is required and neither size of objects nor their intensity with respect to the background need to be restricted [5].

Our analysis of the stop criterion indicates that a fixed threshold δ is generally not feasible since an appropriate value is hard to determine. Even minor changes of δ could lead to poor results, or, at worst, to non-termination of the algorithm. In the future we plan to develop a non-parametric version of SE estimation algorithm. Therefore, a possible approach could be to terminate if a local minimum of Δ_{smooth} is reached. According to our analysis, however, detecting a local minimum of Δ_{smooth} could lead to numerical instability as values tend to be nearly constant. Since $\Delta_{entropy}$ always shows an easy detectable minimum, a better approach would be to terminate if a local minimum of entropy is reached.

References

1. Bergen T, Wittenberg T, Münzenmayer C. Shading correction for endoscopic images using principal color components. Int J CARS. 2016;11(3):397–405.
2. Vovk U, Pernus F, Likar B. A review of methods for correction of intensity inhomogeneity in MRI. IEEE Trans Med Imaging. 2007;26(3):405–421.
3. Likar B, Maintz JBA, Viergever MA, et al. Retrospective shading correction based on entropy minimization. J Microsc. 2000;197(3):285–295.
4. Tomazevic D, Likar B, Pernus F. Comparative evaluation of retrospective shading correction methods. J Microsc. 2002;208(3):212–223.
5. Reyes-Aldasoro CC. Retrospective shading correction algorithm based on signal envelope estimation. Electronics Letters. 2009;45(9):454–456.

Neural Network for Analyzing Prostate Cancer Tissue Microarrays

Problems and Possibilities

Markus Bauer[1,2], Sebastian Zürner[1], Georg Popp[1], Glen Kristiansen[3],
Ulf-Dietrich Braumann[1,2,4]

[1]Fraunhofer Institute for Cell Therapy and Immunology (IZI), Leipzig, Germany
[2]Faculty of Engineering, Leipzig University of Applied Sciences (HTWK), Germany
[3]Institute of Pathology, University Hospital Bonn (UKB), Germany
[4]Inst. f. Med. Informatics, Statistics, and Epidemiology, Leipzig Univ. (UL), Germany
markus.bauer@izi.fraunhofer.de

Abstract. Prostate cancer (PCa) is the dominating malignant tumor for men worldwide and across all ethnic groups. If a carcinoma is being suspected, e.g. due to blood levels, trans-rectal punch biopsies of the prostate will be accomplished, while in case of higher stages of the disease the complete prostate is being surgically removed (radical prostatectomy). In both cases prostate tissue will be prepared into histological sections on glass microscope slides according to certain laboratory protocols, and is finally microscopically inspected by a trained histopathologist. Even though this method is well established, it can lead to various problems because of objectivity deficiencies. In this paper, we present a proof of concept of using Artificial Neural Networks (ANN) for automatically analyzing prostate cancer tissue and rating its malignancy using tissue microarrays (TMAs) of sampled benign and malignant tissue.

1 Introduction

The histomorphological grading of the PCa remains the most important prognostic parameter for the clinical management and is mostly done by the Gleason grading [1, 2] which assesses both the *glandular architecture* and the *pattern of tumor spread* (Gleason grades 1–5). To determine a substantial PCa malignancy grading based on "simple" morphological parameters may appear straightforward, but can be difficult, mainly due to a distinct heterogeneity of the PCa. A main problem of all grading systems in particular is their deficient reproducibility by independent observers [3], in part caused by differences across histology laboratory procedures. For the individual patient this intra- and interobserver variability adds more vagueness with respect to the therapeutic management of his own tumor. All this has led to a variety of previous work on digital microscope image processing in order to objectify PCa malignancy grading. E. g., an approach by Doyle et al. [4] exactly aims at such integration into routine

© Springer Fachmedien Wiesbaden GmbH, ein Teil von Springer Nature 2020
T. Tolxdorff et al. (Hrsg.), *Bildverarbeitung für die Medizin 2020*,
Informatik aktuell, https://doi.org/10.1007/978-3-658-29267-6_4

PCa histopathology, introducing a laborious approach for PCa grading based on hematoxylin & eosin (H&E) stained biopsies. It does textural tissue analysis in sub-cellular resolution, and applies a cascade of supervised trained classifiers in order to dividing into an overall of three malign and four benign tissue types, achieving an accuracy of remarkable 86%. Likewise, the work by Sparks and Madabhushi [5] operates on biopsies, but instead of textural features it focuses on glandular shapes which obtained an accuracy for separating Gleason grades 3 and 4 of 93%. Loeffler et al. [6] have demonstrated in a proof-of-principle study the descriptive potential of two simple geometric measures (shape descriptors) applied to sets of segmented glands within images of 125 PCa tissue sections. Using a classifier based on logistic regression, Gleason grades 3 and 4/5 could be differentiated with an accuracy of approx. 95%. As all such approaches trying to assess explicit glandular or textural features, machine learning approaches had been proposed, such as this by Salman et al. [7], where explicit features from local staining-related histograms and histograms of oriented gradients are being combined, leading to a mean Jaccard index of 0.678. The recent international development of AI based solutions for PCa grading appears quite lively, among them the solution by Arvaniti et al. [8] utilizing the MobileNet approach [9]. Their approach based on tissue microarrays (TMAs) achieved an accuracy of 70% with respect to clinically assigned Gleason grades.

2   Materials and methods

The aim of this work was to replicate an arbitrary measure of malignancy within a set of radical prostatectomy given with the Gleason grade. For analyzing the prostate tissue samples a neural network based supervised-learning algorithm was used.

2.1   Data set & pre-processing

The whole data set used for each experiment contains samples from 303 patients each consisting of two region-of-interest (ROI) images of the referring graded carcinoma, one image of intraepithelial neoplasms, one image of peripheral tissue and one image of benign tissue. The images of intraepithelial neoplasm and peripheral tissue were later dropped as they have been found to be misleading the network instead of training it. The slides have been scanned using a nominal quadratic pixel size of 235 nm. Each whole-slide image has an extent of around 6000 × 6000 pixels. In addition to the microscopy images themselves an arbitrary expert Gleason grading of the primary grades found in each ROI has been used. Because of the large image size of the whole-slide images, directly feeding them to a neural network would result in exploding training times and require an unfeasible amount of computational resources. Besides that, inconsistent color and background shape may be learned by the network. Hence, a pre-processing toolchain creating smaller image patches and minimizing color and background differences has been applied. First of all, from each circular shaped ROI image a square has been cropped by performing a circular Hough transform and extracting valid image coordinates within the detected circle. In addition, images with a too bright luminance channel were dropped to exclude remaining background images from more elliptical samples. The final squares had a measure of around 3300×3300 pixels. In the next step each square was split into a grid of images (:= patches) so that each image has a size of 660×660 pixels, leaving out the remaining images at the borders of each grid row. The created patch's dimensions additionally have been reduced using convolutional downsampling with a Lanczos kernel. Each image of the pre-training data and the new data had been stained using hematoxylin-eosin (H&E) coloring, where the eosin part mainly colors the stromatic parts in red while the hematoxylin is related to the nuclei's blue color. Especially the red stroma color can differ notably between whole-slide images. The staining differences have been found to take a major impact on the classification result, thus a solution to compensate them needed to be applied. In this work the stain-normalization of Vahadane et al. [10] has been used to solve this problem. Using these measures for the first time similar result to Arvaniti et al. [8] could be achieved. From the normalized patches 8 data and test sets were created using the Stratified K-Fold method of scikit-learn [11]. Each set contains around 2000 patches of Gleason grade 0 (benign) to 4 as well as 500 patches of Gleason grade 5. The number of samples has been clipped to balance out the data set. For each class (equal to the Gleason grade) a training-test-split of 10:1 has been used. The created patches have been derived gridwise and are therefore non-overlapping. Furthermore, it should be clarified that the TMA images already contain a high amount of relevant tissue, so the label for each patch has been chosen as the one of the TMA, which will however lead to an inevitable portion of wrong labeled patches. This must however be accepted as more detailed annotations are not available at this point.

2.2   Training process and validation

As it is commonly known, using a network pre-trained on similar data can improve the networks performance as well as speed up the training process notably. Hence, the network and weights of [8] have been used. For training the network further, as well as in the training up until this point, H&E-stained prostate cancer TMA slides have been used. The images fed to the network are the patches described above. To further avoid overfitting effects, besides the pre-processing, data augmentation techniques of rotation, shifting, shearing, stretching and flipping have been applied to the input. The training was done using an ADAM optimizer with a learning rate of 0.0001 and an α parameter of the ANN (a MobileNet) of 0.5. The trained architecture is based on Arvaniti et al. [8]. In addition, each convolutional layer makes use of batch normalization as well as a dropout with a rate of 50 percent. As a final measure against overfitting a weight decay with a rate of 25% has been applied. In addition to the use of the accuracy and loss metric, classification results have been manually checked for plausibility using class activation maps on selected images.

3   Results

The data as presented under Sec. 2 was used to train a neural network. For measuring the networks performance multiple test and training data folds have been used. Given these circumstances we achieved a classification accuracy of 68% in the final cross validation. For training the network multiple approaches have been used that included training on deeper architectures such as InceptionNet-V3 and VGG16, transfer-learning using ImageNet weights and using image patches created by rotating a square inside the circular ROI-image instead of splitting it into a grid. In each of the experiments selecting the grid-based approach for creating the image patches achieved better accuracy than the rotation-based one. Additionally, transfer-learning outperformed the training from scratch by means of accuracy and required training epochs notably. The best results could be achieved by a transfer-learning using the MobileNet architecture with pre-trained weights supplied by Arvaniti et. al. [8]. With this setup the convergence point of the loss and accuracy could be observed at around 50 epochs. As the network had already been pre-trained on images very similar to those used in this work, an initial performance measurement without further training has been done. Using the pre-trained network of Arvaniti et al. [8], an initial accuracy of 41% could be achieved, when using images that had not been stain normalized on purpose, to see how well the network performs on a wide spread color range. When normalizing all of the images to a fixed reference image of the same class taken from Arvaniti et al. [8] and training for 50 epochs, an accuracy of 94% could be achieved. Even though this result seemed to be promising it was not very feasible, as the patches do not only contain related morphological structures but e.g. also benign or stromatic tissue and thus a certain amount of confusion is expected to occur. The overoptimistic classification result is very likely related to the selection of a fixed reference image and the resulting memorizing of its color as a feature. This clearly shows the influence of the staining on the classification result. This assumption could be proven when normalizing all images to a fixed reference image which resulted in a strong confusion of all images with the references grade. As the total compensation of the staining influence has been found to be a very complex pre-processing task no de facto solution could be established due to time constraints of this work. To minimize

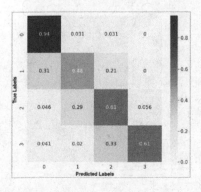

Fig. 1. Confusion matrix of the best fold trained. The labels refer to the primary Gleason grade where 0 equals benign tissue and 1–3 equal Gleason grades 3–5.

the effect as good as possible the training was repeated with reference images that were still related to the same class, but have been chosen randomly. After a further training for 50 epochs on the normalized data, the measured accuracy settled between 58 and 68%. Fig. 1 shows the confusion matrix of this result. For all folds confusion appeared most frequently between neighboring grades. When visualizing the class activation maps (Fig. 2), satisfying results could be achieved as well. For images containing a reasonable amount of basal cell walls the network was paying attention to them as expected. For benign tissue (upper half) the focus obviously lies on the gland walls, which for example can be seen in the top right corner. As well-enveloped gland walls are a tightly coupled morphological characteristic of benign tissue this seems plausible. For the more malignant Gleason grade 4 (lower half), where nuclei can be found separated or in groups larger than usual without a gland-wall-like structure, the network was also capturing this characteristic which can be seen in the bottom area of the image.

4   Discussion

An ANN training based on a relatively small data set of about 300 samples is an inherent challenge. For the present PCa grading application one faces the tension between the complexity of features to be learned and the limited availability of pre-trained models. Useful measures for preventing the network from over-fitting could be found in artificially enlarging the data set as was described above, as well as using batch-normalization, dropout/weight-decay and regularizing the input for neuron activity ranges and batch-standard/mean. Our paper describes that a ANN based approach to do PCa grading is basically transferable, though our results appear slightly worse than in [8]. We conclude from the analysis of our results that this is due to too strong remaining dependency on staining fluctuation inside the TMAs, which is tightly coupled to the process of preparation itself and needs to be tackled before the actual training. Another important fact is that labeling the data, using a supervised approach, still depends heavily on the expert rating in the first place and therefore (i) may be error prone and (ii) may be incomplete. A very recent cutting edge paper by a group from Google

Fig. 2. Network output for benign (top) and carcinoma (bottom) tissue with high (red) and low (blue) activations overlaid.

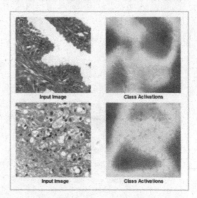

AI labs [12], though 100 million image tiles have been used for training the system, could reach 70% accuracy, similar like [8], and just slightly better than our system. This supports the thesis that problems in front of all arise from manual labeling. All in all we conclude that using ANN for rating malignancy within prostate tissue is a more promising approach than using shape descriptors, as those tend to miss patterns simply because those may have not been identified.

References

1. Gleason DF. Classification of prostatic carcinomas. Cancer Chemotherapy Reports. 1966;50(3):125–128.
2. Bostwick DG. Gleason grading of prostatic needle biopsies. correlation with grade in 316 matched prostatectomies. Am J Surg Pathol. 1994;18(8):796–803.
3. Allsbrook WC, Mangold KA, Johnson MH, et al. Interobserver reproducibility of gleason grading of prostatic carcinoma: urologic pathologists. Hum Pathol. 2001;32(1):74–80.
4. Doyle S, Feldman MD, Shih N, et al. Cascaded discrimination of normal, abnormal, and confounder classes in histopathology: gleason grading of prostate cancer. BMC Bioinformatics. 2012;13(282).
5. Sparks R, Madabhushi A. Statistical shape model for manifold regularization: gleason grading of prostate histology. Comput Vis Image Underst. 2013;117(9):1138–1146.
6. Loeffler M, Greulich L, Scheibe P, et al. Classifying prostate cancer malignancy by quantitative histomorphometry. J Urol. 2012;187(5):1867–1875.
7. Salman S, Ma Z, Mohanty S, et al. A machine learning approach to identify prostate cancer areas in complex histological images. In: Piętka E, Kawa J, Więcławek W, editors. Information Technologies in Biomedicine, Volume 3. vol. 283 of Advances in Intelligent Systems and Computing. Springer International Publishing Switzerland; 2014. p. 295–306.
8. Arvaniti E, Fricker KS, Moret M, et al. Automated gleason grading of prostate cancer tissue microarrays via deep learning. Sci Rep. 2018;8(12054).
9. Howard AG, Zhu M, Chen B, et al. MobileNets: efficient convolutional neural networks for mobile vision applications; 2017. arXiv:1704.04861 [cs.CV].
10. Vahadane A, Peng T, Albarqouni S, et al. Structure-preserved color normalization for histological images. In: 2015 IEEE 12th International Symposium on Biomedical Imaging (ISBI). IEEE; 2015. p. 1–4.
11. Pedregosa F, Varoquaux G, Gramfort A, et al. Scikit-learn: machine learning in python. J Mach Learn Res. 2011;12:2825–2830.
12. Nagpal K, Foote D, Liu Y, et al. Development and validation of a deep learning algorithm for improving gleason scoring of prostate cancer. npj Digital Medicine. 2019;2(48).

Is Crowd-Algorithm Collaboration an Advanced Alternative to Crowd-Sourcing on Cytology Slides?

Christian Marzahl[1,2], Marc Aubreville[1], Christof A. Bertram[3],
Stefan Gerlach[2], Jennifer Maier[1], Jörn Voigt[2], Jenny Hill[4],
Robert Klopfleisch[3], Andreas Maier[1]

[1]Pattern Recognition Lab, Department of Computer Science,
Friedrich-Alexander-Universität
[2]Research & Development Projects, EUROIMMUN Medizinische Labordiagnostika
AG
[3]Institute of Veterinary Pathology, Freie Universität Berlin, Germany
[4]VetPath Laboratory Services, Ascot,Western Australia
c.marzahl@euroimmun.de

Abstract. Modern, state-of-the-art deep learning approaches yield human like performance in numerous object detection and classification tasks. The foundation for their success is the availability of training datasets of substantially high quantity, which are expensive to create, especially in the field of medical imaging. Crowdsourcing has been applied to create large datasets for a broad range of disciplines. This study aims to explore the challenges and opportunities of crowd-algorithm collaboration for the object detection task of grading cytology whole slide images. We compared the classical crowdsourcing performance of twenty participants with their results from crowd-algorithm collaboration. All participants performed both modes in random order on the same twenty images. Additionally, we introduced artificial systematic flaws into the precomputed annotations to estimate a bias towards accepting precomputed annotations. We gathered 9524 annotations on 800 images from twenty participants organised into four groups in concordance to their level of expertise with cytology. The crowd-algorithm mode improved on average the participants' classification accuracy by 7%, the mean average precision by 8% and the inter-observer Fleiss' kappa score by 20%, and reduced the time spent by 31%. However, two thirds of the artificially modified false labels were not recognised as such by the contributors. This study shows that crowd-algorithm collaboration is a promising new approach to generate large datasets when it is ensured that a carefully designed setup eliminates potential biases.

1   Introduction

In recent years, the field of computer vision has experienced tremendous improvements in object detection and classification, largely due to to the availability of

© Springer Fachmedien Wiesbaden GmbH, ein Teil von Springer Nature 2020
T. Tolxdorff et al. (Hrsg.), *Bildverarbeitung für die Medizin 2020*,
Informatik aktuell, https://doi.org/10.1007/978-3-658-29267-6_5

high quality, high quantity labelled image databases and fostered by deep learning technologies. In the medical image domain, the availability of such data
sets is still limited for many tasks, as expert-labelled data sets are expensive to
create. To explore the potential of reducing the human annotation effort while
maintaining expert-level quality, we reviewed a method called crowd-algorithm
collaboration where humans manually correct labels precomputed by an automatic system. In contrast to classical crowdsourcing and its numerous successful
applications [1], this new method of crowdsourcing has been rarely applied to
medical datasets, for example by Maier-Hein et al. [2] and Ganz et al. [3]. In
the present study, we aimed to investigate several research questions regarding
crowd-algorithm collaboration for labelling cytology datasets: First, can crowdsourcing be applied to grade cells and is there a minimum skill level required?
Second, what are the advantages and disadvantages of crowd-algorithm collaboration? Third, can the crowd be fooled by artificially modified annotations
and if so, by what type of modifications? Finally, what would be a promising
design for using crowdsourcing for whole slide image annotation? To achieve our
aims, we carefully designed, performed and evaluated a set of experiments with
crowdsourcing and crowd-algorithm collaboration on a pulmonary haemorrhage
cytology dataset. This dataset was selected because it is a realistic example for
the medical field due to its properties of having a high inter- and intra-observer
variability and only a few examples explaining the grading process in the reference paper [4]. A trained deep learning model to create algorithmic annotations
developed by Marzahl et al. [5] is publicly available making the dataset suitable
for the presented crowd-algorithm collaboration study.

2   Material and methods

Our research group built a dataset of 57 cytological slides of equine bronchoalveolar lavage fluid. The slides were prepared by cytocentrifugation and then stained
to highlight the cellular iron content with Prussian Blue (n=28) or Turnbull's
Blue (n=29), which result in an identical colour pattern. The glass slides were
digitalised using a linear scanner (Aperio ScanScope CS2, Leica Biosystems, Germany) at a magnification of 400× with a resolution of 0.25 $\frac{\mu m}{px}$. Finally, 17 slides
were completely annotated and scored by a veterinary pathologist, according to
M. Y. Doucet and L. Viel [6] into five grades from zero to four. This annotated
part of the dataset containing 78,047 labeled cells ($\mu = 4,591$, $\sigma = 3,389$ per
image, resp.).

2.1   Patch selection

To evaluate the human inter- and intra-observer variability jointly with the influence of precomputed annotations, we extracted twenty 256×256 pixels patches
from the unannotated slides. According to Irshad et al. [6], the crowdsourcing
performance degrades significantly with larger patch sizes. In consequence, we
used the smallest reasonable patch size, which can contain 15 of the largest cells.

Twenty patches with at least 15 cells each contain around 300 hemosiderophages as recommended for grading by Golde et al. [7]. The patches were chosen such that each patch covered all on that whole slide image (WSI) available grades, that only one patch was extracted per WSI, and that the two staining types were equally represented over all patches.

2.2   Label generation

For the crowd-algorithm mode, the labels were generated by the RetinaNet implementation provided from [5] on the same twenty images. To investigate the effect of augmented images, the predictions were modified on some images. On five images, we removed the augmented annotation for one cell. On five other images, we increased all grades by one step. Finally, five images contained standard object detection-caused artefacts like multiple annotations for one cell or false positive hemosiderophages. The augmented images are chosen randomly without replacement.

2.3   Labelling platform

To estimate the effect of human qualification and experience, we divided our twenty contributors equally into four groups according to their qualification and experience with bronchoalveolar lavage (BAL) cytology.

1. No experience in cytology (e.g computer scientist or chemists)
2. Beginner skills in cytology (e.g. biologist in training)
3. Professionals in the field of cytology (e.g. trained biologist)
4. Veterinary pathologist or clinician with a high degree of experience in BAL cytology.

All contributors have provided written consent to participate in this study. We employed the Labelbox [1] platform to host our experiments. Labelbox is a crowd-sourcing platform which focuses on combining human annotations and machine learning methods to create high-quality datasets. Fig. 1 left visualises the Label-Box annotation interface. Anonymity was ensured by checking that no private information is saved in the files' meta-data and that no personal information can be extracted.

2.4   Label experiment design

We designed our experiments with the aim of estimating the effect of computer-aided annotation methods on crowdsourcing. For that purpose, two modes were created in Labelbox: Crowd-algorithm mode, where the contributor is asked to enhance the predictions made by a deep learning system, and annotation mode, where all annotations were performed by the participants without algorithmic support. Each mode started with a trial image to get familiar with the user interface.

---

[1] https://labelbox.com/

3   Results

In total, the twenty contributors made 9524 annotations on 800 images which took around 20 hours. Three veterinary pathologists defined the ground truth by majority vote. Additionally, we compared the contributors' performance with an algorithmic baseline set by a customised RetinaNet model [5].

The crowd-algorithm mode led to significant better results [$F(1,38) = 10.1$, p=0,003] than the annotation mode with an accuracy ranging from 67-89% (μ=74, σ=6) compared to 53-86% (μ=67, σ=7), while the deep learning-based approach alone reached an accuracy of 86% (Fig. 2). The inter-observer Fleiss' kappa score was 0.51 for the annotation mode and 0.71 for the crowd-algorithm mode. In crowd-algorithm mode the elapsed time to complete an image decreased on average from 106 to 74 seconds compared to annotation mode. Simultaneously, the mean average precision (mAP) with an IoU > .5 increased from μ=0.47 (min=0.29, max=0.68, σ=0.09) to μ=0.55 (min=0.47, max=0.78, σ=0.8) and the average precision without grade from μ=0.78 (min=0.47, max=0.91, σ=0.10) to μ=0.92 (min=0.78, max=0.96, σ=0.04) (Fig 2). Additionally, there was no significant performance difference between the groups [$F(3,16) = 0.4715$, p=.7]. If the participants performed the crowd-algorithm task prior to the annotation task, the accuracy variance decreased from 8% (min=53, max=86, μ=68) to 6% (min=59, max=80, μ=67), and the mAP variance decreased from 11% (min=0.29, max=0.68, μ=0.46) to 4% (min=0.44, max=0.59, μ=0.48). The participants found and corrected 74% of the artificially removed cells and 86% of the non-maximum suppression artefacts, but they failed to correct 67% of the cells with artificially increased grade.

The intra-observer cell-based classification accuracy ranged from 56-86% (μ=68, σ=8) with a mean Cohen's kappa score of 0.59. For the object detection performance the mAP ranges from 0.68-0.74 (μ=0.46, σ=0.13) (Fig 1).

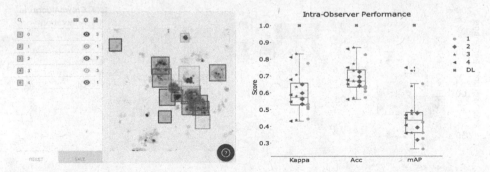

Fig. 1. From left to right: The screenshot shows the Labelbox user interface with the precomputed annotations; On the right, the intra-observer performance for Cohens Kappa, classification accuracy (Acc) and mean average precision (mAP) for the groups of participants and the deep learning approach (DL).

The code for all experiments is available online (https://github.com/ ChristianMarzahl/EIPH_WSI), together with the anonymised participant contributions and the image dataset.

4   Discussion and outlook

Our study shows that the use of precomputed annotations may lead to an increase in accuracy independent of the contributor's skill level, and to a reduction of interaction time by 30%. Remarkably, only the two experts with the highest overall scores (a veterinary pathologist and a cytologist) deteriorated by around two percent in crowd-algorithm mode due to the manifested effect of accepting augmented grades. Although contributors were grouped and selected in concordance to their level of expertise with BAL cytology, there was no apparent difference between the performance of the groups. Additionally, we noticed a training effect when the crowd-algorithm mode was performed first, which was recognisable by a reduced variance and an increased mean average precision in the following annotation mode.

Participants achieved excellent results in the task of correcting non-maximum suppression artefacts or missing cells but failed to correct two thirds of the artificially increased cells. A reason for this could be that the Labelbox user interface adds a shading overlay over each cell altering its visual appearance, which led to an increase in interaction time because contributors often activated and deactivated the shading to better visualize the cell underneath. Furthermore, the task of assigning a grade to cells seems to be more challenging than only

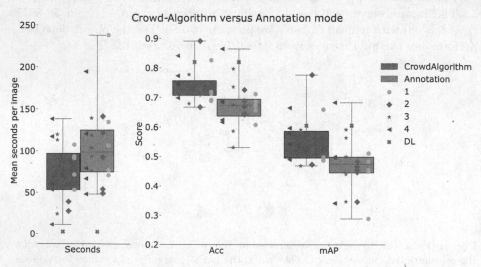

Fig. 2. The crowd-algorithm versus annotation plot compares the increased Acc and mAP jointly with the decreased interaction time between groups for the crowd-algorithm mode. DL represents the deep learning-based scores and the numbers from one to four denote the groups of participats.

identifying them, as shown by the high mAP scores irrespective of the grade. The observed effect towards accepting the augmented grades was independent of the contributor's skill level and should be closely monitored to avoid introducing any unwanted bias into the dataset.

One limitation of this study is that the field of view contained only a limited number of cells, which is not comparable to the usual process of annotating 300 cells freely on a whole slide image. In this case, human performance is expected to decrease. Another drawback of the crowd-algorithm approach is that training data annotated from a pathologist has to be available in a sufficient quantity to train a deep learning-based method.

The insights from this study allow us to effectively use crowd-algorithm collaboration in further work to label large high quality whole slide image datasets. However, the bias towards accepting precomputed grades has to be considered, and the training period of participants has to be extended. In conclusion, we would recommend using crowd-algorithm collaboration for the task of grading pulmonary hemosiderophages only if high quality precomputed annotations are available, and only for the task of correcting object detection and not for finding classification errors.

Acknowledgement. We thank Labelbox for providing us with a education license, and we thank all contributors for making this work possible. CAB gratefully acknowledges financial support received from the Dres. Jutta & Georg Bruns-Stiftung für innovative Veterinärmedizin.

References

1. Ørting S, Doyle A, van Hilten MHA, et al. A survey of crowdsourcing in medical image analysis. arXiv preprint arXiv:190209159. 2019;.
2. Maier-Hein L, Ross T, Gröhl J, et al. Crowd-algorithm collaboration for large-scale endoscopic image annotation with confidence. In: Med Image Comput Comput Assist Interv. Springer; 2016. p. 616–623.
3. Ganz M, Kondermann D, Andrulis J, et al. Crowdsourcing for error detection in cortical surface delineations. Int J Comput Assist Radiol Surg. 2017;12(1):161–166.
4. Doucet MY, Viel L. Alveolar macrophage graded hemosiderin score from bronchoalveolar lavage in horses with exercise-induced pulmonary hemorrhage and controls. J Vet Intern Med. 2002;16(3):281–286.
5. Marzahl C, Aubreville M, Bertram CA, et al. Deep Learning-Based Quantification of Pulmonary Hemosiderophages in Cytology Slides. arXiv preprint arXiv:190804767. 2019;.
6. Irshad H, Montaser-Kouhsari L, Waltz G, et al. Crowdsourcing image annotation for nucleus detection and segmentation in computational pathology: evaluating experts, automated methods, and the crowd. In: Pac Symp Biocomput. World Scientific; 2014. p. 294–305.
7. Golde DW, Drew WL, Klein HZ, et al. Occult pulmonary haemorrhage in leukaemia. Br Med J. 1975;2(5964):166–168.

Abstract: Defence of Mathematical Models for Deep Learning based Registration

Lasse Hansen, Maximilian Blendowski, Mattias P. Heinrich

Institut für Medizinische Informatik, Universität zu Lübeck
hansen@imi.uni-luebeck.de

Deep learning based methods have not reached clinically acceptable results for common medical registration tasks that could be adequately solved using conventional methods. The slower progress compared to image segmentation is due to the lower availability of expert correspondences and the very large learnable parameter space for naive deep learning solutions. We strongly believe that it is necessary and beneficial to integrate conventional optimisation strategies as differentiable modules into deep learning based registration. The process can then be broken down into smaller components (e.g. feature learning and regularisation) that are easier to train and enable explainable network models. In [1], we propose to learn interpretable multi-modal features that can be directly employed using classical iterative registration schemes. The differentiable operations within a supervised descent approach enables us to learn a mapping of the complex multi-modal appearance to a common space. Incorporating keypoint models is vital for state-of-the-art performance in challenging 3D thoracic registration. Deep learning of sparse point cloud matching using graph convolutions was shown in [2] to predict keypoint features and correspondences solely by their inherent geometric structure. Approximate mean-field inference (based on a graphical model) together with densely sampled discrete displacements has been shown to outperform previous work on abdominal CT registration and enabling the learning of large deformation with few labelled scans [3]. Our work demonstrates advantages over state-of-the-art fully-convolutional models and provides an interesting avenue for further research.[1]

References

1. Blendowski M, Heinrich MP. Learning interpretable multi-modal features for alignment with supervised iterative descent. In: MIDL; 2019. p. 73–83.
2. Hansen L, Dittmer D, Heinrich MP. Learning deformable point set registration with regularized dynamic graph CNNs for large lung motion in COPD patients. arXiv preprint arXiv:190907818. 2019;.
3. Heinrich MP. Closing the gap between deep and conventional image registration using probabilistic dense displacement networks. In: MICCAI; 2019. p. 50–58.

---

[1] https://github.com/multimodallearning

© Springer Fachmedien Wiesbaden GmbH, ein Teil von Springer Nature 2020
T. Tolxdorff et al. (Hrsg.), *Bildverarbeitung für die Medizin 2020*,
Informatik aktuell, https://doi.org/10.1007/978-3-658-29267-6_6

Degenerating U-Net on Retinal Vessel Segmentation
What Do We Really Need?

Weilin Fu[1,2], Katharina Breininger[1], Zhaoya Pan[1], Andreas Maier[1,3]

[1] Pattern Recognition Lab, Friedrich-Alexander Universtiy
[2] International Max Planck Research School for Physics of Light (IMPRS-PL)
[3] Erlangen Graduate School in Advanced Optical Technologies (SAOT)
weilin.fu@fau.de

Abstract. Retinal vessel segmentation is an essential step for fundus image analysis. With the recent advances of deep learning technologies, many convolutional neural networks have been applied in this field, including the successful U-Net. In this work, we firstly modify the U-Net with functional blocks aiming to pursue higher performance. The absence of the expected performance boost then lead us to dig into the opposite direction of shrinking the U-Net and exploring the extreme conditions such that its segmentation performance is maintained. Experiment series to simplify the network structure, reduce the network size and restrict the training conditions are designed. Results show that for retinal vessel segmentation on DRIVE database, U-Net does not degenerate until surprisingly acute conditions: one level, one filter in convolutional layers, and one training sample. This experimental discovery is both counter-intuitive and worthwhile. Not only are the extremes of the U-Net explored on a well-studied application, but also one intriguing warning is raised for the research methodology which seeks for marginal performance enhancement regardless of the resource cost.

1 Introduction

Segmentation of retinal vessels is a crucial step in fundus image analysis. It provides information of the distribution, thickness and curvature of the retinal vessels, thus greatly assists early stage diagnosis of circulate system related diseases, such as diabetic retinopathy. Researchers have devoted to this field for decades, and with the development of deep learning technologies [1], many deep networks have been proposed to tackle this problem. For instance, a Convolutional Neural Network (CNN) combined with conditional random field in [2], a network pipeline concatenating a preprocessing net and a vesselness Frangi-Net in [3], and the U-Net [4]. Since published, U-Net has achieved remarkable performance in various fields. Researchers [5] even claim that hyper-parameter tuning the U-Net rather than constructing new CNN architectures is the key

© Springer Fachmedien Wiesbaden GmbH, ein Teil von Springer Nature 2020
T. Tolxdorff et al. (Hrsg.), *Bildverarbeitung für die Medizin 2020*,
Informatik aktuell, https://doi.org/10.1007/978-3-658-29267-6_7

to high performance. However, U-Net generally contains huge amounts of parameters and is resource consuming. Previously, researchers [6] have proposed to prune U-Net levels in the testing phase to reduce the network size. Yet the modifications introduce even more parameters in the training phase, and only one decisive factor of the architecture, the number of levels, is considered.

We work on retinal vessel segmentation on the DRIVE database and start with a three-level U-Net with 16 filters in the input layer. Firstly, we aim to enhance its performance by integrating common deep learning blocks into the architecture. As the expected performance boost is not observed, we propose the assumption that the basic U-Net alone is adequate or even overqualified for the task. To verify this hypothesis, we design an experiment series to compress the basic U-Net. The number of levels, convolutional layers per level, and filters per convolutional layer are reduced respectively. Non-linear activation layers are removed, and the number of training sets are decreased to further delve into the limits of the network training procedure. Results show that surprisingly harsh conditions are required for the U-Net to degenerate, indicating that the default configuration is redundant. Our contributions are two-fold: the minimum U-Net for this task is reported, indicating the possibility of real-time retinal vessel segmentation on mobile devices; and the issue of excessive computational power use is exposed and stressed on.

2   Materials and methods

2.1   Default U-Net configuration

A three-level U-Net with 16 filters in the input layer is used as the baseline architecture as shown in Fig. 1 (a). Batch normalization layers are utilized to stabilize the training process. The deconvolution layers are replaced with upsampling combined with convolution layers to avoid the checkerboard artifact.

2.2   Additive variants

Three popular CNN blocks are utilized to modify the network structure. The dense block [7] is inserted in each level of the encoder path. The side-output layer [2] is employed to provide deep supervision in the decoder path. And the residual block [8] is integrated into the encoder, the bottleneck as well as the decoder. The block structures are illustrated in Fig. 1 (b-d).

2.3   Subtractive variants

The experiment design of the subtractive variants of the U-Net is based on the "control variates" strategy, meaning only one factor is changed from the default configuration in one series. Both the structural and training condition limits of the U-Net are studied in the following experiments:

1. The non-linear activation layers, i.e. the ReLU layers, are removed.

2. The number of convolutional layers in each level decreases to one.
3. The number of filters in the input layer is reduced from 16 to 1.
4. The number of levels decreases step-wise down to one, until the network degenerates into a chain of consecutive convolution layers.
5. The default U-Net is trained with subsets of the training data. The size of the subset is reduced from 16 down to 1 by a factor of 2.

2.4 Database description

All experiments are trained and evaluated on the Digital Retinal Images for Vessel Extraction (DRIVE) database. DRIVE is composed of 40 RGB fundus photographs with the size of 565×584 pixels. All images are provided with manual labels and Field of View (FOV) masks. The database is equally divided into one training and testing set. A subset containing four images is randomly selected from the training set for validation.

The raw images are prepared with a preprocessing pipeline, where the green channels are extracted, the inhomogeneous illumination is balanced with CLAHE, and pixel intensities within the FOV masks are standardized to (-1, 1). The borders of all FOV masks are eroded by four pixels to remove potential border effects and ensure meaningful comparison. Additionally, multiplicative pixel-wise weight maps w are generated from the manual labels to emphasize on thin vessels using the equation: $w = \frac{1}{\alpha \times d}$, where d represents the vessel diameter in the given manual label, and α is manually set to 0.18.

2.5 Experimental details

The loss function in this work is composed of two main parts: weighted focal loss [9] and ℓ_2-norm weight regularizer. The objective function is minimized with the Adam optimizer [10] with a decaying learning rate initialized to 5×10^{-5}. Early stopping is applied according to the validation loss curve. Each batch

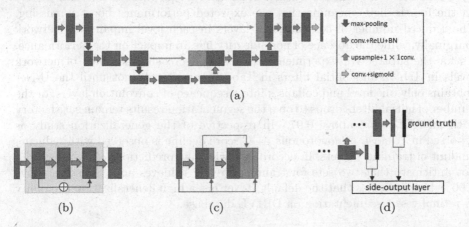

Fig. 1. U-Net (a), residual block (b), dense block (c) and side-output layer (d).

Table 1. Performance w.r.t. structural variants. Additive variants: Ures, Uden, Uside denote the U-Net with residual blocks, U-Net with dense blocks, U-Net with side-output layers; subtractive variants: U-lin, U-1C represent U-Net without ReLU layers and U-Net with one convolutional layer per level, respectively.

Var	Param	AUC	Specificity	Sensitivity	F1 score	Accuracy
U	108 976	.9748±.0005	.9758±.0014	.7941±.0063	.8101±.0010	.9518±.0005
Ures	154 768	.9756±.0005	.9758±.0003	.7994±.0033	.8133±.0017	.9525±.0004
Uden	2 501 067	.9745±.0005	.9742±.0013	.8029±.0035	.8110±.0023	.9515±.0008
Uside	109 072	.9744±.0006	.9757±.0012	.7938±.0060	.8097±.0023	.9517±.0007
U-lin	108 976	.9632±.0014	.9693±.0022	.7874±.0076	.7885±.0021	.9453±.0010
U-1C	49 072	.9722±.0007	.9742±.0007	.7918±.0044	.8043±.0017	.9501±.0004

contains 50 image patches sized 168×168, and data augmentation techniques such as rotation, shearing, additive Gaussian noise and intensity shifting are employed. All experiments are conducted for five times with random initializations to show that the performance is stable and that the conclusion is not dominated by certain specific initialization settings. For subset training experiments, the training sets are selected randomly.

3   Results

The evaluation of each experiment over the five different initialization roll-outs are reported in Tab. 1-4. The mean and standard deviations of five commonly used metrics, namely specificity, sensitivity, F1 score, accuracy and the AUC score are presented. The threshold for binarization is selected such that the F1 score is maximized on the validation sets. The threshold independent AUC score is chosen as the main performance indicator. The output probability maps of the degenerated trials are presented in Fig. 2 (c-f).

Tab. 1 shows that the AUC scores of additive U-Net variants fluctuate merely on the fourth digit, meaning that the expected performance boost is missing. The reduced number of convolutional layers in each level impairs the network marginally, while the absence of non-linearity has an impact on the performance. As for the subtractive experiment series with decreasing numbers of network levels in Tab. 2 and initial filters in Tab. 3, surprisingly not until the U-Net contains only one level and collapses into a sequence of convolution layers, or the number of initial filters drops to one, the segmentation results remain satisfactory with an AUC score above 0.97. In respective of the generalization study as reported in Table 4, a monotonous AUC score decline is observed with reducing amount of training subsets, in accordance with our prediction. However we did not anticipate that two sets for training already achieves an AUC score above 0.96, which indicates that the default U-Net has a high generalization capability in retinal vessel segmentation on DRIVE database.

Table 2. U-Net performance w.r.t. different numbers of levels.

#	Param	AUC	Specificity	Sensitivity	F1 score	Accuracy
2	23 984	.9724±.0003	.9733±.0016	.7970±.0063	.8050±.0013	.9500±.0007
1	7 344	.9625±.0006	.9652±.0014	.7970±.0056	.7832±.0015	.9429±.0006

Table 3. U-Net performance w.r.t. different numbers of initial filters.

#	Param	AUC	Specificity	Sensitivity	F1 score	Accuracy
8	27 352	.9745±.0004	.9754±.0007	.7940±.0035	.8090±.0018	.9514±.0005
4	6 892	.9739±.0003	.9746±.0009	.7962±.0044	.8080±.0010	.9510±.0004
2	1 750	.9708±.0004	.9728±.0005	.7889±.0028	.7986±.0006	.9485±.0001
1	451	.9620±.0010	.9678±.0028	.7776±.0102	.7785±.0029	.9427±.0014

Table 4. U-Net performance w.r.t. various number of training sets.

#	AUC	Specificity	Sensitivity	F1 score	Accuracy
8	.9722±.0007	.9732±.0018	.7961±.0093	.8043±.0021	.9498±.0007
4	.9674±.0009	.9700±.0036	.7926±.0144	.7935±.0013	.9465±.0014
2	.9635±.0034	.9657±.0069	.7919±.0180	.7818±.0091	.9427±.0041
1	.9545±.0064	.9672±.0049	.7508±.0243	.7602±.0173	.9387±.0047

4 Discussion

In this work, we explore extreme U-Net configurations for retinal vessel segmentation, and report the results on DRIVE database. This work is motivated by the observation that additive modifications, such as the dense block, introduce additional parameters yet fail to improve the segmentation performance. Hence, an experiment series to decrease the network size as well as simplifying the network structure is conducted. The results do not follow our expectations. It is understandable that non-linearity, rather than the number of convolutional layers per level, has a stronger impact on the network representation capability. However, we did not expect that U-Net with two levels of 23 984 parameters, and even U-Net with two initial filters of 1 750 parameters can reach an AUC score of over 0.97. Also the generalization ability of U-Net with 108 976 weights with only two training sets, achieving an AUC score above 0.96 is surprising. The minimum set-up needed for the U-Net to generate satisfactory results is small for this particular task.

Our discoveries challenge the trend towards networks with increasingly large numbers of parameters that are trained with often marginal improvements in segmentation performance. They also emphasize that, depending on the task, very few samples are sufficient to train CNNs and achieve generalization on unseen data. One can argue that these results are due to the simplicity of the retinal vessel segmentation. Nevertheless, retinal vessel segmentation may not be the only application in this line of observations. We therefore question research approaches merely focused on performance improvement regardless of excessive

Fig. 2. Probability output of U-Net variants.

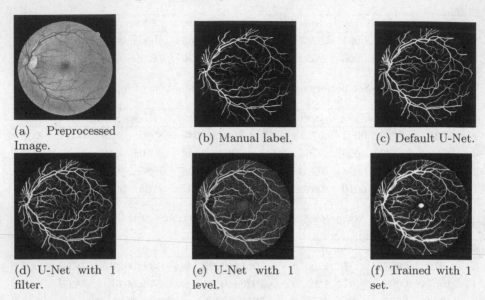

(a)   Preprocessed Image.

(b) Manual label.

(c) Default U-Net.

(d) U-Net with 1 filter.

(e) U-Net with 1 level.

(f) Trained with 1 set.

resource demand. In the future, similar approaches designed under the proposed paradigm could be applied on other tasks to save computational resources.

References

1. Maier A, Syben C, Lasser T, et al. A gentle introduction to deep learning in medical image processing. Zeitschrift für Medizinische Physik. 2019;.
2. Fu H, Xu Y, Wong DWK, et al. Retinal vessel segmentation via deep learning network and fully-connected conditional random fields. In: ISBI; 2016. .
3. Fu W, Breininger K, Schaffert R, et al. A divide-and-conquer approach towards understanding deep networks. MICCAI. 2019;.
4. Ronneberger O, Fischer P, Brox T. U-Net: convolutional networks for biomedical image segmentation. In: MICCAI; 2015. .
5. Isensee F, Petersen J, Klein A, et al. NnU-Net: self-adapting framework for u-net-based medical image segmentation. arXiv:180910486. 2018;.
6. Zhou Z, Siddiquee MMR, et al. Unet++: a nested u-net architecture for medical image segmentation. In: DLMIA; 2018. .
7. Huang G, Liu Z, Van Der Maaten L, et al. Densely connected convolutional networks. In: CVPR; 2017. .
8. He K, Zhang X, Ren S, et al. Deep residual learning for image recognition. In: CVPR; 2016. .
9. Lin TY, Goyal P, Girshick R, et al. Focal loss for dense object detection. In: Proc IEEE Int Conf Comput Vis; 2017. .
10. Kingma DP. Adam: A method for stochastic optimization. arXiv:14126980. 2014;.

COPD Classification in CT Images Using a 3D Convolutional Neural Network

Jalil Ahmed[1], Sulaiman Vesal[1], Felix Durlak[2], Rainer Kaergel[2],
Nishant Ravikumar[1,3], Martine Rémy-Jardin[4], Andreas Maier[1]

[1]Pattern Recognition Lab, Friedrich-Alexander-Universität Erlangen-Nürnberg,
Germany
[2]Siemens Healthcare GmbH, Forchheim, Germany
[3]CISTIB, Centre for Computational Imaging and Simulation Technologies in
Biomedicine, School of Computing, University of Leeds, United Kingdom
[4]CHRU Lille, Département d'Imagerie Thoracique, Lille, France
jalil.ahmed@fau.de

Abstract. Chronic obstructive pulmonary disease (COPD) is a lung disease that is not fully reversible and one of the leading causes of morbidity and mortality in the world. Early detection and diagnosis of COPD can increase the survival rate and reduce the risk of COPD progression in patients. Currently, the primary examination tool to diagnose COPD is spirometry. However, computed tomography (CT) is used for detecting symptoms and sub-type classification of COPD. Using different imaging modalities is a difficult and tedious task even for physicians and is subjective to inter-and intra-observer variations. Hence, developing methods that can automatically classify COPD versus healthy patients is of great interest. In this paper, we propose a 3D deep learning approach to classify COPD and emphysema using volume-wise annotations only. We also demonstrate the impact of transfer learning on the classification of emphysema using knowledge transfer from a pre-trained COPD classification model.

1 Introduction

COPD is a lung disease characterized by chronic obstruction of lung airflow that interferes with normal breathing, and it is not fully reversible [1]. It is considered to be the 4th leading cause of death by 2030 [2]. Generally, COPD is caused by a mixture of two sub-types, emphysema and small airway disease (SAD). Emphysema is the permanent abnormal enlargement of air spaces along with the destruction of their wall without prominent fibrosis. Emphysema is further classified into panlobular, centrilobular, and paraseptal emphysema based on the disease distribution in the lung, shape, and location of the affected area using lung CT images. The pulmonary function test is the gold standard for COPD detection. However, limitations in early detection and the ability of radiographic studies to visualize COPD sub-types have made CT a recent focus in

© Springer Fachmedien Wiesbaden GmbH, ein Teil von Springer Nature 2020
T. Tolxdorff et al. (Hrsg.), *Bildverarbeitung für die Medizin 2020*,
Informatik aktuell, https://doi.org/10.1007/978-3-658-29267-6_8

the diagnosis and categorization of COPD. COPD is often misdiagnosed in early stages because of the similarity of initial symptoms to common illnesses, and lack of significant symptoms until the advanced stage [3]. The shortcomings in the diagnosis are addressed using computer-aided detection (CAD). CAD techniques allow for a reduction in misdiagnosis rate leading to possible prevention of disease progression, complications, improving management, and early mortality.

Automated COPD classification is conventionally approached using traditional machine learning techniques. Recently, deep neural networks are also employed for COPD classification in CT images [4]. The majority of studies use some prior information such as landmark slices [5], regions of interest (ROIs) [6], and meta-data [7] in cooperation with 2D neural networks. In a 2D convolutional neural network (CNN), slices from the CT volume are used as input samples. This leads to inherent failure to leverage context from adjacent slices. These methods also require slice-wise annotations, which is a time-consuming and tedious task. We hypothesize that a solution to this problem is to use a 3D CNN which could overcome limitations for COPD classification using 3D convolutional kernels and volume-wise annotations. A 3D CNN can extract larger spatial context to preserve more discriminative information which subsequently could improve COPD classification.

In this study, we propose a 3D CNN for the volumetric classification of COPD as well as emphysema. We first train our proposed model for the classification of COPD vs. healthy. We then investigate the effects of transfer learning by using features learned during COPD classification and fine-tune the model for emphysema classification.

2   Methods

We utilized VoxResNet [8] which extends deep residual learning to 3D volumetric data. The VoxRes module introduces identity mapping by adding input features with a residual function using a skip connection (Fig. 1(g)). We modified the VoxResNet by removing the auxiliary classifiers and adding fully connected layer for classification task. All the operations in VoxResNet are implemented in 3D to strengthen the volumetric feature representation learning. Fig. 1(h) shows the proposed network architecture. The 2 initial convolutional layers have 32 filters each. Further layers consist of 64 filters each. Instead of a conventional pooling layer approach, after every 2 VoxRes modules, a convolutional layer with stride 2 was added to reduce the feature map size. Each convolutional layer uses a kernel size of $3 \times 3 \times 3$ and is followed by batch normalization and a ReLU activation function. A 3D global-pooling layer with 64 units is used to preserve the 3D information of the last feature map. Afterward, a fully connected layer with the leaky-ReLU activation function is added. We also used an L2-regularizer to prevent sharp learning spikes and achieve a smooth learning curve. The network is implemented in the Keras/TensorFlow framework.

2.1 Data

We trained the proposed model using CT images from two data sets called SI-I and SI-II. In SI-I all the subjects were annotated into different categories based on the Global Initiative for Chronic Obstructive Lung Disease (GOLD) system. We marked all the instances with GOLD stage 0 as healthy and those with GOLD stage 1-4 as COPD cases.

SI-II data set consists of 1000 patients with at least 2 scans per patient. We used the inspiration scan with the soft kernel. SI-II was annotated for emphysema and its potential multiple sub-types after visual assessment by medical experts. The non-emphysema label included patients who were healthy or had respiratory diseases other than emphysema. Sub-types of emphysema are not mutually exclusive. Both data sets were imbalanced. The SI-I data set has a ratio of 3/4 for the healthy vs. COPD classes. SI-II consisted of 573 non-emphysema and 366 emphysema samples. The emphysema sub-types distribution was also imbalanced (panlobular: 4, centrilobular: 96, paraseptal: 32, multiple: 233).

2.1.1 Data Pre-processing: Both data sets were available in the form of DICOM files. Binary lung masks were extracted for SI-I and SI-II using MeVis-Lab [9]. Masking and isometric re-sampling to a voxel size of 1mm^3 resulted in volumes of various sizes in each dimension. Due to memory limitations, we downsampled the volumes to $110 \times 200 \times 200$ pixels for batch processing. The x and y planes were down-sampled using bi-linear interpolation. No interpolation was done in z-axis because COPD could be very small and appear only on few

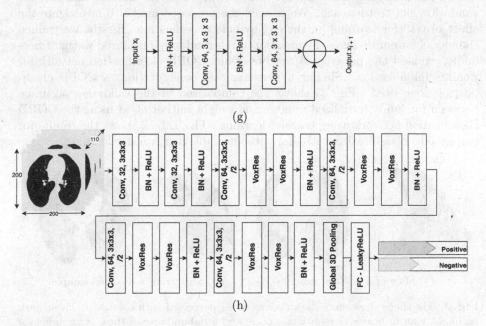

Fig. 1. (a) An illustration of VoxRes module (b) the proposed VoxResNet variant.

slices, and downsampling could remove this information. For a volume with N slices, 110 new slices were created by averaging over $m = \frac{N}{110}$ slices in each new slice. A sample slice from SI-I data set is shown in Fig. 2.

3   Experiments and results

COPD classification aimed to classify COPD vs. healthy, and emphysema classification aimed to distinguish emphysema from non-emphysema. Non-emphysema cases incorporated samples annotated as healthy or any other type of lung disease, such as SAD, lung cancer, or bronchitis etc.

COPD classification performed using the SI-I data set. We employ under-sampling to balance the data set and use 6000 samples for training, 500 samples for validation, and 300 samples for testing. A binary cross-entropy loss function is used with randomly initialized weights. The network was trained using an Adam optimizer with an initial learning rate of 10^{-6}, decay learning rate on plateau factor (α) of 0.9, and a batch size of 2. It was not possible to increase the batch size because of memory limitations. The network was trained until there was no further decrease in the validation loss. The Tab. 1 shows the accuracy achieved by our model for the task of COPD classification along with results published by Gonzalez et al [5], and Hatt et al. [4]

Emphysema vs. non-emphysema classification was performed using the SI-II data set. SI-II was imbalanced therefore the emphysema class was oversampled to balance the classes using data augmentation techniques such as flipping, rotation, and cropping. The data set was split into 80% for training and 10% for validation and testing each. We trained the proposed model to investigate the effect of transfer learning on the emphysema classification. Firstly, we trained the model for emphysema classification using randomly initialized weights. Secondly, we used the pre-trained weights of our COPD classification network for weights initialization. Similar hyperparameter configuration as COPD classification were used. Fig. 3 shows the comparison of the validation accuracy between randomly initialized weights and weight initialization using the COPD classification network using transfer learning. The Tab. 2 shows the results for emphysema classification with and without employing transfer learning.

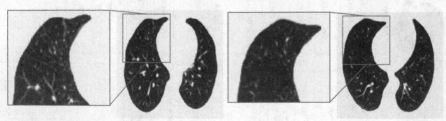

(a) Slice of a healthy sample   (b) Slice from a diseased sample

Fig. 2. The slices show more dark regions when perceived with colormap. These dark regions are an indicator of empty air space, and an abundance of these is an indicator of alveoli enlargement because of COPD.

Table 1. Results for COPD classification.

	Validation	Test	
	Accuracy	*Accuracy*	*AUC*
Gonzalez et al.[5]	N/A	N/A	0.856
Hatt et al.[4]	77.7%	76.2%	N/A
VoxResNet 3D (ours)	79.8%	74.3%	0.820

Table 2. Results for emphysema classification.

	Validation accuracy	Test accuracy
VoxResNet 3D - Transfer learning	78.3 %	70.0 %
VoxResNet 3D - No transfer learning	68.5 %	58.8 %

4 Discussion

The main focus of our work was to study the effects of using a 3D CNN for COPD classification, and effects of using transfer learning for emphysema classification. Current systems for COPD classification use CNN based on 2D kernels [4] [5]. While 2D CNNs have shown success in COPD classification, they intrinsically lose the 3D context [10]. In comparison, 3D kernels are able to learn discriminative features in all 3 spatial dimensions. 2D CNNs also require slice-wise annotations. As diseased lung tissue is not visible in each slice of CT volume, therefore, COPD classification with volume-wise annotations is also a challenging task for 2D CNN because in a complete CT volume annotated as COPD, there may be many slices with only healthy tissue. We aim to overcome these limitations by utilizing a 3D CNN for COPD classification. Our work is not directly comparable to the state-of-the-art systems because of different model parameters, training strategies, and data splits. Gonzalez et al. [5] extract 4 slices using anatomical landmarks to create 2D montages to train a 2D CNN. Hatt et al. [4] divides a single CT volume into 4 different 2D montages by extracting random axial slices and trains a 2D CNN. In comparison, we used complete CT volumes down sampled to $110 \times 200 \times 200$ with volume-wise annotations. We achieved comparable results as shown in Tab. 1 to Hatt et al. [4],

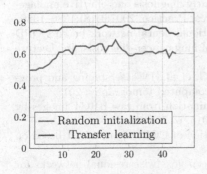

Fig. 3. Validation accuracy comparison of our network between random initialization and transfer learning for emphysema vs. non-emphysema classification.

Gonzalez et al. [5] indicating that 3D CNNs show promising results with limited training data.

For emphysema vs. non-emphysema classification, we compare the performance of randomly initialized weights vs. transfer learning (Fig 3). As shown in Tab. 2, without the use of transfer learning our network achieved 68.5% validation and 58.8% test accuracy. In comparison, with transfer learning, we were able to achieve 78.3% validation and 70.0% test accuracy. A significant increase in performance with transfer learning indicates that features learned by neural networks for COPD classification are also effective in emphysema classification. The transfer learning step included knowledge transfer across different data sets, i.e. SI-I and SI-II, and different tasks, i.e. COPD and emphysema classification.

5   Conclusion

In this paper, we proposed a variant of 3D VoxResNet for COPD and emphysema classification. The model uses volume-wise annotations without any further feature enhancement or addition of meta-data. Our network achieved similar results for the COPD classification. For the emphysema classification, we fine-tuned the COPD classification network, which significantly increased the model performance. As a future work, validating the model on larger and balanced data sets with a thorough comparison with other methods, preferably, using k-fold cross validation is recommended.

Disclaimer. The concepts and information presented in this paper are based on research and are not commercially available.

References

1. Organization WH. Fact Sheet on Chronic Obstructive Pulmonary Disease (COPD);. http://www.who.int/en/news-room/fact-sheets.
2. Mathers CD, Loncar D. Projections of Global Mortality and Burden of Disease from 2002 to 2030. PLOS Medicine. 2006 11;3(11):1–20.
3. Bellamy D, Smith J. Role of primary care in early diagnosis and effective management of COPD. International Journal of Clinical Practice. 2007;61(8):1380–1389.
4. Hatt C, Galban C, Labaki W, et al. Convolutional neural network based COPD and emphysema classifications are predictive of lung cancer diagnosis. In: Lecture Notes in Computer Science; 2018. .
5. Gonzalez G, Ash SY, Vegas-Sánchez-Ferrero G, et al.. Disease staging and prognosis in smokers using deep learning in chest computed tomography; 2018.
6. Karabulut EM, Ibrikci T. Emphysema discrimination from raw HRCT images by convolutional neural networks. In: ELECO; 2015. p. 705–708.
7. Ying J, Dutta J, Guo N, et al. Gold classification of COPDGene cohort based on deep learning. In: ICASSP; 2016. p. 2474–2478.
8. Chen H, Dou Q, Yu L, et al. VoxResNet: Deep voxelwise residual networks for brain segmentation from 3D MR images. NeuroImage. 2018;170:446–455.

9. MeVis Medical Solutions AG. MeVisLab;. Https://www.mevislab.de/.
10. Huang X, Shan J, Vaidya V. Lung nodule detection in CT using 3D convolutional neural networks. In: 2017 IEEE 14th International Symposium on Biomedical Imaging (ISBI 2017); 2017. p. 379–383.

Automatische Detektion von Zwischenorgan-3D-Barrieren in abdominalen CT-Daten

Oliver Mietzner[1], Andre Mastmeyer[2]

[1]Institut für Medizinische Informatik, Universität zu Lübeck
[2]Fakultät für Optik und Mechatronik, Hochschule Aalen
oliver.mietzner@student.uni-luebeck.de

Kurzfassung. Volumenwachstumssegmentierungstechniken sind oftmals mit der Übersegmentierung angrenzender Organe oder Strukturen behaftet. Künstlich eingebrachte Segmentierungsbarrieren als Nebenbedingungen helfen hierbei. Aktuell werden diese Markierungen häufig noch als manuelle Scribbles vom Benutzer i.d.R. mühsam schichtweise erstellt. Hier wird ein neuer vollautomatischer Ansatz zum Finden von virtuellen 3D-Barrieren mit maschinellen Lernmethoden vorgestellt. Die Abstandsfehler zu Referenzbarrieren liegen zwischen 4,9±1,3 und 10,3±3,6 mm.

1   Einleitung

Ein typisches Problem von effizienten Volumenwachstums oder auch GraphCut-Segmentierungen [1], die bspw. für virtuelle 4D-Patientensimulationen [2, 3] benötigt werden [4], ist das Auftreten von Übersegmentierungen eng benachbarter Organen oder Strukturen mit vergleichbaren Intensitäten.

Dieses Risiko kann durch die Verwendung von Barrieren mitigiert werden: Diese virtuelle Wachstums-Barriere wird hier vollautomatisch generiert und ist nicht intensitätsmäßig manifestiert. In der Praxis muss der Anwender die Barrieren mühsam schichtweise präventiv manuell markieren [5]. *Post-hoc* können falsch segmentierte Bereiche durch manuelle oder (halb-)automatische Nachbearbeitung der Label-Karten korrigiert werden[1].

2   Material und Methoden

Die Datenmenge bestand aus 60 abdominalen 3D-CT-Scans und Label-Bildern aus drei verschiedenen Segmentierungswettbewerben: SLIVER07[2], LiTS[3] und

---

[1] http://3dslicer.org, http://itksnap.org
[2] http://sliver07.org
[3] http://competitions.codalab.org/competitions/17094

© Springer Fachmedien Wiesbaden GmbH, ein Teil von Springer Nature 2020
T. Tolxdorff et al. (Hrsg.), *Bildverarbeitung für die Medizin 2020*,
Informatik aktuell, https://doi.org/10.1007/978-3-658-29267-6_9

Abb. 1. Training der RRF und U-Nets: Dem RRF dienten Voxel p und zugehörigen Feature Boxen F_j als Eingabe, um die Distanz der Voxel zur Organ-BB zu lernen. Dem U-Net wurden VOI-Intensitäten und -Masken übergeben [6].

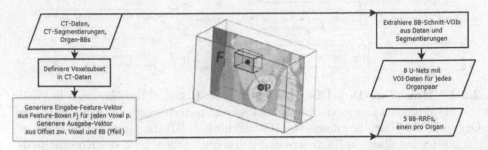

VISCERAL[4]. Die einzelnen Scans unterscheiden sich nicht nur in der Anzahl der Schichten (64-861), dem Field-of-View (FoV), sondern auch in Schichtdicke und Bildrauschen. Die komplette Form der fünf Zielorgane (Leber, rechte Niere, linke Niere, Milz, Bauchspeicheldrüse) musste abgebildet sein. $\binom{5}{2} = 10$ Organ-nahzonen sind theoretisch möglich und werden als Paarungen bezeichnet. Überschneidung der Bounding-Boxen der Paarungen linke Niere:rechte Niere, rechte Niere:Milz und Leber:linke Niere waren praktisch nicht relevant, es wurden nur die verbleibenden sieben Nahzonen untersucht.

Das Ziel unseres neuen Ansatzes ist es, automatisch virtuelle 3D-Barrieren ohne realer Strukturentsprechung zwischen bestimmten Organen in abdominalen CT-Scans zu generieren, die innerhalb festgestellter Überlappungen von Bounding-Boxen (BB) liegen. Wir verwenden zwei verschiedene maschinelle Lernmethoden, um die Barrieren basierend auf Intensitätsmerkmalen vorherzusagen. Die Abbn. 1 und 2 stellen schematisch Training und Anwendung mit Random-Regression-Forests (RRF) und U-Nets dar.

Die Anwendungsgrundidee ist (Abb. 2), einen dedizierten RRF pro Organ zu verwenden, um die BB-Positionen zu schätzen. Im zweiten Schritt, prüfen wir, ob Überschneidungen zwischen den BBen auftreten. Falls eine Überschneidung detektiert wird, erhält ein U-Net, die entsprechende Region als Eingabe und schätzt die Segmentierung der Strukturen innerhalb der Region. Schließlich kann die so entstandene Segmentierung genutzt werden, um eine Barriere zwischen den Strukturen deterministisch zu generieren.

2.1 Datenvorbereitung

Es war regelmäßig notwendig, einige relevante Strukturen (Bauchspeicheldrüse) manuell zu nachzusegmentieren, da diese nicht in den Challenge-Daten enthalten waren. Die neuen Segmentierungen wurden von zwei Experten geprüft.

2.2 Gemeinsam genutzte Methoden in Training und Anwendung

---

[4] http://visceral.eu/closed-benchmarks/anatomy3

Abb. 2. Anwendung der BB- und Barrierendetektion: Flowchart der sequentiellen Anwendung unseres Verfahrens auf ungesehene, abdominale CT-Daten.

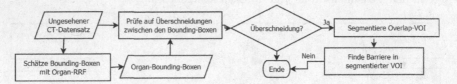

2.2.1 Bounding-Box-Überschneidungen Um eine Barriere zwischen nahen abdominalen Organen grob zu lokalisieren, nutzen wir die Überlappung von Organ-BBen. Hierführ müssen sich die zugehörigen BB-Intervalle auf jeder Koordinaatenachse überschneiden, so daß durch sequentielle Checks der Koordinatenrichtungen eine BB-Schnittmenge entsteht. In diesem Fall wird das resultierende Volume-of-Interest (VOI) auf Barrieren untersucht (Abb. 3(b)).

2.3 Training der Modelle

2.3.1 Trainieren von Random-Forests für die BB-Detektion Für die Schätzung der Koordinaten der BBen, nutzen wir pro Organ einen RRF [6]. Hierbei wird eine 3D-Organ-BB als ein 6D-Vektor $b = (x^L, x^R, y^A, y^P, z^H, z^F)$ in mm definiert. In Training und Anwendung iterieren wir über alle Voxel $p = (x_p, y_p, z_p)$, welche sich in einem bestimmten Radius ($r=5$ cm) zur Scan-Medialachse befinden (Zentrumzylinder). Der Distanzvektor eines solchen Voxels zu jeder der BB-Wände, berechnet durch $d(p) = (x_p - x^L, x_p - x^R, y_p - y^A, y_p - y^P, z_p - z^H, z_p - z^F)$, wird als Ausgabe gelernt. Für die Generierung des Eingabe-Feature-Vektors, nutzen wir im Gegensatz zu [6] nur 50 auf drei Kugelschalen ($r=5$ cm; 2,5 cm; 1,25 cm) gleichmäßig verteilte Feature-Boxen (FB). Diese FBen F_j (Abb. 1) sollen den räumlichen und Intensitätskontext der BBen einfangen. Hierfür wird der Mittelwert der in den FBen enthaltenen Intensäten berechnet und in den Feature-Vektor der Länge 50 eingetragen. Der RRF lernt nun im Training anhand der FBen den Distanzvektor (Ausgabe) zur Referenz-BB.

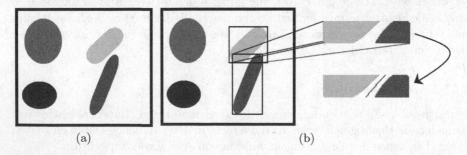

(a)   (b)

Abb. 3. 2D Lageschema und eine BB-Überschneidung: (a) Das Abschätzen der räumlichen Nähe zweier Objekte ist mittels BBen möglich. (b) Falls eine Kollision zwischen BBen detektiert wird, wird mit morphologischen Operatoren eine Trennfläche erstellt.

2.3.2 Training eines U-Net für die semantische VOI-Segmentierung
Die Trainingsgrundlage für unser U-Net bilden die Expertensegmentierungen
und die BB-Überlappungs-VOIs (2.2.1). Die VOIs werden dann genutzt um
lokal die Intensitäts- und Label-Daten zu extrahieren. Als Eingabe erhält das
U-Net somit eine VOI aus den Intensitätsdaten, während die gleiche Region
innerhalb der Label-Daten als Ausgabe genutzt wird. Wir verwenden die U-Net-
Architektur [7], die aus neun Layern mit vier Encoder-Decoder-Schritten besteht.
Für jede der sieben Organpaarungen haben wir je ein. Modell trainiert.

2.4 Anwendung der Modelle

2.4.1 Bounding-Box und Überschneidungsdetektion Die organspezi-
fischen RRFs erkennen zunächst die Organ-BB-Kandidaten. Anschließend wird
mittels Mehrheitsvotierung ein Distanz-Vektor ausgewählt und in einen 6D-BB-
Vektor und somit eine finale organspezifische BB-Schätzung umgerechnet. Ihre
Überschneidungen werden als VOIs für die typischen sieben Organpaarungen,
wie in Abschnitt 2.2.1 beschrieben, berechnet.

2.4.2 Partielle Segmentierung von Organen in BB-Schnittmengen
Nun bekommt das paarabhängige U-Net-Modell die entsprechende VOI als Ein-
gabe. Jede detektierte VOI wird separat segmentiert und zur Erzeugung der
Segmentierungsbarriere mit euklidischer Morphologie verwendet.

2.4.3 Barrierengenerierung Wie in Abb. 3 zu sehen ist, werden die Segmentierungsbarrieren in den VOIs zwischen den Organ BBen erzeugt. Um eine
Barriere zu modellieren, wenden wir morphologische Dilatationen mit symme-
trischen Kernen an. Zunächst wird die Anzahl der vorhandenen Organe im VOI
bestimmt. Es gibt drei Fälle: (1) Keine Barriere entsteht, falls im klassifizierten
Teilbild keine Struktur vorhanden ist, dies tritt vor allem bei konkaven Objek-
ten auf. (2) Falls eine Struktur gefunden wird, dilatieren wir sie heuristisch, bis
sie die Hälfte des VOI-Volumens enthält und extrahieren die Trennfläche zwischen Hintergrund und Objekt als Barriere. Falls das Objekt bereits groß genug
ist, wird nur eine Dilatation (Sicherheitsabstand) durchgeführt. (3) Wenn zwei
oder mehr Objekte vorhanden sind, dilatieren wir alle Objekte, bis jeder Voxel
des VOI eindeutig ge-labelt ist. Die 3D-Barriere wird dann durch die sich be-
rührenden Grenzen der Objekte definiert (Abb. 3(b)). Abb. 4 zeigt eingefügte
3D-Barrieren (grün).

2.5 Evaluation

Es wurde eine fünffache Monte-Carlo-Kreuzvalidierung basierend auf einer 30:20
(trainieren:testen) Datenaufteilung verwendet.
Die resultierenden U-Net-Barrieren wurden gegen Referenzbarrieren anhand von
Oberflächenabständen bewertet, d.h. dem mittleren Oberflächenabstand (MOA)
und Hausdorff-Abstand (HA) [8]. Aus Expertensegmentierungen werden dafür

Tabelle 1. Ergebnistabelle: über der Hauptdiagonale: HA [mm]. Darunter: MOA [mm].

	Leber	Niere links	Niere rechts	Pankreas	Milz
Leber	-	n.v.	29,1±16	19,4±8	20,5±11,4
Niere links	n.v.	-	n.v.	17,2±1,4	21,9±7,4
Niere rechts	6,88±1,4	n.v.	-	19,7±10,4	n.v.
Pankreas	4,9±1,3	5,9±4,5	10±3,6	-	15±7,9
Milz	9,1±3	9,1±0,5	n.v.	9,5±4,2	-

neben Referenz-BBen auch -Barrieren erstellt und für Vergleiche genutzt (Tab. 3).

3 Ergebnisse

Während sich einige BBen sehr häufig überschneiden (Leber:rechte Niere), waren andere selten, so dass die Paarungsanzahlen innerhalb der Trainingsdaten nicht gleich verteilt waren. Abb. 4 zeigt zwei gefundene 3D-Barrieren am Pankreas. Tab. 3 zeigt MOA- und HA-Ergebnisse (Ausreißer) für detektierten vs. Goldstandardbarrieren für die Organpaarungen mit BB-Überschneidungen. Das Training aller benötigten Modelle, dauerte auf einem Intel-i7-Rechner mit einer NVIDIA GTX 1050 GPU 10 Minuten, die Anwendung auf einen ungesehenen Patientendatensatz dauert je nach Größe des Datensatzes zwischen 30 Sekunden und einer Minute.

4 Diskussion

Die Lungenbodenbarrieren oft nicht komplett in den Bilddaten enthaltener, hypodenser Lungen sind trivial generierbar per Volumenwachstum der Lunge sowie morphologischen Operationen und wurden aus dieser Untersuchung ausgespart. Die gefundenen BBen waren vergleichbar mit den Ergebnissen von [6]. Wir haben jedoch andere Daten und ein effizienteres Training mit nur 50 FBen gewählt

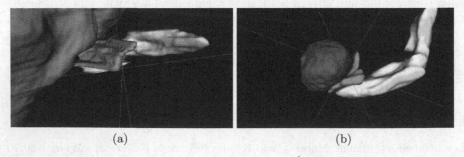

(a)   (b)

Abb. 4. Beispiel einer 3D-Barriere zwischen 2 Organen: (a) PA-Ansicht: Die Organe Leber (lila) und Bauchspeicheldrüse (weiß) werden durch eine Barriere (grün) räumlich getrennt. (b) Ansicht von oben: Die Organe Niere (rot) und Bauchspeicheldrüse (weiß) werden durch eine Barriere (grün) räumlich getrennt.

und zudem größere BBen generiert. Dieser Unterschied kann für die hier vorgestellten weiteren Schritte günstig genutzt werden. Unser Random-Forest bevorzugt extremere Werte für Maximal-/Minimalwerte der BB-Grenzen. Größere 3D-Barrieren sind von Vorteil für die spätere Gesamtbildsegmentierung mit Barrieren. Die lokal-partiellen Segmentierungen aus unseren U-Net-Modellen kann nicht mit anderen Gesamtorgansegmentierungsansätzen verglichen werden, da für die neue Methode keine Vergleichsdaten existieren. Die Barrieren wurden nicht direkt gelernt, da sie nur dünne Strukturen mit wenig Intensitätsinformationen darstellen, was die Robustheit der Modelle in Frage stellen würde. Einige Paarungen ergaben regelmäßig kleine VOIs, die schwer zu segmentieren sind. Dies erklärt die schlechtere Leistung in Tab. 1 einiger Modelle, beispielsweise Leber:Milz mit dem MOA 9,1±3 mm und HA 20,5±11,4 mm. Schwierige Organpaarungen mit der Bauchspeicheldrüse führten oft zu schlechten Ergebnissen mit MOA von 10±3,6 mm und HA 19,7±10,4 mm. Dennoch verursacht eine ungenaue U-Net-Segmentierung nicht zwangsläufig eine unnützliche, virtuelle Barriere, die aufgrund des Abstands zwischen den Organen qualitativ richtig liegen kann. Novum und Unterschied bspw. zum Watershed-Verfahren ist die partielle, d.h. VOI-beschränkte Partitionierung des Bildes. U-Nets in gefundenen Gesamt-BBen organweise anzuwenden ist ein naheliegendes Verfahren, das in dieser Arbeit nicht untersucht wurde. Die zukünftige Arbeit wird sich mit der Barriere-gestützten Gesamtbildsegmentierung befassen.

Danksagung. DFG-Projekt: MA 6791/1-1.

Literaturverzeichnis

1. Mastmeyer A, Fortmeier D, Handels H. Random forest classification of large volume structures for visuo-haptic rendering in CT images. 2016; p. 97842H.
2. Mastmeyer A, Wilms M, Handels H. Interpatient respiratory motion model transfer for virtual reality simulations of liver punctures. Journal of World Society of Computer Graphics - WSCG. 2017;25(1):1–10.
3. Mastmeyer A, Wilms M, Handels H. Population-based respiratory 4D motion atlas construction and its application for VR simulations of liver punctures. In: SPIE Medical Imaging 2018: Image Processing. vol. 10574. International Society for Optics and Photonics; 2018. p. 1057417.
4. Mastmeyer A, Wilms M, Fortmeier D, et al. Real-Time ultrasound simulation for training of US-guided needle insertion in breathing virtual patients. In: Studies in health technology and informatics. vol. 220. IOS Press; 2016. p. 219.
5. Zou Z, Liao SH, Luo SD, et al. Semi-automatic segmentation of femur based on harmonic barrier. Comput Methods Programs Biomed. 2017;143:171 – 184.
6. Criminisi A, Robertson D, Pauly O, et al. Decision forests for computer vision and medical image analysis. London: Springer; 2013.
7. Ronneberger O, Fischer P, Brox T. U-Net: convolutional networks for biomedical image segmentation. Proc MICCAI 2015. 2015; p. 234–241.
8. Taha AA, Hanbury A. Metrics for evaluating 3D medical image segmentation: analysis, selection, and tool. BMC Med Imaging. 2015;15(1):29.

Abstract: Automatic Detection of Cervical Spine Ligaments Origin and Insertion Points

Ibraheem Al-Dhamari, Sabine Bauer, Eva Keller, Dietrich Paulus

Koblenz University, Koblenz, Germany
idhamari@uni-koblenz.de

Creating patient-specific simulation models helps to make customised implant or treatment plans. To create such models, exact locations of the Origin and Insertion Points of the Ligaments (OIPL) are needed. Locating these OIPL is usually done manually and it is a time-consuming procedure. A fast method to detect these OIPL automatically using spine atlas-based segmentation [1] is proposed in this paper [2]. The average detection rate is 96.16% with a standard deviation of 3.45. The required time to detect these points is around 5 seconds. The proposed method can be generalised to detect any other important points or features related to a specific vertebra. The method is implemented as an open-source plugin for 3D Slicer. The method and the datasets are available for a free download from a public server.

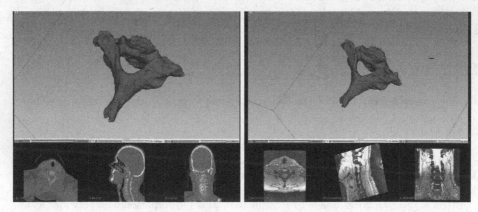

Fig. 1. Samples of detection results of C7 vertebra, left: CT, and right: MRI.

References

1. Al-Dhamari I, Bauer S, Paulus D. In: A M, Th D, H H, et al., editors. Automatic multi-modal cervical spine image atlas segmentation. 101007. Springer Berlin Heidelberg, Berlin Heidelberg; 2018. p. 303–308.
2. AL-Dhamari I, Bauer S, Keller E, et al. Automatic detection of cervical spine ligaments origin and insertion points. In: 2019 IEEE 16th International Symposium on Biomedical Imaging (ISBI 2019); 2019. p. 48–51.

© Springer Fachmedien Wiesbaden GmbH, ein Teil von Springer Nature 2020
T. Tolxdorff et al. (Hrsg.), *Bildverarbeitung für die Medizin 2020*,
Informatik aktuell, https://doi.org/10.1007/978-3-658-29267-6_10

Abstract: Recognition of AML Blast Cells in a Curated Single-Cell Dataset of Leukocyte Morphologies Using Deep Convolutional Neural Networks

Christian Matek[1,2], Simone Schwarz[2], Karsten Spiekermann[2,3,4], Carsten Marr[1]

[1]Institute of Computational Biology, Helmholtz Zentrum München - German Research Center for Environmental Health, Neuherberg, Germany
[2]Laboratory of Leukemia Diagnostics, Department of Medicine III, University Hospital, LMU Munich, Munich, Germany
[3]German Cancer Consortium (DKTK)
[4]German Cancer Research Center (DKFZ), Heidelberg, Germany

c.matek@med.uni-muenchen.de

Reliable recognition and microscopic differentiation of malignant and non-malignant leukocytes from peripheral blood smears is a key task of cytological diagnostics in hematology [1]. Having been practised for well over a century, cytomorphological analysis is still today routinely performed by human examiners using optical microscopes, a process that can be tedious, time-consuming, and suffering from considerable intra-and inter-rater variability [2]. Our work aims to provide a more quantitative and robust decision-aid for the differentiation of single blood cells in general and recognition of blast cells characteristic for Acute Myeloid Leukemia (AML) in particular. As a data source, we digitised the monolayer region of Pappenheim-stained peripheral blood smears from 100 patients diagnosed with AML at LMU University Hospital in 2014-2017, as well as 100 samples from controls without signs of hematological malignancy. The scanned regions were annotated into a 15-category classification scheme by staff experienced in routine cytomorphological diagnostics on a single-leukocyte level. Intra- and inter-rater variability was determined by multiple re-annotations. The resulting annotated dataset contains over 18,000 single- cell images and has been made publicly available on The Cancer Imaging Archive [3]. Using our dataset, we trained and evaluated multiple Convolutional Neural Networks (CNNs) on the cytomorphological recognition task [4]. Using the ResNeXt network [5], we observe very good classification performance for most relevant cytomorphological classes. For the clinically relevant questions if a given cell belongs into a blast category or is atypical, performance of the network is on the same level as that of an independent human examiner performing single-cell classification. Finally, we analyse the importance of specific single-cell image regions to the classification decision of our network, hence shedding light on the inner workings of the network.

© Springer Fachmedien Wiesbaden GmbH, ein Teil von Springer Nature 2020
T. Tolxdorff et al. (Hrsg.), *Bildverarbeitung für die Medizin 2020*,
Informatik aktuell, https://doi.org/10.1007/978-3-658-29267-6_11

References

1. Bain BJ. Diagnosis from the blood smear. N Eng J Med. 2005;353:498–507.
2. Fuentes-Arderiu X, Dot-Bach D. Measurement uncertainty in manual differential leukocyte counting. Clin Chem Lab Med. 2009;47:112–115.
3. Matek C, Schwarz S, Marr C, et al.. A Single-cell morphological dataset of leukocytes from AML patients and non-malignant controls.; 2019. Cancer Imaging Archive.
4. Matek C, Schwarz S, Spiekermann ea. Human-level recognition of blast cells in acute myeloid leukemia with convolutional neural networks. Nature Mach Intell. 2019;(1):538–544.
5. Xie S, Girshick R, Dollár P, et al. Aggregated residual transformations for deep neural networks. Proc IEEE CVPR. 2017;.

Fully Automated Segmentation of the Psoas Major Muscle in Clinical CT Scans

Marcin Kopaczka[1], Richard Lindenpütz[1], Daniel Truhn[1,2],
Maximilian Schulze-Hagen[2], Dorit Merhof[1]

[1] Institute of Imaging and Computer Vision, RWTH Aachen University
[2] Klinik für Diagnostische und Interventionelle Radiologie, Uniklinik Aachen
marcin.kopaczka@lfb.rwth-aachen.de

Abstract. Clinical studies have shown that skeletal muscle mass, sarcopenia and muscle atrophy can be used as predictive indicators for morbidity and mortality after various surgical procedures and in different medical treatment methods. At the same time, the major psoas muscle has been has been used as a tool to assess total muscle volume. From the image processing side it has the advantage of being one of the few muscles that are not surrounded by other muscles at all times, thereby allowing simpler segmentation than in other muscles. The muscle is fully visible on abdominal CT scans, which are for example performed in clinical workups before surgery. Therefore, automatic analysis of the psoas major muscle in routine CT scans would aid in the assessment of sarcopenia without the need for additional scans or examinations. To this end, we present a method for fully automated segmentation of the psoas major muscle in abdominal CT scans using a combination of methods for semantic segmentation and shape analysis. Our method outperforms available approaches for this task, additionally we show a good correlation between muscle volume and population parameters in different clinical datasets.

1 Introduction and previous work

Sarcopenia, the age-related degenerative loss of skeletal muscular mass, has been associated with a number of harmful outcomes. In the surgical scenario, several studies have shown that sarcopenia negatively impacts the outcome of a number of surgical procedures. Therefore, assessing the level of sarcopenia before surgery has effect on treatment decisions. The European Working Group on Sarcopenia (EWGSOP) demands that the diagnosis of sarcopenia should be made in the presence of low muscle mass and either generally low muscle strength or low physical performance. The quantification of muscle mass requires dedicated examinations such as dual-energy X-ray absorptiometry (DEXA), bioelectrical impedance analysis (BIA) or whole body scans using MRI or CT. The latter two often require manual muscle segmentations or semi-automated software approaches. At the same time, abdominal CTs are commonly performed in clinical

© Springer Fachmedien Wiesbaden GmbH, ein Teil von Springer Nature 2020
T. Tolxdorff et al. (Hrsg.), *Bildverarbeitung für die Medizin 2020*,
Informatik aktuell, https://doi.org/10.1007/978-3-658-29267-6_12

workups before surgery, for treatment planning or general medical assessment. The psoas major muscle is fully visible on abdominal CTs, additionally several studies have shown that the area of the psoas muscle in axial CT slices is correlated with surgical outcome and sarcopenia. Ultimately an automated analysis of the psoas muscle could facilitate the assessment of sarcopenia in routine CT scans and could potentially render dedicated examinations, such as DEXA or BIA obsolete. To this end, we introduce and evaluate a method for the fully automated segmentation and analysis of the psoas major muscle in clinical CT scans that quantitatively outperforms available methods previously presented for this task. Additionally, we evaluate segmentation results by performing qualitative studies on different patient cohorts, showing that muscle volume reported by our algorithm allows performing analysis of CT data for sarcopeny assessment in a clinical scenario.

Decicated methods for the segmentation of the psoas major muscle have been presented in [1], where a set of shape priors built from quadratic functions was fitted to the muscle in coronal slices after the centerline of the muscle had been extracted. In [2], the authors also detect the centerline of the muscle and subsequently perform a graph cut segmentation following the centerline on axial slices. Next to those dedicated approaches, a number of abdominal multi-organ segmentation methods that also include the psoas muscle have been presented, namely in [3], [4] and [5]. In all approaches, the psoas muscle is not analyzed in its entirety. Instead only the lumbar section of the muscle is assessed since this part of the muscle that is seems relevant for clinical analysis.

2   Materials and methods

In this section, all components that have been used to design the final algorithm are introduced.

2.1   Materials

The data used for algorithm development consisted of 30 abdominal CT scans in which the central part of the psoas major muscle had been manually segmented by radiologists. Since the central part of the muscle is the most relevant for any assessment, the lower end was not segmented consistently. Therefore, our aim was to develop a method that can cope with incomplete manual segmentations.

2.2   Single-pass methods

The methods described here use the unprocessed input volume for muscle segmentation and process it either as a whole in 3D or slice by slice in 2D. The methods used for single-pass segmentation are a 2D and a 3D U-Net [6] [7], different DenseNet variants [8] and the original FCN [9]. All data was converted to 8 bit unsigned integers with a windowing of -55 to +200 HU to capture both fat and muscle densities. The 2D approaches were trained and validated on all axial slices that contained a segmentation mask which was resampled to a size of 512 x 512 pixels. For the 3D segmentation, all data was resampled to a voxel size of 256 x 256 pixels and a voxel z-size of 4 mm, as this is was the dominant resolution in the provided data. Since the annotations were not always covering the whole muscle, the 3D U-Net was trained on slabs of 16 and 32 slices containing annotations that were sampled from the input volumes.

2.3   Refining the initial segmentation

While the single-pass methods already yield a segmentation accuracy comparable to the best published methods for segmenting the psoas muscle (See Sec. 3.1 for evaluation results), these can be further refined by additional segmentation stages. The refined methods aim at improving segmentations produced by a single-pass method as described in the previous section, taking advantage of the fact that these algorithms already provide a valid prior regarding muscle position and shape. Since the center part of the muscle is surrounded by retroperitoneal fatty tissue it is easily detectable. The lower (kaudal) part of the muscle belly coherents with the iliac muscle and is thus harder to differentiate. As this region contributes to the overall psoas muscle mass to a lower degree, it was neglected in this study.

2.3.1   Detecting the area of interest
For comparable assessment, a consistent part of the muscle must be analyzed in all scans. In order to remain consistent with existing literature and after consultations with radiologists it was decided that the slices located up to 5 cm above and below the slice in which the psoas muscle has its largest area should be analyzed, since the largest part of the muscle mass is concentrated in this area. To define the area of interest, the total area of left and right psoas muscle in each slice as reported by the single-pass segmentation are computed and the slice with largest area is selected as center slice. Subsequently, the slices with a distance of up to 5 cm from the center are selected and forwarded to the refinement stage.

2.3.2   Local refinement methods with semantic segmentation networks
We trained a set of different fully connected networks to perform local segmentations of regions of interest (ROIs) defined by the initial segmentation. To this end, all right muscles were mirrored to allow training a single architecture for both left and right muscle. Subsequently, ROIs were defined as square subimages of the input slice with their center at the center of the segmentation result reported by the initial segmentation. Different sizes of the bounding boxes were evaluated, with larger boxes yielding increased contextual information. We evaluated the performance on input sizes of 128, 160 and 256 pixels that were cropped from the original CT slices. We combined three individual slices into a multicahnnel image to perform a 2.5D segmentation in the semantic networks, this approach yielded slightly better results than processing single slices exclusively.

2.3.3   Local refinement methods with shape contstraints We applied a shape-constrained segmentation method by applying patch-based feature-based active appearance models (AAMs) [10] to the data. HOG, DSIFT and Fast DSIFT were used as feature descriptors. To acquire the points required for point-based registration from the segmentation masks, the boundary of the segmentation mask in each slice was represented with 72 equidistantly arranged landmark points. Subsequently, a total of 1898 slices from the center areas of the muscles in the training set were selected to build the AAMs. The AAMs were initialized using three different methods: by providing the bounding box of the initial segmentation result and starting with the AAM's mean shape as initial shape (Box-AAM), by using the boundary of the initial segmentation result as initial shape (Boundary-AAM) and by performing fitting on the center slice and subsequently using the result of the AAM fitting and propagating it to the next unsegmented slice above or below the current slice (Propagation-AAM). Fig. 1 shows how the methods for single-pass segmentation and local improvement are combined into the full segmentation pipeline.

3   Experiments and results

We evaluate the segmentation performance of the described methods and analyze how well the segmentations provided by our algorithm can be used to perform prediction of clinical markers.

3.1   Segmentation performance

We evaluated the semantic segmentation methods for predicting the lumbar segment of the psoas muscle on a set of 30 CT scans and a total of 700 axial slices showing the whole scanned area. The methods were validated using five-fold cross validation. Segmentation results are shown in Table 1. Based on these

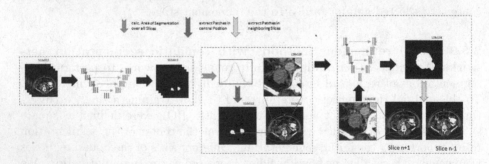

Fig. 1. Our proposed multi-pass algorithm. Initial segmentations on are provided by processing uncropped axial CT slices in a fully convolutional network. The slice with the largest psoas area is selected as center of the lumbar section and a set of slices above and below are forwarded to the refinement stage that processes subimages and the segmentations cropped around the initially segmented psoas muscle.

Table 1. Dice coefficients of the implemented single-pass segmentation methods. The best performing multi-pass method from the literature (Graph Cut) is given for comparison.

2D U-Net	3D U-Net 16	3D U-Net 32	DenseNet 67	DenseNet 103	Graph Cut
0.607	0.881	0.889	0.851	0.850	0.87

Table 2. Dice coefficients of the segmentations after applying the different refinement methods.

Box-AAM	Boundary-AAM	Propagation-AAM	2D DenseNet 56	2.5D DenseNet 56
0.850	0.880	0.927	0.928	0.932

results, the DenseNet 2 has been chosen as the initial segmentation method for single-pass segmentation that can be followed by further refinement steps.

The refinement results of the methods presented in Sec. 2.3.2 are shown in table 2. All proposed methods additionally increase the performance. When using shape-constrained methods, the Propagation-AAM delivers best performance, however results show that a second pass of DenseNet on a local scale yields best overall results. The feature extractor of the AAMs was a fast DSIFT descriptor, the other feature descriptors yielded lower results and are not shown here due to space constraints.

4   Discussion

Even the single-pass segmentation methods yield results that are comparable with the best published methods presented for segmentation of the psoas major muscle. however, it should be noted that the results could not be compared directly since the datasets used for the other methods were not publicly available. The local refinement allows further improvement of the segmentation. While adding a shape constraint enhances the segmentation performance, using two passes of DenseNet segmentation on global and local scale yielded the best results. An analysis of the volumes computed from our segmentation results shows that they are well correlated with clinical markers.

5   Conclusion

We have presented a method for fully automated segmentation of the psoas major muscle in abdominal CT scans. Our method detects the main muscle volume with high reliability by performing a multi-step segmentation where initial results provided by a deep neural network are refined by a second segmentation on local sub-images by applying a shape constraint or forwarding them to a second, locally trained neural network. Future work will include further analysis of the clinical relevance of automated segmentation of the psoas major muscle and also incorporating all presented methods into a single, end-to-end trainable solution.

References

1. Kamiya N, Zhou X, Chen H, et al. Automated segmentation of psoas major muscle in x-ray CT images by use of a shape model: preliminary study. Radiological physics and technology. 2012;5(1):5–14.
2. Inoue T, Kitamura Y, Li Y, et al. Psoas major muscle segmentation using higher-order shape prior. In: International MICCAI Workshop on Medical Computer Vision. Springer; 2015. p. 116–124.
3. Hu P, Huo Y, Kong D, et al. Automated characterization of body composition and frailty with clinically acquired CT. In: International Workshop and Challenge on Computational Methods and Clinical Applications in Musculoskeletal Imaging. Springer; 2017. p. 25–35.
4. Heinrich MP, Blendowski M. Multi-organ segmentation using vantage point forests and binary context features. In: International Conference on Medical Image Computing and Computer-Assisted Intervention. Springer; 2016. p. 598–606.
5. Meesters S, Yokota F, Okada T, et al. Multi atlas-based muscle segmentation in abdominal CT images with varying field of view; 2012. .
6. Ronneberger O, Fischer P, Brox T. U-net: convolutional networks for biomedical image segmentation. In: International Conference on Medical image computing and computer-assisted intervention. Springer; 2015. p. 234–241.
7. Çiçek Ö, Abdulkadir A, Lienkamp SS, et al. 3D U-Net: learning dense volumetric segmentation from sparse annotation. In: International conference on medical image computing and computer-assisted intervention. Springer; 2016. p. 424–432.
8. Jégou S, Drozdzal M, Vazquez D, et al. The one hundred layers tiramisu: fully convolutional densenets for semantic segmentation. In: Proceedings of the IEEE Conference on Computer Vision and Pattern Recognition Workshops; 2017. p. 11–19.
9. Long J, Shelhamer E, Darrell T. Fully convolutional networks for semantic segmentation. In: Proceedings of the IEEE conference on computer vision and pattern recognition; 2015. p. 3431–3440.
10. Antonakos E, Alabort-i Medina J, Tzimiropoulos G, et al. Feature-based Lucas–Kanade and active appearance models. IEEE Transactions on Image Processing. 2015;24(9):2617–2632.

Automated Segmentation of the Locus Coeruleus from Neuromelanin-Sensitive 3T MRI Using Deep Convolutional Neural Networks

Max Dünnwald[1,2], Matthew J. Betts[3,4], Alessandro Sciarra[1], Emrah Düzel[3,4,5], Steffen Oeltze-Jafra[1,6]

[1]Department of Neurology, Otto-von-Guericke University Magdeburg (OVGU)
[2]Faculty of Computer Science, OVGU
[3]German Center for Neurodegenerative Diseases (DZNE), Magdeburg
[4]Institute of Cognitive Neurology and Dementia Research, OVGU
[5]Institute of Cognitive Neuroscience, University College London
[6]Center for Behavioral Brain Sciences (CBBS), OVGU
max.duennwald@med.ovgu.de

Abstract. The locus coeruleus (LC) is a small brain structure in the brainstem that may play an important role in the pathogenesis of Alzheimer's Disease (AD) and Parkinson's Disease (PD). The majority of studies to date have relied on using manual segmentation methods to segment the LC, which is time consuming and leads to substantial interindividual variability across raters. Automated segmentation approaches might be less error-prone leading to a higher consistency in Magnetic Resonance Imaging (MRI) contrast assessments of the LC across scans and studies. The objective of this study was to investigate whether a convolutional neural network (CNN)-based automated segmentation method allows for reliably delineating the LC in in vivo MR images. The obtained results indicate performance superior to the inter-rater agreement, i.e. approximately 70% Dice similarity coefficient (DSC).

1 Introduction

The LC is a nucleus located alongside the fourth ventricle in the pons. This small nucleus in the brainstem is the major source of noradrenaline modulation in the brain and is involved in a variety of important brain functions such as memory, learning, attention and arousal. Recently, it has attracted increasing interest since it may also play an important role in the pathogenesis of neurodegenerative disorders such as PD [1] and AD [2, 3].

Similar to the substantia nigra (SN), the LC contains large amounts of neuromelanin (NM) - a pigmented polymer that results from the oxidation of catecholamines such as noradrenaline in the LC. This allows for in vivo visualization of the LC using neuromelanin sensitive MRI (NMs-MRI), e.g.,

© Springer Fachmedien Wiesbaden GmbH, ein Teil von Springer Nature 2020
T. Tolxdorff et al. (Hrsg.), *Bildverarbeitung für die Medizin 2020*,
Informatik aktuell, https://doi.org/10.1007/978-3-658-29267-6_13

T_1-weighted Fast Low Angle Shot (FLASH) imaging [4] and Magnetization Transfer (MT)-weighted imaging as recently reviewed [5].

A reliable segmentation is often the prerequisite for the extraction of (potential) biomarkers, e.g., contrast ratios between the LC and a reference region, which are used for further analyses of the characteristics of this structure in different cohorts (for instance subjects with AD, PD or healthy controls). For the analysis of larger cohorts, a manual segmentation approach is unfeasible, since it is tedious, time consuming and may be prone to errors [6]. Instead, automated segmentation approaches are required. To date, few methods have been published for the segmentation of the LC. The existing approaches are similar to those used for the segmentation of the SN [7] and sometimes have been applied to both structures [6, 8].

Several methods dependent purely on the intensity of the voxels. For instance, the localization of a region of interest (ROI) based on landmarks found in histological analyses and the subsequent application of an intensity threshold within the specified volume [6, 9] were proposed. This approach is inherently biased towards high intensity voxels which may pose a problem when applied to pathological cases where the signal intensity is typically decreased and the resulting contrast ratios in relation to a reference region might be overestimated. Alternatively, a fixed-numbered set of 10-connected brightest voxels can be chosen from within the ROI [10, 11]. Besides, different atlas registration-based approaches have been developed [8, 12]. However, they strongly depend on the quality of the registration output and are computationally expensive due to the required multiple co-registrations.

Recently, CNNs have been successfully applied to the automated segmentation of the SN [7]. Since SN and LC show similar imaging characteristics, we investigate here a CNN approach for LC segmentation.

2   Materials and methods

2.1   Data and manual segmentations

For this study, the same data set as in [4] was employed. It consists of T_1-weighted FLASH 3T MRI scans of 82 healthy subjects: 25 younger (22-30 years old; 13 male, 12 female) and 57 older adults (61-80 years; 19 male, 38 female). The images were acquired with an isotropic voxel size of 0.75mm. Prior to delineation of the LC, they were upsampled by means of a sinc filter to an isotropic resolution of 0.375mm. Furthermore, a bias field correction was applied. We refer the reader to [4] for more details on the characteristics of the data set.

The inter-rater agreement was determined for this study based on manual segmentations from two independent raters, rater 1 (R1) and rater 2 (R2). The DSC is on average 0.495 ± 0.158 and 0.457 ± 0.155 for the left and right LC, respectively, which is comparable to the 0.499 reported in [8], but lower than the approximately 0.6 (left LC) and 0.55 (right LC) from [12]. These relatively low values underline the difficulty of the segmentation task. The comparison with the inter-rater agreement of the SN of around 0.7 [8] indicates that LC segmentation might be even more challenging.

2.2 Network model

Inspired by results obtained for SN segmentation [7], we applied a U-Net-like [13] network. However, to address the even smaller size of the LC (as compared to the SN), we employed an architecture similar to 3D-U-Net [14], which exploits information in neighboring slices. The network is composed of blocks that each contain two convolutional layers (kernel size of $3 \times 3 \times 3$) which are each followed by a ReLU activation and a batch normalization layer. Three of such blocks form the contracting path, one is used for the bottom and another three blocks make up the expansive path. The downsampling is carried out by MaxPooling ($2 \times 2 \times 2$) and the upsampling using transposed convolutional layers.

The subjects were separated into 10 subsets and a 10-fold cross validation has been carried out in order to assess the potential of our network for LC segmentation. In every iteration, one of the 10 subsets was left out as test set while the others composed the training set. This was repeated until every subset was once used for testing. All evaluation values in the results section have been computed based on the segmentation masks resulting from the test iteration of each subset. For the training, patches of the size $64 \times 64 \times 64$ voxels were chosen as the input to the network. These were extracted randomly from all over the whole-brain volumes. However, the probability of a patch containing the LC was set to 50% to avoid a negative bias. Other forms of data augmentation such as rotation and scaling were not applied to avoid further interpolation of the data. The fuzzy DSC [15] was used as a loss function and Adam (learning rate 0.001, $\beta_1 = 0.9$, $\beta_2 = 0.999$) was chosen as the optimization scheme. The networks were trained for 250 epochs where for each epoch, 10 random patches were extracted from each subject in the training subsets. The manual segmentations of R1 were used as ground truth for the training. When applying the network to the subjects in the test set, overlapping (by half of the patch size) patches were extracted and processed by the network. The resulting masks were combined by creating their union.

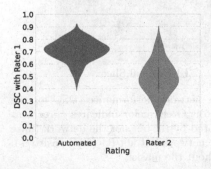

Fig. 1. Violinplots comparing the obtained DSCs of the proposed method with the masks of R1 and the inter-rater agreement (between R1 and R2).

An investigation of preliminary results revealed that the network tends to segment very small regions outside of the brainstem in some of the subjects. Due to the tiny size of these false positive regions, they did not have a noticeable impact on the DSC or the median intensity contrast ratios. However, the maximum intensity was mostly located in these voxels and therefore, caused erroneous maximum intensity contrast ratios as will be shown later. To address this issue, we applied two simple post-processing steps to the network's masks: First, some of the most outer slices of the volume were removed (fixed number across all subjects to roughly narrow down the region) and second, all connected segments with a size smaller than 50 voxels were disregarded. An alternative post-processing could be the application of a mask of the brainstem, which can be generated by popular tools like FSL [16] or using another CNN as demonstrated in a method for SN segmentation [7].

3   Results

The average DSCs of the network's masks and the segmentations of R1 for the left, right LC and the combination of both are 0.711 ± 0.096, 0.697 ± 0.091 and 0.705 ± 0.082. These values are higher than both, the inter-rater agreement (left LC: 0.501 ± 0.148, right LC: 0.463 ± 0.147, both: 0.485 ± 0.135), which can be seen in Fig. 1, as well as the results of a recently proposed atlas registration-based approach [8] (0.404 ± 0.141). However, latter comparison is to be taken with a grain of salt as [8] was evaluated on a different dataset. When compared to the masks created by R2, the network performs comparable to the inter-rater agreement: 0.499 ± 0.119 (left LC), 0.467 ± 0.126 (right LC) and 0.486 ± 0.108 (combined). Fig. 2 shows the example of an average network result.

Furthermore, the contrast ratios between the masks of the LC and a reference region within the pons were calculated. Contrast ratios are an important element in analyzing LC properties [4], which is why the influence of the automatic LC segmentations on these values was evaluated. Hence, the intra-class correlation (ICC) with a confidence level of 0.95 was determined between the contrast ratios based on manual (R1) and automatic LC masks (each in relation to the same

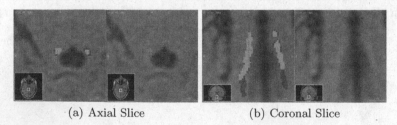

(a) Axial Slice   (b) Coronal Slice

Fig. 2. Selected slices of an example of average network performance (DSC for the left LC: 0.706, right LC: 0.683, combined: 0.696). Green color indicates agreement between network and R1, red voxels were segmented by R1 but not the network (false negatives) and blue voxels were segmented by the network but not R1 (false positives). On the right, the respective section is shown without the masks.

reference region [4]). For the median intensity contrast ratios, ICCs of 0.893 (left LC) and 0.871 (right LC) could be achieved. The maximum intensity contrast ratios are in a similar range with ICCs of 0.842 (left LC) and 0.974 (right LC). Without the previously described post-processing, the ICCs of the maximum ratios were -0.008 (left LC) and -0.014 (right LC).

4   Discussion

We applied a 3D-U-Net-like CNN for segmenting the LC in T_1-weighted FLASH NMs-MRI data. The obtained DSC and ICC values indicate a good correlation between the network and R1 as well as a performace in the range of the inter-rater agreement when compared to R2. Together, this indicates the high potential of the proposed method as an alternative to manual delineation. Small-sized false positive regions outside of the brainstem produced by the network can be addressed using different simple post-processing techniques.

However, several interesting aspects remain to be investigated in future work, for instance, an extensive evaluation of different network architectures, 2D instead of 3D input, and a direct comparison to the current state-of-the-art atlas registration-based LC segmentation methods. Furthermore, methods for the avoidance of the above-mentioned erroneous regions outside of the brainstem need to be addressed in more detail. To fully automate the LC analysis process as a whole, automatic delineation of the reference regions is also needed.

Considering that the performance of the proposed approach is already in the range or above the inter-rater agreement, we plan to set the focus of further investigations to the evaluation and improvement of the robustness of this method rather than to the increase of the performance. In particular, the robustness with respect to cohorts of subjects that show pathologies such as AD and PD and the resulting changes in the LC are of interest. Their investigation poses a challenge since they are characterized by a loss in signal intensity due to less NM in the LC region. Also, the robustness against domain shift in terms of different acquisition techniques such as the different MRI sequences suitable for LC imaging as well as methods for handling and leveraging the ambiguities of the masks created by different raters will be investigated in our future work.

Acknowledgement. This work received funding from the federal state of Saxony-Anhalt, Germany (Project I 88). Matthew J. Betts is supported by the Human Brain Project (SP3 WP 3.3.1).

References

1. Braak H, Tredici KD, Rüb U, et al. Staging of brain pathology related to sporadic parkinson's disease. Neurobiol Aging. 2003;24(2):197 – 211.
2. Braak H, Thal DR, Ghebremedhin E, et al. Stages of the pathologic process in alzheimer disease: age categories from 1 to 100 years. Journal of Neuropathology & Experimental Neurology. 2011;70(11):960–969.

3. Stratmann K, Heinsen H, Korf HW, et al. Precortical phase of alzheimer's disease (AD)-Related tau cytoskeletal pathology. Brain Pathology. 2016;26(3):371–386.
4. Betts MJ, Cardenas-Blanco A, Kanowski M, et al. In vivo MRI assessment of the human locus coeruleus along its rostrocaudal extent in young and older adults. Neuroimage. 2017;163:150 – 159.
5. Liu KY, Marijatta F, Hämmerer D, et al. Magnetic resonance imaging of the human locus coeruleus: a systematic review. Neurosci Biobehav Review. 2017;83:325 – 355.
6. Chen X, Huddleston DE, Langley J, et al. Simultaneous imaging of locus coeruleus and substantia nigra with a quantitative neuromelanin MRI approach. Magn Reson Imaging. 2014;32(10):1301 – 1306.
7. Le Berre A, Kamagata K, Otsuka Y, et al. Convolutional neural network-based segmentation can help in assessing the substantia nigra in neuromelanin MRI. Neuroradiology. 2019;61(12):1387–1395.
8. Ariz M, Abad RC, Castellanos G, et al. Dynamic atlas-based segmentation and quantification of neuromelanin-rich brainstem structures in parkinson disease. IEEE Trans Med Imaging. 2019;38(3):813–823.
9. Langley J, Huddleston DE, Liu CJ, et al. Reproducibility of locus coeruleus and substantia nigra imaging with neuromelanin sensitive MRI. Magnetic Res Mat Phys, Biol Medi. 2017;30(2):121–125.
10. García-Lorenzo D, Longo-Dos Santos C, Ewenczyk C, et al. The coeruleus/subcoeruleus complex in rapid eye movement sleep behaviour disorders in parkinson's disease. Brain. 2013;136(7):2120–2129.
11. Olivieri P, Lagarde J, Lehericy S, et al. Early alteration of the locus coeruleus in phenotypic variants of alzheimer's disease. Ann Clin Transl Neurol. 2019;6(7):1345–1351.
12. Rong Ye, Claire O'Callaghan, Catarina Rua, et al.. Imaging the locus coeruleus in parkinson's disease with ultra-high 7t MRI; 2019. Website. Available from: https://ww5.aievolution.com/hbm1901/index.cfm?do=abs.viewAbs&abs=4579.
13. Ronneberger O, Fischer P, Brox T. U-Net: convolutional networks for biomedical image segmentation. Proc - MICCAI 2015. 2015; p. 234–241.
14. Çiçek Ö, Abdulkadir A, Lienkamp SS, et al. 3D u-net: learning dense volumetric segmentation from sparse annotation. Medical Image Computing and Computer-Assisted Intervention – MICCAI 2016. 2016; p. 424–432.
15. Milletari F, Navab N, Ahmadi S. V-Net: fully convolutional neural networks for volumetric medical image segmentation. CoRR. 2016;abs/1606.04797. Available from: http://arxiv.org/abs/1606.04797.
16. Woolrich MW, Jbabdi S, Patenaude B, et al. Bayesian analysis of neuroimaging data in FSL. Neuroimage. 2009;45(1, Supplement 1):S173 – S186.

Multi-Channel Volumetric Neural Network for Knee Cartilage Segmentation in Cone-Beam CT

Jennifer Maier[1,2], Luis Carlos Rivera Monroy[1], Christopher Syben[1], Yejin Jeon[3], Jang-Hwan Choi[3], Mary Elizabeth Hall[4], Marc Levenston[4], Garry Gold[4], Rebecca Fahrig[5], Andreas Maier[1]

[1]Pattern Recognition Lab, Friedrich-Alexander-Universität Erlangen-Nürnberg (FAU), Erlangen, Germany
[2]Machine Learning and Data Analytics Lab, Friedrich-Alexander-Universität Erlangen-Nürnberg (FAU), Erlangen, Germany
[3]College of Engineering, Ewha Womans University, Seoul, Korea
[4]Stanford University, Stanford, California, USA
[5]Siemens Healthcare GmbH, Erlangen, Germany
jennifer.maier@fau.de

Abstract. Analyzing knee cartilage thickness and strain under load can help to further the understanding of the effects of diseases like Osteoarthritis. A precise segmentation of the cartilage is a necessary prerequisite for this analysis. This segmentation task has mainly been addressed in Magnetic Resonance Imaging, and was rarely investigated on contrast-enhanced Computed Tomography, where contrast agent visualizes the border between femoral and tibial cartilage. To overcome the main drawback of manual segmentation, namely its high time investment, we propose to use a 3D Convolutional Neural Network for this task. The presented architecture consists of a V-Net with SeLu activation, and a Tversky loss function. Due to the high imbalance between very few cartilage pixels and many background pixels, a high false positive rate is to be expected. To reduce this rate, the two largest segmented point clouds are extracted using a connected component analysis, since they most likely represent the medial and lateral tibial cartilage surfaces. The resulting segmentations are compared to manual segmentations, and achieve on average a recall of 0.69, which confirms the feasibility of this approach.

1 Introduction

Patients suffering from Osteoarthritis (OA) experience pain in their joints due to the degeneration of cartilage and bones. To better understand how OA is affecting the knee joint, it can be analyzed under load, because it then shows different mechanical properties compared to the unloaded case [1]. This analysis can be realized using weight-bearing *in-vivo* cone-beam computed tomography

© Springer Fachmedien Wiesbaden GmbH, ein Teil von Springer Nature 2020
T. Tolxdorff et al. (Hrsg.), *Bildverarbeitung für die Medizin 2020*,
Informatik aktuell, https://doi.org/10.1007/978-3-658-29267-6_14

(CBCT) acquisitions with injected contrast agent visualizing the thin line between femoral and tibial cartilage (Fig. 1a).

A prerequisite for the analysis of cartilage is a prior segmentation of the knee's structures. The segmentation of cartilage resp. its surface has mainly been investigated in Magnetic Resonance (MR) acquisitions [2]. Since the conventional manual labeling of cartilage in CBCT is very time consuming, (semi-) automatic approaches using machine learning have been developed. Acetabular cartilage in the hip joint was segmented using a shape-based approach and prior knowledge [3], or by applying a seed-growing algorithm [4], both exploiting the specific shape of the hip joint. Regarding the segmentation of the thin contrast agent line in knee CBCT, Myller et al. [5] were one of the first to apply a semi-automatic approach based on model registration and intensity changes. Their approach yielded good results on high resolution unloaded CT images segmenting the whole femoral and cartilage surface.

In contrast to this, this work aims to segment only the region of the contrast agent line where femoral and tibial cartilage are in contact. Consequently, the main challenge is the high imbalance in the data between the small contrast agent line and the large background. We propose an automatic segmentation based on a 3D volumetric convolutional neural network. The network is trained and evaluated on manual segmentations of contrast enhanced knee CBCT volumes. Since the resulting segmentations contain many false positives as expected due to the high class imbalance, a post processing step of extracting the largest connected point clouds is applied.

2   Materials and methods

2.1   Data

The dataset used in this work was acquired under an IRB-approved protocol, containing in total 40 CBCT scans of 8 subjects in a supine (s) or weight-bearing (w) position. The C-arm (Artis Zeego, Siemens Healthcare GmbH, Erlangen, Germany) acquired 496 (s)/248 (w) projections of size 1240×960 pixels with

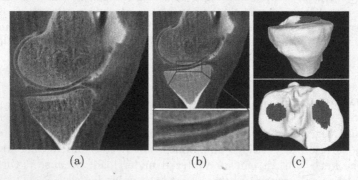

(a)   (b)   (c)

Fig. 1. Example volume and segmentation. (a) Contrast-enhanced gray-scale image. (b) Ground truth segmentation of bone and cartilage (red), zoomed image below. (c) 3D visualization of the segmentation in sagittal (top) and axial (bottom) view.

isotropic pixel size of 0.308 mm on a calibrated vertical (s)/horizontal (w) trajectory. Contrast agent was injected in the knee to visualize the outline of soft tissues. The reconstructions had a size of 512^3 voxels with an isotopic spacing of 0.2 mm.

The tibia and the thin contrast agent line where tibial and femoral cartilage are in contact were manually segmented slice by slice in the sagittal view by an expert (Fig. 1b, c). In total, only 0.18% of all voxels belonged to the cartilage surface (= positive voxels), resulting in a high imbalance in the annotations.

The dataset was divided into 70%−10%−20% for the training/validation/test group, with no subject being represented in both training/validation and test. Due to GPU memory restrictions, the data had to be sub-divided into smaller volumetric patches of size 100^3. To address the high class imbalance, for training and validation the data was oversampled by using 70% patches that have a randomly picked positive voxel in the center, and 30% all negative patches. Four patches per volume were extracted for training and validation, and data augmentation was applied to the training patches with random rotations of 90°, 180°, and 270°. For testing, the whole volumes were divided into disjoint patches.

2.2   Multi-channel volumetric neural network

The architecture we used was a VNet [6], an extension of UNet for volumetric data (Fig. 2). It takes advantage of 3D convolutions, fully connected connec-

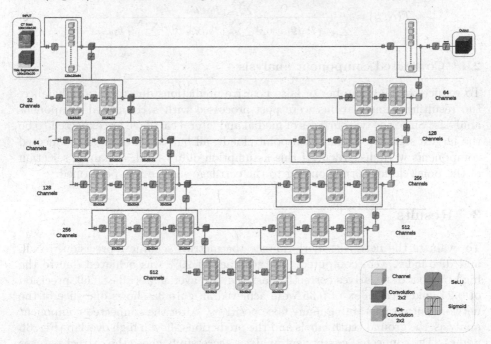

Fig. 2. Proposed architecture: Adapted VNet with SeLu activation. + represents an element-wise sum, x depicts a convolution.

tions and modified types of residual connections. Introducing skip connections between encoder and decoder path produced results correctly located and at the same time with more confidence in the prediction. The number of convolutions and several stages were adapted to the task of cartilage segmentation. SeLu was used as the activation function showing a stable and relatively fast convergence. Finally, AMSGrad was chosen as the optimization scheme, since it outperformed the ADAM traditionally used on VNet. AMSGrad proved that adding the concept of memory for a highly imbalanced dataset produced better results and a faster convergence [7]. To avoid overfitting, dropout was added with a value of 60%.

2.3   Loss function

The Tversky index [8] described by Equation 1 was chosen as loss function since it is able to work with highly imbalanced data. p_{ni}, p_{pi} represent the negative and positive voxels of the prediction, g_{ni}, g_{pi} are the negative and positive voxels in the ground truth annotation. Tversky directly takes into account the relation between False Positive (FP) and False Negatives (FN) predictions and proposes parameters α and β to manage the trade-off between both errors. For this specific case, the highest performance was achieved using $\alpha = 0.4$ and $\beta = 0.6$

$$T(\alpha, \beta) = \frac{\sum_{i=1}^{N} p_{ni} g_{ni}}{\sum_{i=1}^{N} p_{ni} g_{ni} + \alpha \sum_{i=1}^{N} p_{ni} g_{pi} + \beta \sum_{i=1}^{N} p_{pi} g_{ni}} \tag{1}$$

2.4   Connected component analysis

To reduce the high number of false positive predictions due to data imbalance, the resulting segmentations were post-processed with a connected component analysis. Since the two surfaces of medial and lateral cartilage are expected to be the largest segmented connected point clouds, all but the two largest connected components were discarded. If this assumption didn't hold, a manual selection of the point clouds corresponding to the cartilage surface was performed.

3   Results

To evaluate the network's performance the metrics accuracy, precision, recall, and dice index were computed. An accuracy of 99% was achieved due to the high number of negatives correctly classified. An average recall of 0.69, precision of 0.24, and dice index of 0.35 were achieved. Figure 3a shows one slice of the network output containing many false positives. After the connected component analysis, the ground truth labels and the predictions show a high overlap (Fig. 3b and c). The connected component analysis successfully chose the correct patches in most of the test cases, and only one had to be adapted manually.

4 Discussion

The proposed network shows promising results for the task of knee cartilage surface segmentation. Despite the use of oversampling and Tversky loss, the high imbalance still led to a high false positive rate. Using mainly patches containing positive voxels for training led the model to learn that even patches in the periphery of the knee joint should contain positive voxels (Fig. 3a). Since these peripheral false segmentations are small and closely connected, the connected component analysis applied in post-processing was able to remove them and predict the desired cartilage segmentation in a stable way (Fig. 3b). Only the false positives in the segmentation's proximity could not be removed (Fig. 3c).

We see the connected component post-processing step as an intermediate solution. In future, we want to investigate an enhancement of the network using the prior knowledge about the segmentation being a 1D continuous line in the sagittal view. This can be achieved following the learning with known operators paradigm [9] by including either the connected component analysis or a polynomial fitting step directly into the network.

An additional reason for the high false positive rate is the current way of dividing the volume into patches, thereby restraining the network from learning the spatial relation of the cartilage contact area between femur and tibia. The border between patches can even be seen in the resulting segmentation (Fig. 3c). The reason for dividing the volume into patches is the hardware limitation due to the large size of medical data. A solution with bigger patches or even the full volume could be achieved using reversible networks as proposed in [10].

Note that the manual segmentations used as ground truth are one pixel thin lines in the sagittal view, meaning that a 1-pixel shift directly results in false predictions. However, the contrast agent in the cartilage contact area is in most cases multiple pixels thick, leading the network to predict a point cloud instead of only a thin line (Fig. 3b). The consequence of this is directly observable in our reported metrics with a very low precision due to many false positives, but also with a good recall because most of the true labels are contained in the

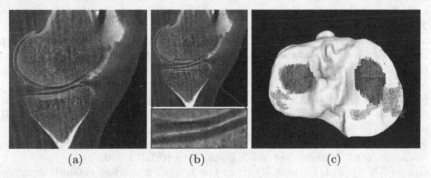

(a)   (b)   (c)

Fig. 3. (a) Sagittal slice overlaid with network output (blue). (b) Overlay of ground truth (red) and final output (blue) in a sagittal slice, overlap marked in yellow. (c) 3D view of ground truth (red) and final output (blue).

predicted point clouds. As these metrics are used to compute the loss function and therefore guide the training, we hope that the enrichment of the network with prior knowledge or a polynomial fitting can stabilize the training and overcome this instability.

The presented results confirm the complexity of this highly imbalanced task, but show promising results towards a fully automatic cartilage segmentation in CBCT. Even though there are still many false positives in the final segmentation (Fig. 3c), the proposed method can help to facilitate and accelerate the process of analyzing cartilage thickness in the clinical field.

Acknowledgement. This work was supported by the Research Training Group 1773 Heterogeneous Image Systems, funded by the German Research Foundation (DFG). Further, the authors acknowledge funding support from NIH 5R01AR065248-03 and NIH Shared Instrument Grant No. S10 RR026714 supporting the zeego@StanfordLab.

References

1. Powers CM, Ward SR, Fredericson M, et al. Patellofemoral kinematics during weight-bearing and non-weight-bearing knee extension in persons with lateral subluxation of the patella: a preliminary study. J Orthop Sports Phys Ther. 2003;33(11):677–685.
2. Raj A, Vishwanathan S, Ajani B, et al. Automatic knee cartilage segmentation using fully volumetric convolutional neural networks for evaluation of osteoarthritis. In: ISBI 2018. IEEE; 2018. p. 851–854.
3. Tabrizi PR, Zoroofi RA, Yokota F, et al. Shape-based acetabular cartilage segmentation: application to CT and MRI datasets. Int J Comput Assist Radiol Surg. 2016;11(7):1247–1265.
4. Baniasadipour A, Zoroofi RA, Sato Y, et al. A fully automated method for segmentation and thickness map estimation of femoral and acetabular cartilages in 3D CT images of the hip. In: ISPA 2007; 2007. p. 92–97.
5. Myller KAH, Honkanen JTJ, Jurvelin JS, et al. Method for segmentation of knee articular cartilages based on contrast-enhanced CT images. Ann Biomed Eng. 2018;46(11):1756–1767.
6. Milletari F, Navab N, Ahmadi S. V-Net: fully convolutional neural networks for volumetric medical image segmentation. In: 3DV 2016; 2016. p. 565–571.
7. Duchi J, Hazan E, Singer Y. Adaptive subgradient methods for online learning and stochastic optimization. J Mach Learn Res. 2011;12(Jul):2121–2159.
8. Salehi SSM, Erdogmus D, Gholipour A. Tversky loss function for image segmentation using 3D fully convolutional deep networks. In: MLMI 2017. Springer; 2017. p. 379–387.
9. Maier AK, Syben C, Stimpel B, et al. Learning with known operators reduces maximum error bounds. Nat Mach Intell. 2019;1(8):373–380.
10. Gomez AN, Ren M, Urtasun R, et al. The reversible residual network: backpropagation without storing activations. In: Adv Neural Inf Process Syst; 2017. p. 2214–2224.

Abstract: WeLineation
STAPLE-Based Crowdsourcing for Image Segmentation

Malte Jauer[1], Saksham Goel[2], Yash Sharma[2], Thomas M. Deserno[1]

[1]Peter L. Reichertz Institute for Medical Informatics of TU Braunschweig and
Hannover Medical School
[2]Indian Institute of Technology Bombay
malte-levin.jauer@plri.de

WeLineation [1] is a web-based platform supporting scientists of various domains to obtain segmentations, which are close to ground truth (GT) references. A set of image data accompanied by a written task instruction can be uploaded, users can be invited or subscribe to join in. After passing a guided tutorial of pre-segmented example images, users can provide segmentations. The Simultaneous Truth and Performance Level Estimation (STAPLE) algorithm generates estimated ground truth segmentation masks and evaluates the users performance continuously in the backend. As a proof of concept, a test-study with 75 photographs of human eyes was performed by 44 users, collecting 2060 segmentation masks with a total of 52826 vertices along the mask contour. The number of inexperienced users required to establish a reliable STAPLE-based GT and the number of vertices the user's shall place were investigated [2]. Between 27 and 37 segmentation masks were obtained per image. Requiring an error rate lower than 2%, same segmentation performance is obtained with 13 experienced and 22 rather inexperienced users. More than 10 vertices shall be placed on the delineation contour in order to reach an accuracy larger than 95%. In average, a vertex along the segmentation contour shall be placed every 81 pixels. The results indicate that knowledge about the users segmentation performance can reduce the number of segmentation masks per image, which are needed to estimate reliable GT. Therefore, gathering user performance parameters during a crowdsourcing study and applying this information to the assignment process is recommended. In this way, benefits in the cost-effectiveness of a crowdsourcing segmentation study can be achieved.

References

1. Goel S, Sharma Y, Jauer ML, et al. WeLineation: crowdsourcing delineations for reliable ground truth estimation. Proc SPIE. 2020;11318. (in press).
2. Jauer ML, Goel S, Sharma Y, et al. STAPLE performance assessed on crowdsourced sclera segmentations. Proc SPIE. 2020;11318. (in press).

© Springer Fachmedien Wiesbaden GmbH, ein Teil von Springer Nature 2020
T. Tolxdorff et al. (Hrsg.), *Bildverarbeitung für die Medizin 2020*,
Informatik aktuell, https://doi.org/10.1007/978-3-658-29267-6_15

Abstract: Fully Automated Deep Learning Pipeline for Adipose Tissue Segmentation on Abdominal Dixon MRI

Santiago Estrada[1], Ran Lu[1], Sailesh Conjeti[1], Ximena Orozco[1], Joana Panos[1], Monique M.B Breteler[1,2], Martin Reuter[1,3]

[1]German Center for Neurodegenerative Diseases (DZNE), Germany
[2]IMBIE, Faculty of Medicine, University of Bonn, Bonn, Germany
[3]Department of Radiology, Harvard Medical School, Boston MA, USA
santiago.estrada@dzne.de

The accurate quantification of visceral and subcutaneous adipose tissue (VAT and SAT) has become a mayor interest worldwide, given that these tissue types represent an important risk factor of metabolic disorders. Currently, the gold standard for measuring volumes of VAT and SAT is the manual segmentation of abdominal fat images from 3D Dixon magnetic resonance (MR) scans – a very expensive and time-consuming process. To this end, we recently proposed Fat-SegNet [1] a fully automated pipeline to accurately segment adipose tissue inside a consistent anatomically defined abdominal region. The proposed pipeline is based on our competitive dense fully convolutional network (CDFNet): A new 2D F-CNN architecture that promotes feature selectivity within a network by introducing maximum attention through a maxout activation unit [2]. We show that the proposed network architecture (CDFNet) improves segmentation performance and simultaneously reduces the number of required training parameters. FatSegNet produces highly accurate segmentation results (Dice Scores) on SAT compared to inter-rater variability (0.975 vs. 0.982) and outperforms manual raters on the more challenging task of VAT segmentation (0.850 vs. 0.788). VAT is a more fine-grained compartment with large shape variation. The pipeline additionally demonstrates very high test-retest reliability (ICC VAT 0.998 and SAT 0.996). Overall, FatSegNet generalizes well to different body shapes, sensitively replicates known VAT and SAT volume effects in the Rhineland Study (a large prospective cohort study), and permits localized analysis of fat compartments.

References

1. Estrada S, Lu R, Conjeti S, et al. FatSegNet: A Fully Automated Deep Learning Pipeline for Adipose Tissue Segmentation on Abdominal Dixon MRI. Journal of Magnetic Resonance Imaging. 2019;.
2. Goodfellow IJ, Warde-Farley D, Mirza M, et al. Maxout networks. In: Proceedings of the 30th International Conference on International Conference on Machine Learning-Volume 28. Atlanta,USA: JMLR. org; 2013. p. III–1319.

© Springer Fachmedien Wiesbaden GmbH, ein Teil von Springer Nature 2020
T. Tolxdorff et al. (Hrsg.), *Bildverarbeitung für die Medizin 2020*,
Informatik aktuell, https://doi.org/10.1007/978-3-658-29267-6_16

Semantic Lung Segmentation Using Convolutional Neural Networks

Ching-Sheng Chang[1,2], Jin-Fa Lin[2], Ming-Ching Lee[3], Christoph Palm[1,4]

[1]Regensburg Medical Image Computing (ReMIC)
Ostbayerische Technische Hochschule Regensburg (OTH Regensburg)
[2]Department of Information and Communication Engineering
Chaoyang University of Technology, Taiwan (CYUT)
[3]Division of Thoracic Surgery, Department of Surgery
Taichung Veterans General Hospital, Taichung, Taiwan
[4]Regensburg Center of Biomedical Engineering (RCBE)
OTH Regensburg and Regensburg University
christoph.palm@oth-regensburg.de

Abstract. Chest X-Ray (CXR) images as part of a non-invasive diagnosis method are commonly used in today's medical workflow. In traditional methods, physicians usually use their experience to interpret CXR images, however, there is a large interobserver variance. Computer vision may be used as a standard for assisted diagnosis. In this study, we applied an encoder-decoder neural network architecture for automatic lung region detection. We compared a three-class approach (left lung, right lung, background) and a two-class approach (lung, background). The differentiation of left and right lungs as direct result of a semantic segmentation on basis of neural nets rather than post-processing a lung-background segmentation is done here for the first time. Our evaluation was done on the NIH Chest X-ray dataset, from which 1736 images were extracted and manually annotated. We achieved 94.9% mIoU and 92% mIoU as segmentation quality measures for the two-class-model and the three-class-model, respectively. This result is very promising for the segmentation of lung regions having the simultaneous classification of left and right lung in mind.

1 Introduction

Chest X-Ray (CXR) is a very effective imaging method used extensively in the initial diagnosis of pulmonary diseases. With the help of computer vision techniques, physicians may be able to increase accuracy and reproducibility in diagnosis. Previous studies indicate that lung regions can be effectively detected, which is an essential step for further processing [1]. The lung region detection may be part of a computer-aided diagnosis procedure tackling the problem of recovery status assessment before and after surgery in the clinical disease of

© Springer Fachmedien Wiesbaden GmbH, ein Teil von Springer Nature 2020
T. Tolxdorff et al. (Hrsg.), *Bildverarbeitung für die Medizin 2020*,
Informatik aktuell, https://doi.org/10.1007/978-3-658-29267-6_17

empyema. Recently, deep learning methods for medical imaging tasks have increased in importance. Hence, we propose an automatic lung region detection method using an encoder-decoder deep learning approach.

1.1 Background

Empyema is a result of pus accumulation within an existing lung cavity. This requires physicians to perform an invasive surgical procedure to clean the pus. After surgery, the alveoli can inflate again. Thus, physicians are able to diagnose the recovery status of the patient via the size of lung regions in CXR images (Fig. 1) to determine the success of surgery. A key limitation of the current diagnosis is that there is no quantitative reference value to explain the recovery of a patient. This study proposes an automatic lung segmentation procedure to provide the pre- and post-operation lung region sizes.

2 Material and method

Current methods on lung field segmentation based on rules, intensity-thresholding, edge-detection [2] and machine learning [3]. In each method, we constantly pursue precision and segmentation speed but still have some restrictions [1]. In the last years, neural networks were used intensively in medical semantic object segmentation. Examples of currently well-known methods are U-Net, SegNet, Mask-RCNN, and DeepLab. In this study, we decided on the architecture of DeepLab$v3^+$ [4] which is well known as state-of-art in the PASCAL VOC 2012 dataset.

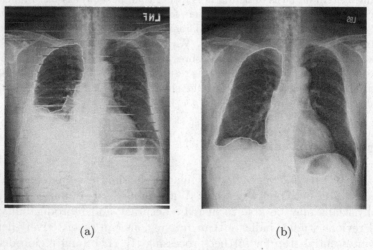

(a)   (b)

Fig. 1. Examples of pre-operative (a) and post-operative (b) CXR images. Each lung region is manually labelled by a physician (contour in green).

2.1 Image database and pre-processing

Our work is based on an images as part of the NIH Chest X-ray dataset [5]. It contains 112,120 frontal-view X-ray images from 30,805 patients in 1024×1024 resolution, showing 14 common thoracic pathologies like Atelectasis, Consolidation, Infiltration, Pneumothorax, Edema, Empyema, Fibrosis, Effusion, Pneumonia, Pleural thickening, and Cardiomegaly. A random selection of 1736 samples was labelled by physicians of Taichung Veterans General Hospital. Due to the disease of empyema three labels are necessary: left lung, right lung, and background (Fig. 2). Note, that additionally, a two-label database (lung and background) was compiled from this to enable comparison experiments. To use DeepLab$v3^+$ [4], the images were downsized to 513×513 pixels as a pre-processing step.

2.2 Encoder-Decoder nets with atrous convolutions

The well-known semantic segmentation architectures such as U-Net, SegNet, and DeepLab have an Encoder-Decoder structure using Convolutional Neural Networks. These architectures encode multi-scale contextual information by hierarchical features and effective fields-of-view. Then, they capture sharper object boundaries by decoding gradually while recovering the spatial information. For our study, we decided to use DeepLab architecture [4] as a model to train our dataset. DeepLab$v3^+$ integrates DeepLab, Encoder-Decoder and Atrous Convolution. This architecture has the characteristic of fast training and high precision.

2.2.1 Atrous convolutions increase the field of view at the same kernel computational cost. In standard convolutions, each input is passed through a 3×3 single-channel filter with nine weights. Atrous convolutions introduce another parameter to convolutional layers called the dilation rate. This defines the spacing between the values in a kernel. A 3×3 kernel with a dilation rate of

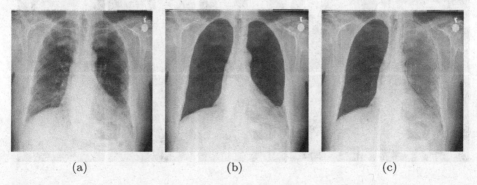

       (a)   (b)   (c)

Fig. 2. Examples of labelled dataset images. (a) Original CXR image, (b) both lung parts are annotated with the same label, (c) both lung parts are annotated with different labels.

2 will have the same field of view as a 5×5 kernel, while still using nine weights. Therefore a multi-scale information is extracted very efficiently without frequent spatial downsampling.

2.3   Training and evaluation process

We used the annotated lung images in two different kinds of experimental setting: Firstly, the annotations for the left and the right lung were treated as two different classes yielding a three-class approach together with the background. Second, both lung annoatations were handeled as one class yielding a two-class approach. For evaluation, the CXR image dataset (Sec. 2.1) was split into 1254 training and 482 testing samples. The performance is measured in terms of pixel intersection-over-union averaged across the classes (mIoU). We employed the learning rate as 0.007, crop size 513×513, fine-tuning batch normalization parameters when output stride is 16, and random scale data augmentation during training. Cross entropy was used as loss function during training.

3   Results

We achieved promising results for the three-class-model and the two-class-model with 92% mIoU and 94.9% mIoU, respectively (Fig. 3). However, we found that there are some limits to CXR image lung segmentation. To give more insight into these failures, we want to show some typical cases:

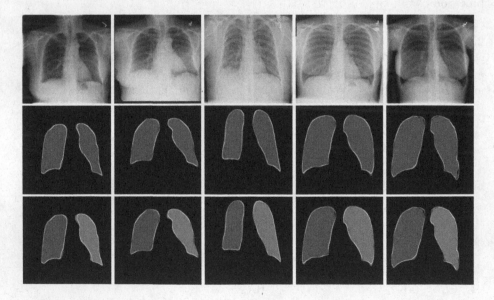

Fig. 3. Segmentation results of CXR images (manual delineation in green). The upper row shows original images. Using our two-class-model and our three-class-model, the results are shown in the middle row and in the last row, respectively.

Fig. 4. Failure examples of two-class segmentation: (a) poor image quality, (b) incomplete lung regions, (c) shadow effect of stomach air, (d, e) artificial objects within the lung regions.

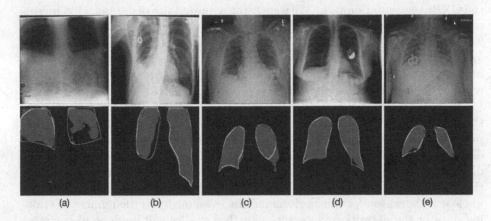

- Poor quality images cause decreased lung details, which are too dark to be identified properly (Fig. 1(a)).
- The lung region is not captured completely (Fig. 1(b)).
- Air inside the stomach will affect the result of recognition because air appears similar to regions below the lung (Fig. 1(c)).
- Artificial objects like instruments or wires will affect the segmentation results (Figs. 1(d), 1(e)).

Especially for the three-class-model we found some errors taking the left and right lung differentiation into account. Interestingly, these errors are strongly limited to the semantics of left and right lung rather than segmentation errors according to the lung-background delineation (Fig. 5).

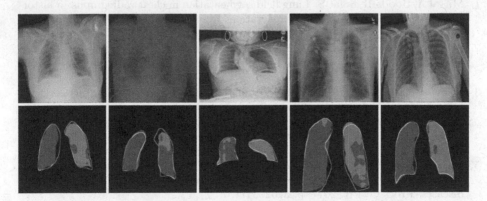

Fig. 5. Failure examples of three-class segmentation. While the lungs are well separated from the background, the left and right lung differentiation failed here.

4   Discussion and conclusion

We have shown that Encoder-Decoder neural networks can be effectively used for the CXRs segmentation task. We were using a limited size of dataset 1736 images to train the network model. Nevertheless, we achieved promising results with 94.9% mIoU and 92% mIoU for the two-class-model and the three-class-model approach on the same data, respectively. After segmenting the regions, this model is able to the calculate pixel size of the lung area and, hence, might reduce the diagnosis time and artificial error of physician.

A recent work of Solovyev et al. [3] applied several different networks for the lung semantic segmentation task such as UNet, LinkNet, PSPNet, and their proposed Feature Pyramid Network (FPN). They achieved on the same basic dataset (NIH Chest X-ray dataset [5]) but with a lower number of training data (421 images) a result of 92% mIoU. Therefore, our study outperformed the state-of-the-art approach of FPN using DeepLab$v3^+$. However, it remains unclear if the reason for this performance increase might be the number of training data or the network architecture. Further studies will be done to get more information about this issue.

The comparison between two-class-segmentation and three-class-segmentation showed, that DeepLab$v3^+$ was able to distinguish between the left and right lungs quite well. This unexpected performance will be studied further to get more insight into the features learned.

Acknowledgement. This work was supported by grants from the Taichung Veterans General Hospital and Chaoyang University of Technology (TCVGH-CYUT1088803) Taichung, Taiwan, Republic of China.

References

1. Mittal A, Hooda R, Sofat S. Lung field segmentation in chest radiographs: a historical review, current status, and expectations from deep learning. IET Image Proc. 2017;11(11):937–952.
2. Li X, Luo S, Hu Q, et al. Automatic lung field segmentation in x-ray radiographs using statistical shape and appearance models. J Med Imaging Health Inform. 2016 04;6:338–348.
3. Solovyev R, Melekhov I, Lesonen T, et al. Bayesian feature pyramid networks for automatic multi-label segmentation of chest x-rays and assessment of cardio-thoratic ratio. arXiv e-prints. 2019 Aug;.
4. Chen LC, Zhu Y, Papandreou G, et al. Encoder-decoder with atrous separable convolution for semantic image segmentation. Procs ECCV. 2018 September;.
5. Wang X, Peng Y, Lu L, et al. ChestX-ray8: hospital-scale chest x-ray database and benchmarks on weakly-supervised classification and localization of common thorax diseases. Procs CVPR. 2017; p. 3462–3471.

Abstract: MITK-ModelFit

Generic Open-Source Framework for Model Fitting

Ina Kompan[1], Charlotte Debus[2], Michael Ingrisch[3], Klaus Maier-Hein[1],
Amir Abdollahi[4], Marco Nolden[1], Ralf Floca[1]

[1]Division of Medical Image Computing, German Cancer Research Center DKFZ,
Heidelberg, Germany
[2]Simulation and Software Technology, Department of High-Performance Computing,
German Aerospace Center, Cologne, Germany
[3]Department of Radiology, University Hospital Munich,
Ludwig-Maximilians-University Munich, Germany
[4]Translational Radiation Oncology, German Cancer Research Center DKFZ,
Heidelberg, Germany
i.kompan@dkfz-heidelberg.de

Model fitting is employed in numerous medical imaging applications for quantitative parameter estimation. Prominent examples include pharmacokinetic modelling of dynamic contrast-enhanced (DCE) MRI data and apparent diffusion coefficient calculations. There are many fitting tools available, however most of them are limited to a special purpose and do not allow for own development and extension. In this work, we present MITK-ModelFit [1], a truly open-source and operating-system-independent fitting framework embedded as a package into the medical imaging interaction toolkit (MITK). The MITK-integration allows for easy data import/export and inclusion into workflows using pre-and post-processing steps such as segmentation and registration. MITK-ModelFit provides ready-to-use libraries for fitting, fit quality evaluation and result visualization. The software design was chosen such that the framework is highly adaptable to various use-cases and easily extendable for developers. The abstraction between model, data and fit representation makes the framework easily adaptable to any fitting task, independent of modality, fitting domain, fitting strategy or applied model. Further it achieves a high versatility regarding the support of different fitting workflows. As an example, an extensive toolbox for pharmacokinetic analysis of DCE MRI data is available with both, interactive and automatized batch processing workflows.

References

1. Floca R, Debus C, Ingrisch M, et al. MITK-ModelFit: A generic open-source framework for model fits and their exploration in medical imaging - design, implementation and application on the example of DCE-MRI. BMC Bioinformatics. 2019;20(21).

© Springer Fachmedien Wiesbaden GmbH, ein Teil von Springer Nature 2020
T. Tolxdorff et al. (Hrsg.), *Bildverarbeitung für die Medizin 2020*,
Informatik aktuell, https://doi.org/10.1007/978-3-658-29267-6_18

Compressed Sensing for Optical Coherence Tomography Angiography Volume Generation

Lennart Husvogt[1,2], Stefan B. Ploner[1], Daniel Stromer[1],
Julia Schottenhamml[1], Eric Moult[2], James G. Fujimoto[2], Andreas Maier[1]

[1]Pattern Recognition Lab, Friedrich-Alexander-Universität Erlangen-Nürnberg
[2]Biomedical Optical Imaging and Biophotonics Group, MIT, Cambridge, USA
lennart.husvogt@fau.de

Abstract. Optical coherence tomography angiography (OCTA) is an increasingly popular modality for imaging of the retinal vasculature. Repeated optical coherence tomography (OCT) scans of the retina allow the computation of motion contrast to display the retinal vasculature. To the best of our knowledge, we present the first application of compressed sensing for the generation of OCTA volumes. Using a probabilistic signal model for the computation of OCTA volumes and a 3D median filter, it is possible to perform compressed sensing reconstruction of OCTA volumes while suppressing noise. The presented approach was tested on a ground truth, averaged from ten individual OCTA volumes. Average reductions of the mean squared error of 9.67% were achieved when comparing reconstructed OCTA images to the stand-alone application of a 3D median filter.

1 Introduction

Optical coherence tomography (OCT) is a widely used standard imaging modality in ophthalmology. It is non-invasive and provides 3D volumes of scattering tissue with micrometer resolution. Increases in imaging speed have led to the development of OCT angiography (OCTA) [1]. For OCTA, tissue is scanned multiple times. This allows to calculate motion contrast within the tissue which reveals areas of blood flow [2]. Use of OCTA has been continually increasing since it provides several advantages over previously available imaging methods such as fluorescein angiography (FA). FA requires the injection of a contrast agent which is invasive and carries the risk of anaphylactic shock and death in a small number of patients [3]. The availability of a non-invasive method for the imaging of retinal blood vessels promises to be advantageous for the early diagnosis of common ophthalmic diseases, such as diabetic retinopathy (DR) and age-related macular degeneration (AMD). Weaknesses include OCTA's susceptibility to artifacts induced by patient motion during acquisition. Although algorithms exist to mitigate these effects [4]. Another source of noise in OCTA is speckle noise in OCT volumes from which OCTA is computed [2].

© Springer Fachmedien Wiesbaden GmbH, ein Teil von Springer Nature 2020
T. Tolxdorff et al. (Hrsg.), *Bildverarbeitung für die Medizin 2020*,
Informatik aktuell, https://doi.org/10.1007/978-3-658-29267-6_19

To the best of our knowledge, denoising of OCTA images is usually performed by applying basic filters such as a median filter. Thus, there is considerable opportunity to find new ways of generating and filtering OCTA volumes to improve image quality. One possible approach for the generation and denoising of OCTA volumes is compressed sensing (CS) [5]. It has been successfully used in other areas of medical imaging, including computed tomography and magnetic resonance imaging. CS led to the reduction of X-ray dose and imaging time respectively [6, 7]. CS exploits the fact that many signals are sparse, i.e. they exhibit redundancies in a certain base. This can allow reconstructions of signals from a reduced number of measurements or denoising of signals using the available number of measurements.

To apply CS to a reconstruction/denoising problem, a rigorous mathematical derivation of the signal model is needed. Ploner et al. presented such derivations for two formulas commonly used for the generation of OCTA volumes: speckle variance and amplitude decorrelation [8]. In this paper we propose a CS reconstruction method based on that work. CS in OCT itself is not new, there have been proposals in the past to use CS for OCT image generation [9]. However, we present, to the best of our knowledge, the first application of CS for the reconstruction of OCTA volumes.

2   Materials and methods

If $a_{\mathbf{p},i}$ is a series of OCT intensities at volume position $\mathbf{p} \in \mathbb{R}^3$, speckle variance (SV) at the same location is defined as

$$\sigma_{\mathrm{SV},\mathbf{p}}^2 = \frac{1}{N} \sum_{i=1}^{N} (a_{\mathbf{p},i} - \mu_{\mathbf{p}})^2 \tag{1}$$

with N being the number of measurements, $i \in [1, 2, \ldots, N]$, and $\mu_{\mathbf{p}}$ being the mean of all $a_{\mathbf{p},i}$. Ploner et al. used a maximum log-likelihood estimation in their derivation to show that Eq. 1 applies when the log-likelihood $\log L_{\mathrm{SV}}$ is at a maximum. This derivation yields the gradient

$$\frac{d \log L_{\mathrm{SV}}}{d\sigma_{\mathrm{SV},\mathbf{p}}^2} = \frac{-N \cdot \sigma_{\mathrm{SV},\mathbf{p}}^2 + \sum_{i=1}^{N} (a_{\mathbf{p},i} - \mu_{\mathbf{p}})^2}{2\sigma_{\mathrm{SV},\mathbf{p}}^4} \tag{2}$$

which can be used to find $\sigma_{\mathrm{SV},\mathbf{p}}^2$ given a current estimate for it [8].

2.1   Algorithm

From now on, we will denote an OCTA volume, containing $\sigma_{\mathrm{SV},\mathbf{p}}^2$ as $\mathbf{x}$ and the repeated scans of an OCT volume as $\mathbf{y}$. We then define a data consistency term

$$\operatorname*{argmin}_{\hat{\mathbf{x}}} \mathrm{D}(\mathbf{x}, \mathbf{y}) = -\frac{1}{2} \|\mathrm{L}_{\mathrm{SV}}(\mathbf{x}, \mathbf{y})\|_2^2 \tag{3}$$

Algorithmus 1 Listing of the CS OCTA reconstruction algorithm.

Objective: Minimize $D(\mathbf{x}, \mathbf{y}) = -\frac{1}{2}\|L_{SV}(\mathbf{x}, \mathbf{y})\|_2^2$ with respect to $\mathbf{x}$
Input: Supply the following components and parameters:

- Step size λ
- Regularizer R and its parameters
- Total number of iterations N_{iter} and number of iterations N_{reg} for the regularizer

Initialization: Initialize $\mathbf{x}_0$ using the speckle variance formula in Eq. 1.
Loop:

- Update the OCTA volume $\mathbf{x}_{k+1} = \mathbf{x}_k + \lambda \nabla L_{SV}(\mathbf{x}_k)$.
- Every N_{reg} iterations apply the regularizer $\mathbf{x}_{k+1} = R(\mathbf{x}_k)$.

End of Loop
Result: The output $\hat{\mathbf{x}}$

---

with $\hat{\mathbf{x}}$ being the OCTA volume we seek to reconstruct. $L_{SV}(\mathbf{x}, \mathbf{y})$ is the likelihood defined in [8]. The objective is to find an angiography volume $\hat{\mathbf{x}}$ maximizing the probabilities that fit the observations $\mathbf{y}$ by minimizing the term in Eq. 3. Minimization is performed via the Landweber iteration, while the gradient in Eq. 2 allows to find this minimum. This reconstruction approach is also called *maximum a posteriori estimation* [10].

By adding a 3D median filter as regularizer, we can perform a CS reconstruction of OCTA volumes. Not only does a median filter perform denoising, but it also acts as a L_1 estimator because applying a median filter to $\mathbf{x}$ minimizes its L_1 norm [11]. This, in turn, *enforces sparsity in image domain*. Furthermore, Romano et al. showed that the L_1 norm can serve as an effective regularizer for image denosing in their regularization by denoising approach [12]. In this work, we propose the use of a 3D median filter with a kernel size of $3 \times 3 \times 3$ voxel as regularizer. In our experiments, the regularizer was applied to the data every ten iterations. Convergence of the reconstruction can be detected by computing the mean squared error between the current reconstruction result and the input volume. If the error does not change anymore, convergence has been reached. The complete algorithm is listed in Alg. 1.

2.2 Data

To evaluate the presented method, the right eye of a 28 year old, male, healthy volunteer was imaged and ten scans were acquired. The scanned field size is 3×3mm. 500 B-scans were acquired, and each B-scan was repeatedly scanned five times to facilitate the computation of OCTA volumes. Every B-scan contains 500 A-scans. A prototype swept-source OCT system was used for acquiring the scans [2]. Because every B-scan in a single scan is scanned five times, a single scan is thus sufficient to compute an OCTA volume. By computing the speckle variance OCTA volume of each scan and using a non-rigid registration method, an averaged volume, merged from ten OCTA volumes was generated [4]. This low-noise, high signal-to-noise ratio merged volume serves as ground

Table 1. Mean squared error results for eight of the ten test scans. Two scans were omitted, because of severe motion artifacts.

scan	1	2	3	4	5	6	7	8
MSE	1.30	0.35	1.19	0.54	0.83	0.79	1.47	1.23
improvement	11.36%	8.44%	11.82%	7.02%	10.79%	13.16%	8.76%	5.98%

truth. The presented algorithm was applied to single scans, and the resulting OCTA volumes compared against the ground truth. OCTA volumes are usually displayed as en face images. For this, the retinal pigment epithelium and the inner nerve fiber layer were segmented [13]. The volume between these two layers was then projected using a 90th percentile projection. The ensuing en face projection shows the blood vessels and capillaries of the retinal vasculature. Results of the reconstruction process are projected as well and compared to the en face projection of the ground truth data.

Reconstruction was performed on eight of the ten individual scans, because two scans exhibited motion artifacts that made a comparison to the ground truth unfeasible.

3 Results

Quantitative results of the reconstruction of the first scan are shown in Fig. 1, which shows the decrease in mean squared error over the reconstruction iterations. Qualitative results and details for the same scan are shown in Fig. 2 and show a reduction of noise in the areas between capillaries. Tab. 1 shows quantitative results for all test scans.

4 Discussion

The plot in Fig. 1 and the results in Tab. 1 demonstrate a reduction in the mean squared error of all scans used in the experiment. On average, the mean

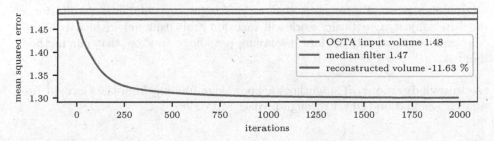

Fig. 1. Mean squared error between ground truth and and the reconstructed en face projection (blue line) of the first out of ten scans. The red line shows the error for the original speckle variance OCTA projection. The green line shows the error of the projected speckle variance volume after 3D median filtering.

Fig. 2. Qualitative results for scan one showing 3 × 3mm speckle variance en face projections. The dashed boxes show enlargements from the marked areas in the en face images. Columns from left to right: ground truth projection, raw speckle variance projection, after application of a 3D median filter, and after 1002 iterations of the reconstruction algorithm. Although it increases the error slightly, performing more reconstruction steps after the last regularization step, slightly increases contrast in the image.

ground truth   initial OCTA projection   median filter   after 1002 iterations

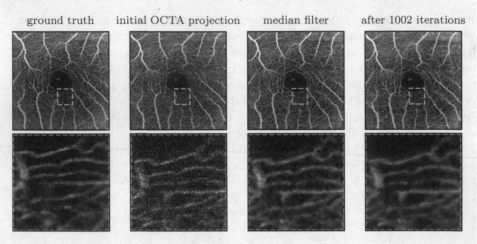

squared error is reduced by 9.67% compared to the median filtered result. The qualitative results in Fig. 2 also show an improvement in image quality. The initial projection exhibits some noise when compared to the ground truth and the reconstructed projections. Noise is reduced by the application of a 3D median filter, but noise, especially in the areas between the capillaries, is still visible. The reconstruction results after 1002 iterations shows further reduction in noise. Vessels and areas in-between appear more consistent.

We showed for the first time that it is possible to use CS for the generation of OCTA volumes. By minimizing a data consistency term while regularizing it with a 3D median filter, we show that our method outperforms a standard 3D median filter. Please note, that at this point, we only show results for a healthy subject. Our future work will focus on evaluating new regularizers and the evaluation on patient data displaying pathology to show that our method holds.

Acknowledgement. The authors acknowledge funding from the German Research Foundation (DFG) through project MA 4898/12-1.

References

1. Husvogt L, Ploner S, Maier A. Optical coherence tomography. In: Medical imaging systems. Springer, Cham; 2018. p. 251–261.

2. Choi W, Moult EM, Waheed NK, et al. Ultrahigh-speed, swept-source optical coherence tomography angiography in nonexudative age-related macular degeneration with geographic atrophy. Ophthalmology. 2015;122(12):2532–2544.
3. Novais EA, Adhi M, Moult EM, et al. Choroidal neovascularization analyzed on ultrahigh-speed swept-source optical coherence tomography angiography compared to spectral-domain optical coherence tomography angiography. Am J Ophthalmol. 2016;164:80–88.
4. Ploner SB, Kraus MF, Husvogt L, et al. 3-D OCT motion correction efficiently enhanced with OCT angiography. In: Investigative ophthalmology & visual science. vol. 59. The Association for Research in Vision and Ophthalmology; 2018. p. 3922.
5. Candès E, Wakin M. An introduction to compressive sampling. IEEE Signal Process Mag. 2008;.
6. Sidky EY, Pan X. Image reconstruction in circular cone-beam computed tomography by constrained, total-variation minimization. Phys Med Biol. 2008;53(17):4777–4807.
7. Lustig M, Donoho D, Pauly JM. Sparse MRI: the application of compressed sensing for rapid MR imaging. Magn Reson Med. 2007;.
8. Ploner SB, Riess C, Schottenhamml J, et al. A joint probabilistic model for speckle variance, amplitude decorrelation and interframe variance (IFV) optical coherence tomography angiography. In: Bildverarbeitung für die Medizin 2018. 211279. Springer Berlin Heidelberg; 2018. p. 98–102.
9. Liu X, Kang JU. Compressive SD-OCT: the application of compressed sensing in spectral domain optical coherence tomography. Opt Express. 2010;18(21):22010–22019.
10. Manhart MT, Kowarschik M, Fieselmann A, et al. Dynamic iterative reconstruction for interventional 4-d c-arm CT perfusion imaging. IEEE Trans Med Imaging. 2013;32(7):1336–1348.
11. Lopuhaa HP, Rousseeuw PJ. Breakdown points of affine equivariant estimators of multivariate location and covariance matrices. The Annals of Statistics. 1991;19(1):229–248.
12. Romano Y, Elad M, Milanfar P. The little engine that could: regularization by denoising (RED). SIAM J Imaging Sci. 2016;10(4):1804–1844.
13. Schottenhamml J, Moult EM, Novais EA, et al. OCT-OCTA segmentation. In: Bildverarbeitung für die Medizin 2018. Berlin, Heidelberg: Springer Vieweg, Berlin, Heidelberg; 2018. p. 284.

Reproduzierbare Kalibrierung von elektromagnetischen Feldverzerrungen

Experimente mit einem miniaturisierten Feldgenerator, befestigt an einer Ultraschallsonde

Florian Hennig[1], Florian Pfiz[1], Diana Mîndroc-Filimon[3], Lena Maier-Hein[3], Bünyamin Pekdemir[3], Alexander Seitel[3], Alfred Michael Franz[2,3]

[1]Institut für Medizintechnik und Mechatronik, Technische Hochschule Ulm
[2]Institut für Informatik, Technische Hochschule Ulm
[3]Abteilung Computer-assistierte Medizinische Interventionen, DKFZ Heidelberg
`alfred.franz@thu.de`

Kurzfassung. Elektromagnetisches (EM) Tracking ist beeinflusst von Störeinflüssen durch metallische und EM Materialien im Trackingvolumen, wie sie in vielen Anwendungen in der Medizin vorkommen. Eine Kompensation derartiger Störungen ist insbesondere dann möglich, wenn diese von statischer Natur sind, wie beispielsweise im Fall eines kleinen EM Feldgenerators (FG) der fest mit einer mobilen Bildgebung verbunden ist. In dieser Arbeit wurde eine Vorrichtung zur reproduzierbaren Kalibrierung solcher Aufbauten entwickelt und für den Anwendungsfall eines an einer Ultraschallsonde befestigten FGs experimentell validiert. Mit einer interpolationsbasierten Kalibrierungsmethode zeigte sich eine deutliche, reproduzierbare Reduktion der Feldverzerrung sowohl im Bereich unterhalb der Sonde, als auch in den erstmals untersuchten Seitenbereichen. Der mittlere Fehler der untersuchten 5 cm Distanzen konnte von 1,6 mm auf 0,5 mm reduziert werden.

1 Einleitung

Elektromagnetisches (EM) Tracking ist eine vielversprechende Technologie um medizinische Instrumente auch ohne freie Sichtlinie im Körper des Patienten zu lokalisieren [1]. Hierzu werden kleine Sensoren in die Instumente integriert. Ein von einem externen Feldgenerator (FG) emittiertes EM Feld wird durch diese Sensoren gemessen. Dadurch kann die Pose innerhalb eines als Trackingvolumen bezeichneten Bereichs bestimmt werden. EM Tracking kann jedoch leicht durch metallische oder EM Materialien im Trackingvolumen gestört werden, was zu einer mangelnden Robustheit führt. Daher setzten sich Medizinprodukte mit EM Trackingsystemen bisher in der klinischen Praxis häufig nicht durch.

Insbesondere wenn die Störungen des EM Trackings von statischer Natur sind, können diese jedoch durch Kalibrierung kompensiert werden. Punktbasierte [2] oder interpolationsbasierte [3] Kalibrierungsmethoden wurden hierfür

© Springer Fachmedien Wiesbaden GmbH, ein Teil von Springer Nature 2020
T. Tolxdorff et al. (Hrsg.), *Bildverarbeitung für die Medizin 2020*,
Informatik aktuell, https://doi.org/10.1007/978-3-658-29267-6_20

bereits erfolgreich eingesetzt. Zur Kalibrierung müssen üblicherweise unverzerrte Referenzdaten, beispielsweise von einem optischen Trackingsystem, im benötigten Trackingvolumen aufgezeichnet werden. Eine Herausforderung ist dabei eine gleichmäßige und reproduzierbare Abdeckung des Volumens mit Messpunkten.

Derartige Kalibrierungsmethoden können vor allem dann hilfreich sein, wenn ein kleiner EM FG mit einer mobilen Bildgebung verbunden wird. Ein Beispiel hierfür ist die Kombination des kleinen TX1 FG der Firma Polhemus Inc. (Colchester, Vermont, USA) mit einer Ultraschall(US)-Sonde, wie in Abb. 1a) gezeigt. Dieser Aufbau ermöglicht bei US-geführten Punktionen die Visualisierung von Instrument und Einstichpfad [4]. Mittels Kalibrierung könnten durch die US-Sonde verursachte Feldverzerrungen kompensiert werden, was bisher jedoch noch nicht untersucht wurde.

Ziel dieses Projekts ist daher die Entwicklung einer Vorrichtung, die die reproduzierbare Kalibrierung von Feldverzerrungen bei handlichen Aufbauten ermöglicht. Exemplarisch soll diese Vorrichtung zur Kalibrierung der in Abb. 1a) gezeigten Kombination von EM FG und US-Sonde mittels einer interpolationsbasierten Methode genutzt werden. Neben dem Hauptbereich unter der Sonde sollen erstmals auch die Seitenbereiche untersucht werden. Im Rahmen dieser Versuche soll ein Kalibrierraster ermittelt werden, welches eine zuverlässige Fehlerreduktion ermöglicht. Für dieses Raster soll die Reproduzierbarkeit bei mehreren Kalibrierungsdurchläufen untersucht werden.

2 Material und Methoden

Das vorgeschlagene Kalibrierungsverfahren mittels der entwickelten Vorrichtung umfasst folgende Schritte: (1) Aufnahme von verzerrten und unverzerrten Werten im gesamten Trackingvolumen, (2) Berechnung der Verzerrungskompensation und (3) Anwendung der Verzerrungskompensation auf neue Daten.

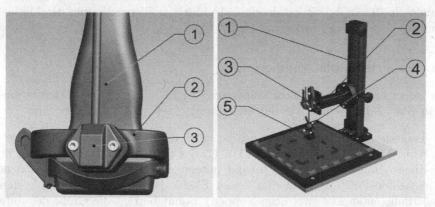

Abb. 1. US-Sonde GE 11L (1) mit Halterung (2) und Polhemus TX1 Feldgenerator (3). Setup zur Kalibrierung. Linearführung mit Höhenverstellung (1), Haltearm für US-Sonde (2), US-Sonde mit FG und opt. Referenzmarker (3), EM Sensor mit opt. Referenzmarker (4), Legoadapter zum Stecken der Kalibrierungspositionen (5).

2.1 Messung der Feldverzerrung

Für die Kalibrierung werden optische Marker so am EM FG und Sensor befestigt, dass über beide Verfahren die aktuelle Position des Sensors in Relation zum FG ermittelt werden kann. Das Setup zur Kalibrierung ist in Abb. 1b) dargestellt. Dabei wird optisches Tracking als Referenz angewandt, da dieses deutlich genauere Messwerte liefert als das zu kalibrierende EM Trackingsystem und gegenüber materialbedingten Störungen unempfindlich ist [5].

Um den Trackingraum möglichst gleichmäßig zu erfassen, wurde die in Abb. 1b) gezeigte Vorrichtung zur Platzierung von Sensor und Referenzmarker entwickelt. Sie ist vollständig metallfrei und flexibel auf verschiedene US-Sonden anwendbar. Der untersuchbare Koordinatenraum beträgt ca. 30 cm x 30 cm x 30 cm. Die Kalibrierpositionen werden in der x-y-Ebene auf eine in die Vorrichtung integrierte Lego-Platte gesteckt. Lego eignet sich aufgrund der angeforderten Flexibilität des Kalibrierbereichs und der hohen Fertigungsgenauigkeit gut für diesen Einsatzzweck [6]. Die Position auf der z-Achse ist mittels einer Linearführung stufenlos verstellbar.

Der Haltearm der Sonde erlaubt eine Drehung von 90 Grad, sowohl mit als auch gegen den Uhrzeigersinn („Rechtsdrehung"bzw. „Linksdrehung"). Somit ist eine Kalibrierung der Seitenbereiche möglich. Die verwendete US-Sonde wird in einer Universalhalterung am äußeren Ende des Haltearms fixiert und befindet sich dadurch mittig über dem Kalibrierbereich. Die Position des Sensors wird mithilfe eines Adapters auf der Lego-Platte fixiert.

2.2 Kalibrierungsmethode

Zur Kalibrierung kommt die multiquadratische Interpolationsmethode von Hardy *et al.* zum Einsatz [7]. Sie liefert eine über die Messpunkte interpolierte Korrekturfunktion mit der neue Positionsmessungen korrigiert werden können. In dieser Arbeit wurde eine MATLAB Implementierung der Methode genutzt.

2.3 Experimentelle Validierung

Der Versuchsaufbau mit einem Polhemus TX1 FG und einer GE 11L US-Sonde ist in Abb. 1 dargestellt. Aus der Zielsetzung ergeben sich drei Versuche:

– *Versuch 1:* Zur Ermittlung eines geeigneten Kalibrierrasters wurden die in Abb. 2 dargestellten Sets von 11 x 11, 6 x 6 und 3 x 3 Positionen auf drei Ebenen mit jeweils 4 cm Abstand untersucht. Der Abstand zwischen den einzelnen Positionen innerhalb einer Ebene des 11 x 11 Sets betrug dabei 16 mm (entspricht zwei Lego-Noppen). Somit beträgt die Größe des untersuchten Volumens 16 cm x 16 cm x 8 cm. Der Abstand von EM-Sensor zu FG betrug auf der obersten Ebene 8 cm. Die Subsets wurden aus dem 11 x 11 Set durch Auslassen jeder zweiten (6 x 6 Set) bzw. jeder zweiten, dritten und vierten Spalte und Zeile (3 x 3 Set) gewonnen.

– *Versuch 2:* Dieses Vorgehen wurde im zweiten Versuch für beide Seitenbereiche der Sonde wiederholt. Dadurch wurde die Möglichkeit einer Kalibrierung der Seitenbereiche untersucht.
– *Versuch 3:* Die Reproduzierbarkeit der Kalibrierung wurde untersucht, indem die Messung aus Versuch 1 mit dem 6 x 6 Kalibrierraster zwei weitere Male wiederholt wurde.

Die Evaluation der Kalibrierungen wurde mit dem Hummel-Protokoll [8] durchgeführt. Dazu wurden zusätzliche Messungen auf einer Plexiglasplatte mit hochgenauen Bohrungen im Abstand von jeweils 50 mm durchgeführt. Es wurden 4 x 3 = 12 Messpunkte auf der Platte genutzt, wobei die Messungen auf zwei Ebenen mit 5 cm Abstand stattfanden. Für jede Ebene wurden die 17 mittels EM Tracking gemessenen Distanzen zwischen den Messpunkten vor und nach Anwendung der Korrekturfunktion mit der Referenz von 50 mm verglichen. Der mittlere Fehler über 2 * 17 = 34 Distanzen dient als Maß für die Trackinggenauigkeit. Die Punktewolke der Evaluationsmessungen liegt, wie in Abb. 2 dargestellt, innerhalb der Punktewolke der Kalibrierungsmessungen, um eine Extrapolation der Korrekturfunktion zu vermeiden.

3 Ergebnisse

Wie in Abb. 3 dargestellt, konnten die durch die Feldverzerrung hervorgerufenen mittleren Fehler von durchschnittlich 1,6 mm durch Kalibrierung auf durchschnittlich 0,5 mm (11 x 11 Raster) und 0,6 mm (6 x 6 Raster) reduziert werden. Der Maximalfehler konnte von 5,2 mm auf 1,3 mm (11 x 11) bzw. 1,7 mm (6 x 6) gesenkt werden. Die Kalibrierung mittels 3 x 3 Raster hingegen sorgte sogar für eine Erhöhung des Fehlers. Die Kalibrierung mit 11 x 11 Raster in drei Ebenen dauerte ca. eine Stunde. Das 6 x 6 Raster benötigte deutlich weniger Zeit.

Diese Ergebnisse ließen sich sowohl für die Hauptausrichtung, als auch für beide Seitenbereiche feststellen. Bei einer deutlich höheren Ausgangsverzerrung des Feldes in den Seitenbereichen (mittlerer Fehler 2,2 mm für Linksdrehung, 2,3 mm für Rechtsdrehung) wurde mit dem 11 x 11 Raster verglichen mit der Hauptausrichtung ein niedrigerer mittlerer Fehler nach der Kalibrierung erzielt (0,4 mm für Linksdrehung, 0,3 mm für Rechtsdrehung).

Bei Versuch 3 betrugen die mittleren Fehler 0,62 mm, 0,61 mm und 0,59 mm. Die Standardabweichung der drei Messungen von 0,016 mm entsprach etwa 2,7 %

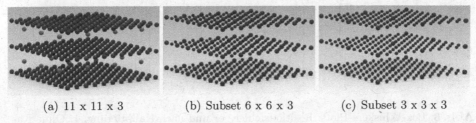

(a) 11 x 11 x 3   (b) Subset 6 x 6 x 3   (c) Subset 3 x 3 x 3

Abb. 2. Kalibrierungspunktewolken (verwendete Punkte rot) mit Evaluationspunkten 4 x 3 x 2 (in gelb).

des mittleren Fehlers. Die Varianz zwischen den Messungen war somit deutlich geringer als die Varianz innerhalb des Feldes.

4 Diskussion

Die entwickelte Vorrichtung ermöglicht die Kalibrierung eines EM FGs, der statisch mit einem Objekt, wie der getesteten US-Sonde, verbunden ist. Der mittlere Trackingfehler konnte im Fall der US-Sonde deutlich von 1,6 mm auf 0,5 mm reduziert werden. Von den untersuchten Kalibrierrastern zeigt sich das 6 x 6 Raster mit einem Fehler von 0,6 mm als guter Kompromiss zwischen Aufwand und Nutzen. Die Vorrichtung erlaubt ausführlichere Experimente zur Ermittlung von etwaigen besseren Kalibrierrastern, was im Rahmen zukünftiger Arbeiten genauer untersucht werden kann.

Die Seitenbereiche der Sonde lassen sich mit der entwickelten Vorrichtung ebenfalls kalibrieren. Die dort erzielten Verbesserungen sind wie bei der Hauptausrichtung deutlich zu sehen (Fehler vor/nach Kalibrierung: 2,2 mm / 0,4 mm (links); 2,3 mm / 0,3 mm (rechts)). Eine gleichzeitige Kalibrierung aller untersuchten Seiten ergab an den Übergängen zwischen den Seiten starke lokale Fehler. Es liegt nahe, dass diese Fehler durch die Aufzeichnung von zusätzlichen Punkten in den Übergangsbereichen reduziert werden können.

In dieser Arbeit wurde nur die Trackingposition kalibriert, je nach Anwendungsfall könnte jedoch auch eine Kalibrierung der Orientierung nötig sein. Hierzu müsste die Sensorhalterung in verschiedenen Achsen drehbar gemacht und die Implementierung des Kalibrierungsalgorithmus entsprechend ergänzt werden.

Erste Versuche zeigten, dass Validierungsmessungen mit optischen oder geometrisch durch Lego festgelegten Referenzwerten ebenfalls möglich sind. Hierfür sind allerdings ausführlichere Untersuchungen notwendig, weshalb für die vorgestellten Ergebnisse das etablierte Hummel-Protokoll angewandt wurde.

Aufgrund von Einschränkungen durch die Geometrie der Vorrichtung und Line-Of-Sight-Problemen durch die optische Referenzmessung können Verzerrungen in unmittelbarer Nähe der Sonde aktuell nicht kalibriert werden. Ist für

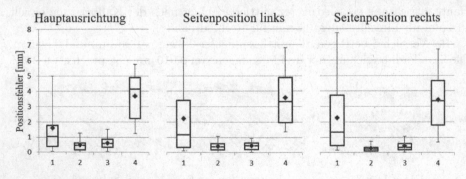

Abb. 3. Box-Whiskers-Plots: Positionsfehler vor und nach Kalibrierung. 1. Ohne Kalibrierung 2. 11 x 11 Raster 3. 6 x 6 Raster 4. 3 x 3 Raster (Whiskers 2,5 % und 97,5 % Quantil; zusätzlich Mittelwerte als Raute).

eine spezielle Anwendung die Genauigkeit in unmittelbarer Nähe der Sonde relevant, wird empfohlen die Geometrie durch Änderung der Bauteile „Haltearm"und „Halterung"anzupassen oder andere Referenzwerte (z.B. geometrisch durch Lego-Raster) zu verwenden.

Außerdem wurde im Rahmen dieser Arbeit nur eine US-Sonde getestet. Die Halterung ist für die Aufnahme von Sonden mit ähnlichen Abmessungen geeignet. Um die Ergebnisse weiter zu validieren, werden deshalb weitere Untersuchungen mit anderen Sonden empfohlen.

Zusammenfassend ermöglicht die vorgestellte Kalibriermethode, in Kombination mit der entwickelten Vorrichtung, eine reproduzierbare Kalibrierung der statischen Feldverzerrungen. Aus den untersuchten Kalibrierrastern wurde ein auf Nutzen und Aufwand bei der Versuchsdurchführung optimiertes Raster ermittelt und für die Seitenbereiche der Sonde ebenfalls bestätigt. Resultierende mittlere Fehler befinden sich im Submillimeterbereich und die Genauigkeit sollte damit für viele Anwendungen ausreichen.

Danksagung. Das diesem Paper zugrundeliegende Vorhaben wurde mit Mitteln des Bundesministeriums für Bildung und Forschung unter dem Förderkennzeichen 03VP03251 gefördert. Wir bedanken uns zudem bei Herrn Thomas Szimeth von der Technischen Hochschule Ulm für die Unterstützung.

Literaturverzeichnis

1. Franz AM, Haidegger T, Birkfellner W, et al. Electromagnetic tracking in medicine—a review of technology, validation, and applications. IEEE Trans Med Imaging. 2014 Aug;33(8):1702–1725.
2. Birkfellner W, Watzinger F, Wanschitz F, et al. Calibration of tracking systems in a surgical environment. IEEE Trans on Medical Imaging. 1998;17(5):737–742.
3. Himberg H, Motai Y, Bradley A. Interpolation volume calibration: a multisensor calibration technique for electromagnetic trackers. IEEE Trans on Robotics. 2012;28(5):1120–1130.
4. Franz AM, Seitel A, Bopp N, et al. First clinical use of the EchoTrack guidance approach for radiofrequency ablation of thyroid gland nodules. Int J Comput Assist Radiol Surg. 2017 Jun;12(6):931–940.
5. Sorriento A, Porfido MB, Mazzoleni S, et al. Optical and electromagnetic tracking systems for biomedical applications: a critical review on potentialities and limitations. IEEE Rev Biomed Eng. 2019 Sep;.
6. Kugler D, Krumb H, Bredemann J, et al. High-precision evaluation of electromagnetic tracking. Int J Comput Assist Radiol Surg. 2019 Jul;14(7):1127–1135.
7. Hardy RL. Multiquadric equations of topography and other irregular surfaces. Journal of Geophysical Research (1896-1977). 1971;76(8):1905–1915.
8. Hummel JB, Bax MR, Figl ML, et al. Design and application of an assessment protocol for electromagnetic tracking systems. Med Phys. 2005;32(7):2371–2379.

Deep Learning-Based Denoising of Mammographic Images Using Physics-Driven Data Augmentation

Dominik Eckert[1], Sulaiman Vesal[1], Ludwig Ritschl[2], Steffen Kappler[2], Andreas Maier[1]

[1] Pattern Recognition Lab, Friedrich-Alexander-Universität Erlangen-Nürnberg, Germany
[2] Siemens Healthcare GmbH, Forchheim, Germany
dominik.17.eckert@fau.de

Abstract. Mammography is using low-energy X-rays to screen the human breast and is utilized by radiologists to detect breast cancer. Typically radiologists require a mammogram with impeccable image quality for an accurate diagnosis. In this study, we propose a deep learning method based on Convolutional Neural Networks (CNNs) for mammogram denoising to improve the image quality. We first enhance the noise level and employ Anscombe Transformation (AT) to transform Poisson noise to white Gaussian noise. With this data augmentation, a deep residual network is trained to learn the noise map of the noisy images. We show, that the proposed method can remove not only simulated but also real noise. Furthermore, we also compare our results with state-of-the-art denoising methods, such as BM3D and DNCNN. In an early investigation, we achieved qualitatively better mammogram denoising results.

1 Introduction

According to the World Health Organization (WHO), cancer is the second leading cause of death globally and is responsible for 9.6 million deaths in 2018 [1]. Among these, breast cancer is the leading cause of women's deaths and accounts for 15 percent of its [1].

One of the most widely used modalities for breast cancer detection is mammography. It is using low-energy X-rays to screen the human breast and helps the radiologist to detect breast cancer in an early stage. For an accurate diagnosis, impeccable image quality is required. This is due to the complexity of mammograms, and the small size of microcalcifications, which are essential for breast cancer detection. Denoising the mammogram is one approach to improve quality. Unlike in the research field of computer vision, few attempts have been made to use convolutional neural networks (CNN's) to reduce the noise in mammograms [2, 3]. In [4], they used a CNN with 17 layers and the MIAS-mini(MMM)

© Springer Fachmedien Wiesbaden GmbH, ein Teil von Springer Nature 2020
T. Tolxdorff et al. (Hrsg.), *Bildverarbeitung für die Medizin 2020*,
Informatik aktuell, https://doi.org/10.1007/978-3-658-29267-6_21

data set for training. To date, we are not aware of works aiming at the correct physical modelling of noise reduction in deep learning following ideas the ones presented in [5].

In this paper, we investigate the feasibility of CNNs for denoising mammograms. This does not only include the development and training of an adequate network, but also the examination of detail preservation since the latter one is crucial for breast cancer detection. We propose a deep residual network, which could denoise the mammogram images with high accuracy.

2   Material and methods

Because of the quantum nature of light, photons arrive at random times. This leads to an uncertainty about the received signal, which can be modeled with a Poisson distribution, where each pixel value z depends on the arrival rate λ of the photons. The distribution can be described as the following

$$P(z|\lambda) = \frac{\lambda^z e^{-\lambda}}{z!} \tag{1}$$

Therefore the detector receives a noisy X-ray image Y, which can be decomposed in a noise-free signal $\mu(Z)$ and the noise V, so that $Y = \mu(Z) + V$ holds. Where $\mu(Z_{i,j})$ is the mean of a pixel value. This study aims to train a network to estimate the noise V, by feeding it the noisy image Y [6].

2.1   Data and augmentation

We use a data set of 125 Full-Field Digital Mammograms (FFDMs), which was provided by our industry partner. The X-ray images are prepared as shown in Fig. 1. In the first step, the real number of photons is calculated out of the pixel values. In the second step, a dose reduction is simulated by generation of more noise, followed by a transformation of the signal-dependent Poisson noise using the Anscombe transformation to white Gaussian noise [7]. To model the Poisson noise reasonably, we exploit the linear dependency of pixel value z of the real number of photons λ by a factor k to get λ. It employs, that $z = k \cdot \lambda$ holds. Since k is unknown, it has to be obtained, by dividing the variance of z over the mean of z

$$\frac{\text{var}(z)}{\text{mean}(z)} = \frac{k^2 \cdot \text{var}(\lambda)}{k \cdot \text{mean}(\lambda)} = k \tag{2}$$

To simulate more noise on the ground truth images, the arrival rate of λ of the photons will be scaled down by a factor α using the following equation

$$P(Z|\alpha\lambda) = \frac{\alpha\lambda^Z \cdot e^{-\alpha\lambda}}{Z!} \tag{3}$$

This results in a new mean $\mu = \alpha\lambda$ and variance $\sigma^2 = \alpha\lambda$. Now the Anscombe transformation can be applied to transform the signal-dependent Poisson noise

Fig. 1. Data augmentation pipeline for FFDM images.

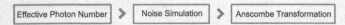

to signal independent white Gaussian noise with a standard deviation of one [7]

$$A : z \to 2\sqrt{z + \frac{3}{8}} \tag{4}$$

2.2 Network architecture

We use a residual network, as shown in Fig. 2. The first layer consists of a convolution layer with 64 kernels of size 3×3 and a ReLU activation function. The middle part of the network consists of fifteen residual blocks. Each block is composed of three convolution layers with 64 kernels of the size of 3×3 and followed by a Batch Normalization and a ReLu. We choose 3 convolution layers in a row for each residual block, to ensure that the information contained in the receptive field is high enough for each residual block. The same padding is used for all layers, and the skip connection can be molded by convolution with 64 Kernels of size 1×1. This setup leads to a network with 1.700.000 trainable parameters.

2.2.1 Loss Function

For image denoising with deep learning, often a Mean Square Error (MSE) is used as a loss function [8]. Since small details are crucial for cancer detection, we propose a new loss function based on MSE and ReLU activation function. This loss penalizes noise overestimation more heavily than noise underestimation, as noise overestimation leads to detail losses. This new loss is defined as

$$\text{ReLU-L} = \text{MSE} + \frac{1}{N} \sum_{i=0}^{N} \text{ReLU}[(-\text{sign}(\hat{V}_i) \cdot (V_i - \hat{V}_i)]^2 \tag{5}$$

where V is the true pixels and $\hat{V}$ is the estimated noise.
As argued by Zhao et al. [8], MSE is not the best choice to use as a loss function, because of its difference to human perception. For this reason, they use a combination of the Structural Similarity Index (SSIM) with MSE. To improve the performance, even more, we combine the SSIM with our new defined ReLU-L.

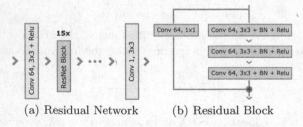

(a) Residual Network   (b) Residual Block

Fig. 2. Residual Network Architecture.

2.2.2   Training For training, the X-ray images are cropped to patches of size 64×64. We used 100 images for training and 25 for validation which leads to 40.000 patches for training and 10.000 patches for validation. For training the network, we use Adam optimizer with a learning rate of 0.0001. The noise is simulated by the means of a dose reduction of 80%. To ensure that the network never sees the same noise twice, the noise is simulated at each iteration. The training of the network takes 125 epochs before it is stopped.

3   Experiments and results

3.1   Denoising of simulated noise and performance comparison

We evaluated the denoising capacity of our residual network on X-ray images with a simulated dose reduction of 80%. The denoised images are shown in Fig. 3. In Tab. 1, we show the PSNR, SSIM and the standard deviation (σ_{image}) of the different outputs of the denoising methods. We also indicate the σ_{image}, because the noise reduction goes below the noise level of the GT. Therefore, one should consider that MSE and PSNR do not reflect entirely the noise reduction anymore. For a better visibility, we present the results of a small area of the original image, which contains two microcalcifications.

The result of the residual network compared against a Gaussian filter with $\sigma = 1$ and the state-of-the-art algorithm BM3D [9]. For both algorithms, we perform the same noise simulation and make use of the Anscombe transformation.

In Singh et al. [4], they trained a CNN with 17 layers similar to Zhang et al. [6]. They downsample the training images to a size of 512×512 and simulate Gaussian noise with $\sigma = 25$. Initially, we retrained this network similar to Singh et al., but instead of scaling down our images of size 3518×2800, we use patches of size 512×512 for training. In a second attempt, we retrained the 17 layer CNN of Zhang et al. [6] with our method. This includes Poisson noise, Anscombe transformation, and MSE + SSIM loss and refers to it as DNCNN.

The σ_{image} of the GT Image is 0.042. All methods produce results with smaller σ_{image} than the GT. However, the results of the Gaussian filter and DNCNN have the highest σ_{image} value (0.41), and the Gaussian filter tends to blur the image (Fig. 3d). This is not the case with the BM3D model (Fig. 3e). Alternatively, the output is over smoothed and artifacts introduced, but microcalcifications are still visible. Fig. 3 (f) shows the output, when employing the trained network of Singh et al. It can be seen that microcalcifications are almost lost because of image averaging. We assume, that a noise level of $\sigma = 25$ is extremely high for training images of our data set. Because of their wide intensity range, many details are suppressed with that noise level. Consequently, the network is not able to learn detailed features anymore. The same network trained with our method produces satisfactory results but reduces the visibility of some microcalcifications (Fig. 3h). Using our proposed network and methods, microcalcifications are still clearly visible and no additional artifacts are introduced. This is also reflected in the highest PSNR and SSIM of 36.18 and 0.841,

Table 1. Performance comparison between our proposed method and other denoising methods.

Methods	PSNR	SSIM	σ_{image}
Noisy	30.94	0.64	0.057
Gaussian filter	35.48	0.815	0.041
BM3D [9]	35.49	0.801	*0.038*
Singh et al. [4]	33.50	0.781	*0.038*
DnCnn [6]	36.08	0.840	0.041
DeResNet (ours)	*36.18*	*0.841*	0.040

respectively. In the last image (Fig. 3a), we show the difference between the GT and the denoised image with ResNet. One can see those small microcalcifications appear in the left lower corner of the difference image. Hence, the network has difficulties in distinguishing them from noise.

3.2   Denoising real-world noise

We further evaluate the denoising capability of our proposed method on real-world noise. Fig. 3 demonstrate the noisy and the denoised FFDM image. It appears that the network denoise the real noise as good as simulated noise. Similar to simulated noise, microcalcifications are visible, and no additional artifacts introduced in the images. The σ_{image} value is also significantly low in compare to actual low dose FFDM.

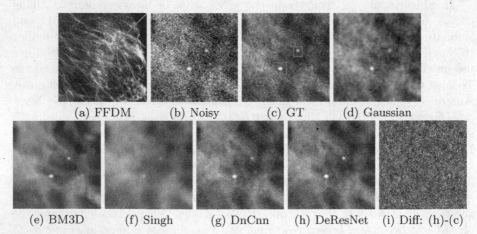

(a) FFDM   (b) Noisy   (c) GT   (d) Gaussian

(e) BM3D   (f) Singh   (g) DnCnn   (h) DeResNet   (i) Diff: (h)-(c)

Fig. 3. Results of different denoising methods. Microcalcifications are marked with an orange square in the GT and the difference image. Two are still clearly visible in the results of the ResNet. The smaller ones are not distinguished from noise by the DeResNet and therefore appear in the difference image. They are also not detectable for the human eye in the noisy image.

Fig. 4. Denoising on real-world noise: Low Dose FFDM, $\sigma_{image} = 0.0442$ (left), Denoised FFDM, $\sigma_{image} = 0.0302$ (right).

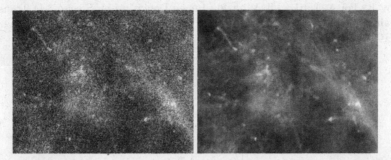

4   Conclusion

In this paper, we introduced a deep learning-based method for mammogram denoising, which significantly enhanced the image quality. Our proposed method outperformed state-of-the-art methods such as BM3D, DnCnn, and Singh et al. This was shown on a visual example and proved by comparing the PSNR and SSIM values with other methods. However, information which is lost in the noise, can not be restored by the network. One should be careful, by reducing the dose, especially if a high degree of detail is demanded.

Disclaimer. The concepts and information presented in this paper are based on research and are not commercially available.

References

1. Bray F, Ferlay J, Soerjomataram I, et al. Global cancer statistics 2018: GLOBO-CAN estimates of incidence and mortality worldwide for 36 cancers in 185 countries. CA: A Cancer Journal for Clinicians. 2018;68(6):394–424. Available from: https://onlinelibrary.wiley.com/doi/abs/10.3322/caac.21492.
2. Abdelhafiz D, Yang C, Ammar RA, et al. Deep convolutional neural networks for mammography: advances, challenges and applications. In: BMC Bioinformatics; 2019. .
3. Joseph AM, John MG, Dhas AS. Mammogram image denoising filters: A comparative study. In: Proc ICEDSS; 2017. p. 184–189.
4. Singh G, Mittal A, Aggarwal N. Deep convolution neural network based denoiser for mammographic images. In: Singh M, Gupta PK, Tyagi V, et al., editors. Advances in Computing and Data Sciences. Singapore: Springer Singapore; 2019. p. 177–187.
5. Maier A, Syben C, Stimpel B, et al. Learning with known operators reduces maximum error bounds. Nature Machine Intelligence. 2019;2019(1):373–380.
6. Zhang K, Zuo W, Chen Y, et al. Beyond a Gaussian Denoiser: Residual Learning of Deep CNN for Image Denoising. IEEE Transactions on Image Processing. 2017 July;26(7):3142–3155.
7. Anscombe FJ. The Transformation of Poisson, Binomial and Negative-Binomial Data. Biometrika. 1948 dec;35(3/4):246.

8. Zhao H, Gallo O, Frosio I, et al. Loss Functions for Image Restoration With Neural Networks. IEEE Transactions on Computational Imaging. 2017 March;3(1).

9. Dabov K, Foi A, Katkovnik V, et al. Image Denoising by Sparse 3-D Transform-Domain Collaborative Filtering. IEEE Transactions on Image Processing. 2007 Aug;16(8):2080–2095.

Video Anomaly Detection in Post-Procedural Use of Laparoscopic Videos

Wolfgang Reiter[1]

[1]Wintegral GmbH, München, Germany
wolfgang.reiter@wintegral.net

Abstract. Endoscopic surgery leads to large amounts of recordings that have to either be stored completely or postprocessed to extract relevant frames. These recordings regularly contain long out-of-body scenes. This paper proposes to apply anomaly detection methods to detect these irrelevant scenes. A conditional generative adversarial networks (GAN) architecture is used to predict future video frames and classify these predictions with an anomaly score. To avoid the successful prediction of anomalous frames due to the good generalization capability of convolutional neural networks (CNNs) we enhance the optimization process with a negative training phase. The experimental results demonstrate promising results for out-of-body sequence detection with the proposed approach. The enhanced GAN training framework can improve the results of the prediction framework by a large margin. The negative training phase reduces the number of false negative (FN) predictions and is shown to counteract a common problem in anomaly detection methods based on convolutional neural networks (CNNs). The good performance in standard metrics also shows the suitability for clinical use.

1 Introduction

Laparoscopic recordings often show intraoperative out-of-body scenes or long irrelevant parts at the beginning or end. These scenes are insignificant to the treatment but may indicate problems if they happen too often. Removing the endoscope from the body to clean the endoscopic lense may be necessitated by impaired vision caused by insufficient white balancing or lens fogging. Removing or highlighting these scenes can assist post-procedural use by saving storage space or by speeding up the manual frame extraction. The detection of intraoperative out-of-body scenes may also serve as quality measure of the surgical procedure.

Prior work uses RGB colorspace features to detect out-of-body frames in colonoscopy [1], or HSV colorspace features in laparoscopic recordings [2]. Both methods rely on the conjecture that in-body and out-of-body frames show distinct color distributions. We posit that this assumption is too simple and that there are many situations where it is not met: blue instruments, specular reflections, out-of-body closeup shots or operating theatres decorated with different

© Springer Fachmedien Wiesbaden GmbH, ein Teil von Springer Nature 2020
T. Tolxdorff et al. (Hrsg.), *Bildverarbeitung für die Medizin 2020*,
Informatik aktuell, https://doi.org/10.1007/978-3-658-29267-6_22

colors. To overcome these problems we reformulate the problem as anomaly detection: finding patterns in data, that diverge from expected behavior [3]. Anomalies are characterized by their rare occurence and a dynamicity in appearance with unbounded variations. A taxonomy of video anomaly detection methods is provided in [4]: Reconstruction error based models that learn a representation from which nonanomalous samples can be reconstructed. Predictive models, which interpret the consecutive video frames as a time series to predict future frames. And generative models, like GANs [5], which learn to generate images following a specific distribution. Our approach builds on the method presented in [6]: the prediction of a single future frame from multiple past frames is learned with a GAN. Predictive modelling is used to overcome problems in reconstruction error based models, anomalous images are being reconstructed as well as nonanomalous images, because of the good generalization. This solves the problem only partially: predictive models rely on the same error metric to rate the quality of a prediction, and can predict a realistic image given enough anomalous past frames. To improve the discrimination of longer anomalous events we add a negative learning phase [7] to the GAN framework.

The contribution of this work is the detection of out-of-body scenes in laparoscopic with predictive modeling. To the best of our knowledge this is the first use of a negative learning constraint with GANs and the first application of this method on complex surgical procedures.

2   Materials and methods

The proposed architecture is depicted in Fig. 2. Following the method presented in [8], a generative model G receives t consecutive video frames $(x_1, \ldots x_t)$ as input and it produces a prediction $\hat{x}_{t+1}$ of the future frame x_{t+1} as output. The choice of U-Net [9] as generator is motivated by the high localization precision that is achieved by passing high resolution features between the contracting and the expanding part of the model by means of skip connections. As described

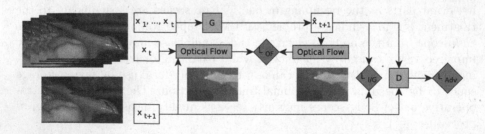

Fig. 1. Our proposed network: computational blocks are shown in blue, input and output tensors on white background and the optimized objectives in red. The images to the left show exemplary input for the generative model, the images in the middle display the calculated optical flow for these inputs.

in [10], we employ two loss functions to improve the appearance of the generated images. The intensity loss L_I constrains pixels in RGB colorspace to be similar to the ground truth. It is calculated with the squared ℓ_2 loss between the predicted future frame and the ground truth frame

$$L_I(\hat{x}, x) = \|\hat{x} - x\|_2^2 \tag{1}$$

The second loss term L_G penalises differences in the image gradients to increase the edge precision in the generated image. It adds the differences of image gradients for ground truth and predicted frames in horizontal and vertical direction. The computation over all pixels with spatial indices i and j is given by

$$L_G(\hat{x}, x) = \sum_{i,j} \||\hat{x}_{i,j} - \hat{x}_{i-1,j}| - |x_{i,j} - x_{i-1,j}|\|_1 \\ + \||\hat{x}_{i,j} - \hat{x}_{i,j-1}| - |x_{i,j} - x_{i,j-1}|\|_1 \tag{2}$$

To emphasize the importance of coherent object and camera movements in a video we follow [6] and add a motion constraint. This objective uses the optical flow between x_t and both versions of the future frame, $\hat{x}_{t+1}$ and x_{t+1}, to constrain the predicted movement to be near the actual movement. A pretrained version of Flownet [11] f, with fixed weights, is used to approximate the dense optical flow

$$L_{OF} = \|f(\hat{x}_{t+1}, x_t) - f(x_{t+1}, x_t)\|_1 \tag{3}$$

The constraints on gradient and motion promise an improved discrimination of the generated features, due to the differences of typical in-body and out-of-body frames: In-body scenes rarely contain any sharp edges apart from instruments, where out-of-body frames may show furniture or technical equipment with distinct shapes. Visible movement while in-body, which mostly shows camera or instrument movements in front of a living background, should be distinguishable from movement in out-of-body scenes.

To classify the predicted frames as anomaly we adopt the peak signal to noise ratio (PSNR) as image similarity metric as described in [10]

$$PSNR(\hat{x}, x) = 10 * log_{10}\left(\frac{1}{\frac{1}{N}\sum_{i=0}^{N}(x_i - \hat{x}_i)^2}\right) \tag{4}$$

2.1   Adversial training in a GAN framework

Optimization in a GAN framework can be an additional means to improve the sharpness of the generated images [10]: the ℓ_2 loss which is used to enforce nearness in RGB space leads to prediction of average frames $x_{avg} = (x + \hat{x})/2$. While x_{avg} minimizes the objective function, it is no realistic prediction of the next frame. A discriminator in a GAN framework can be used to discern these unrealistic frames and provide an incentive to learn better predictions. In this framework two models are trained at the same time, discriminator D and generator G: D produces a single scalar as output, trained to classify the input as real or fake and G learns to generate output that is labeled as real by D. As in [6] we use the PatchGAN discriminator [8]: it only looks at patches of the input image by reducing its receptive field. This effectively leads to only high-frequency details being modelled in the discriminator, while the intensity loss term is relied upon for low-frequency correctness [8]. As an additional benefit this optimization results in less computational overhead. We adopt this GAN framework in a training process with two alternating steps. D performs one optimizer pass on a minibatch of training samples. The weights of D are optimized to classify a predicted frame as fake and the ground truth as real without updating G

$$L_D = (D(x) - 1)^2 + (D(\hat{x}) - 0)^2 \tag{5}$$

Next, G is modified to generate output that is classified as real by D. Now only the parameters of G are modified and those of D stay fixed. The objective of this training step is a linear combination of the objectives with weighting coefficients

$$L = \lambda_I * L_I + \lambda_G * L_G + \lambda_{OF} * L_{OF} + \lambda_{Adv} * L_{Adv} \tag{6}$$

Where L_{Adv} serves as a hint to the generator how to fool the discriminator into labeling its output as real

$$L_{Adv} = (D(\hat{x}) - 1)^2 \tag{7}$$

2.2   Negative training phase to limit the generative abilities

To avoid the prediction of a frame from an anomalous distribution given anomalous frames as input we follow the approach in [7], where the reconstruction abilities of an autoencoder based anomaly detection algorithm are limited with a negative training phase. Negative training modifies the parameters of the autoencoder to unlearn the reconstruction of anomalous patterns. This limits the input distribution that can be reconstructed to the distribution of the nonanomalous training samples. The proposed method optimizes the autoencoder with two alternating steps: (1) minimize the squared ℓ_2 loss between reconstruction $\hat{x}$ and nonanomalous input x, (2) maximize the same metric for an input frame from the anomaly distribution y and its reconstruction $\hat{y}$. With both training steps optimizing the same parameters. The positive learning phase follows the gradient descent and the negative phase its ascent which eventually leads to an equilibrium where anomalous data cannot be reconstructed.

We transfer this algorithm to the GAN framework by interpreting the intensity loss as positive learning signal. This leads to the following equation that must be optimized for all negative data samples N to maximize the distance of predicted samples in intensity space

$$max \sum_{i}^{N} L_I(\hat{y}_i, y_i) \tag{8}$$

The success of this optimization should lead to a decrease of false negative (FN) anomaly predictions, i.e. the number of anomaly samples successfully predicted due to enough past anomaly frames.

3   Results

Endoscopic recordings of 41 laparoscopic cholecystectomy surgeries, provided by our clinical partners, have been used in this study. They show surgeries by different surgeons in multiple hospitals. 90771 Frames were extracted at 1fps and annotated as belonging to one of two classes: classes in-body(0) and out-of-body(1) with a ratio of $\frac{50}{1}$. The dataset was split into three parts along the video boundaries while keeping the class ratio: a training set with 33 videos, a validation set for model selection and a test set to evaluate the generalization error, both with 4 videos. We trained two different models to confirm our hypothesis, with (M_{neg}) and without (M) the negative learning phase. $t=4$ consecutive input frames were sampled from a random video for one training step, since most anomaly sequences are at least 5 seconds long. Hyperparameters were chosen with the validation set. Loss coefficients λ_I and λ_G showed the best results when set to one, λ_{OF} when set to two. These three values proofed to be insensitive to small changes. λ_{Adv} had to be increased to at least 0.5 to prevent learning failure. Adam optimizer was used to optimize the networks with learning rate schedules: start with $2*10^{-4}$, decrease to $2*10^{-5}$ after 100000 steps. Reducing the learning rate for the negative learning phase to a value lower than the generator's was necessary to avoid vanishing gradient: $2*10^{-5}$, $2*10^{-6}$, $2*10^{-7}$ with decrease at steps 30000 and 90000. Batchsize was set to 8, training process converged after 120000 steps. Input images were rid of their black border, cropped and resized to half size and normalized to $[-1, 1]$.

As a baseline we also provide the metrics of an out-of-body indicator (M_{hue}) based on the hue distribution [2] of the HSV colorspace. And a ResNet50-based Convolutional Network trained for binary classification, M_{CNN}.

3.1   Validation

Performance evaluation of anomaly detection methods requires metrics that take class imbalance into account. The Matthews correlation coefficient (MCC)

$$\frac{TP*TN - FP*FN}{\sqrt{(TP+FP)*(TP+FN)*(TN+FP)*(TN+FN)}} \tag{9}$$

is calculated from all four relevant numbers, true positives (TPs), true negatives (TNs), false positives (FPs) and false negatives (FNs). It ranges from *[-1,1]* with 0 being equal to a completely random prediction. The resulting metrics calculated on the test set are shown in table 1. M_{neg} performs notably better than M and M_{hue} in all metrics: Recall shows a large increase, which indicates a decrease in FN, Precision is less discriminative it shows a slight increase due to more FP samples. The MCC encodes the same information in a single index number. While M_{CNN} has very good recall and precision, the MCC value shows, by taking class imbalance into account, that it is not better than random guessing.

Table 1. Evaluation of regularly trained model M, model M_{neg} with extra negative training phase and baseline methods M_{hue} and M_{CNN}.

Model	MCC	Recall	Precision
M_{hue}	0.605	0.469	0.806
M	0.341	0.174	0.704
M_{neg}	0.821	0.779	0.876
M_{CNN}	0.038	0.911	0.981

4   Discussion

We have demonstrated that anomaly detection with GANs can be used to detect out-of-body scenes in recordings of endoscopic surgeries. Furthermore, we have shown the applicability of an additional negative training phase in the GAN Framework. Experimental results show that the used predictive GAN Framework is impaired by the generalization abilities of deep neural networks just like reconstruction error based models. We provide empirical evidence showing large improvements of this problem with the enhanced training procedure. The good performance on laparoscopic recordings suggests the clinical use of the method.

References

1. Stanek SR, Tavanapong W, Wong J, et al. Automatic real-time detection of endoscopic procedures using temporal features. Computer methods and programs in biomedicine. 2012;108(2):524–535.
2. Münzer B, Schoeffmann K, Böszörmenyi L. Relevance segmentation of laparoscopic videos. In: Proc ISM. IEEE; 2013. p. 84–91.
3. Chandola V, Banerjee A, Kumar V. Anomaly detection: A survey. ACM computing surveys (CSUR). 2009;41(3):15.
4. Kiran B, Thomas D, Parakkal R. An overview of deep learning based methods for unsupervised and semi-supervised anomaly detection in videos. Journal of Imaging. 2018;4(2):36.
5. Goodfellow I, Pouget-Abadie J, Mirza M, et al. Generative Adversarial Nets. In: Proc NIPS 27. Curran Associates, Inc.; 2014. p. 2672–2680.
6. Liu W, Luo W, Lian D, et al. Future frame prediction for anomaly detection–a new baseline. In: Proc CVPR; 2018. p. 6536–6545.
7. Munawar A, Vinayavekhin P, De Magistris G. Limiting the reconstruction capability of generative neural network using negative learning. In: Proc MLSP. IEEE; 2017. p. 1–6.
8. Isola P, Zhu JY, Zhou T, et al. Image-to-image translation with conditional adversarial networks. In: Proc CVPR; 2017. p. 1125–1134.
9. Ronneberger O, Fischer P, Brox T. U-net: Convolutional networks for biomedical image segmentation. In: Proc MICCAI. Springer; 2015. p. 234–241.
10. Mathieu M, Couprie C, LeCun Y. Deep multi-scale video prediction beyond mean square error. arXiv preprint arXiv:151105440. 2015;.
11. Dosovitskiy A, Fischer P, Ilg E, et al. Flownet: Learning optical flow with convolutional networks. In: Proc ICCV; 2015. p. 2758–2766.

Entropy-Based SVM Classifier for Automatic Detection of Motion Artifacts in Clinical MRI

Chandrakanth Jayachandran Preetha[1,2], Hendrik Mattern[1], Medha Juneja[2], Johannes Vogt[2], Oliver Speck[1,3,4], Thomas Hartkens[2]

[1]Department of Biomedical Magnetic Resonance,
Otto-von-Guericke-Universität Magdeburg
[2]Imaging Innovations, medneo GmbH, Berlin
[3]German Center for Neurodegenerative Disease, Magdeburg, Germany
[4]Leibniz Institute for Neurobiology, Magdeburg, Germany
chandrakanth.jayachandran@st.ovgu.de

Abstract. The extended acquisition time of Magnetic Resonance Imaging (MRI) makes it susceptible to image artifacts caused by subject motion. Artifact presence reduces diagnostic confidence and it could also necessitate a re-scan or an additional examination in extreme cases. Automatic artifact detection at the modality could improve the efficiency, reliability and reproducibility of image quality verification. It could also prevent patient recall for additional examination due to unsatisfactory image quality. In this study we evaluate a machine learning method for the automatic detection of motion artifacts in order to instantly recognise problematic acquisitions before the patient has left the scanner. The paper proposes the use of local entropy estimation in the feature extraction stage of the chosen Support Vector Machine (SVM) classifier. Availability of sufficiently large training data set is one of the main constraints in training machine learning models. In order to enable training a model that could detect motion artifacts of varying severity, the paper also proposes a framework for generation of synthetic motion artifatcs in head MRI. On a per-slices basis, the implemented SVM classifier achieved an accuracy of 93.5% in the detection of motion artifacts in clinical MR images.

1 Introduction

Compromised image quality due to motion artifacts can make interpretation difficult and reduce diagnostic confidence. A recent study [1] conducted to determine the prevalence, severity and cost of patient motion during clinical MR examinations found that motion artifacts are a frequent cause of image quality degradation and resulted in repeated scans, affecting about 20% of all examinations in the study. The study estimated that motion artifact-induced costs can approach $ 115,000 per scanner per year. Timely detection of motion corrupted images would help to reduce costs related to patient recalls arising from unsatisfactory image quality.

© Springer Fachmedien Wiesbaden GmbH, ein Teil von Springer Nature 2020
T. Tolxdorff et al. (Hrsg.), *Bildverarbeitung für die Medizin 2020*,
Informatik aktuell, https://doi.org/10.1007/978-3-658-29267-6_23

Besides visual inspection, an automatic detection of image artifact at the modality can assist the radiographer to identify acquisitions of low quality and enables him/her to initiate a re-acquisition while the patient is still in the scanner [2]. An automated tool for artifact detection could also facilitate standardization of image quality and contribute to improvement in diagnostic confidence.

Learning-based methods for detection of motion artifacts in MR images have been extensively investigated. Trends in computer vision have heavily influenced quality assessment techniques for medical image data. Lorch et al. [3] proposed an automated, reference-free method for detection of motion artifacts using a machine learning approach based on decision forests. Many deep learning based approaches [4, 5] have also been investigated for the detection of motion artifatcs in MRI. While these studies have demonstrated effective methods for detection of motion artifacts in synthetic images or artifacts produced by deliberate subject motion, the robustness of these methods in detecting artifacts caused by natural patient motion needs to be further investigated. The transferability of these methods to different imaging protocols also needs to be verified.

We propose an entropy based SVM classifier for the detection of motion artifacts in clinical MR images at the modality. Manual annotation of images for developing data-driven classification methods is time consuming and requires experts' valuable time. The paper also proposes a motion simulation framework which can generate synthetic images with varying levels of motion artifacts for training the proposed SVM model. The ability to create proper synthetic examples could enable experimentational studies on artifact detection with small data sets, reduce the dependence on manual data labelling, alleviate the class-imbalance problem and improve artifact detection in real data.

2   Materials and methods

2.1   Motion simulation framework and image data preparation

Patient motion is simulated as rigid body motion with six degrees of freedom, allowing 3D object translation and rotation. The motion corruption framework induces motion artifacts with the help of affine transformations of the original image volume. It is assumed that the image volume is aligned with the physical coordinate and therefore both have the same orientation and center. The image volume undergoes repeated affine transformation based on the 3D motion data provided in the form of a 4×4 transformation matrix, simulating rigid body motion. As shown in Fig. 1, affine transformation followed by FFT is applied several times on the same image to generate k-space data corresponding to a corrupted image. Finally, a motion corrupted sequence is obtained from the manipulated k-space by the application of 2D FFT.

The range of parameters for the 3D affine transformation of the image volume for motion artifact generation was heuristically determined. The values were then sampled from a zero-mean normal distribution. The origin of the image volume was translated up to a maximum of 4 mm and rotation was restricted to 5 degree. The k-space regions affected by signal corruption due to motion is chosen randomly from the total range of phase encoding steps (similar to the approach adopted by Johnson et al. [6]).

The MRI data set used for training the model consisted of 8 T1-weighted and 7 T2-weighted sequences of the head identified as artifact free by an MR expert. From these images an equal number of motion corrupted images were generated using the motion simulation framework illustrated in Fig. 1. The positive examples in the training data set were obtained from these image volumes. The test data consisted of 3 T1-weighted images and 14 T2-weighted sequences which were inspected and rated by an expert using a framework for image quality feedback [2]. Labels were assigned to the whole volume to make the annotation task easier for the expert. The training and test image volumes were first resampled to a fixed voxel spacing of $0.5 \times 0.5 \times 1.5\ mm^3$ and subsequently resized such that the individual slices were of size 320×320 (maintaining uniform voxel spacing in the axial direction). 2D slices from the original and synthetically generated sequences in the training data set were compared using SSIM and in cases where the SSIM value was more than 0.95, the images were excluded from the training data set. A total of 440 images were used for training, out of which half of the examples were motion corrupted. 170 slices were used for testing, with 10 middle slices extracted from each of the test sequences.

2.2   SVM classifier

Entropy minimization is applied in iterative motion compensation methods for MR images [7]. It is based on the idea that a motion blurred image will have more gray values to represent than a motion-free image. Local entropy estimation can be performed on a pixel neighbourhood using an entropy filter to produce a feature map. The application of entropy filter would enable detection of subtle

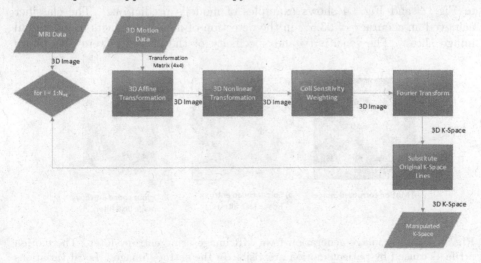

Fig. 1. Algorithm for simulation of motion artifacts in MR images

variations in the local gray level distribution. Entropy images were generated from the slices extracted from the training data set of motion corrupted and motion-free MR images using an entropy filter of size 2×2 (Fig.2). The use of small kernel size reveals local intensity variations. The resultant feature maps are flattened and Principal Component Analysis (PCA) is applied on the training data set for dimensionality reduction. The first 76 components which explain 95% of the total variance are retained.

A soft-margin non-linear SVM model was chosen for the classification task. The model uses a radial basis function (RBF) as the kernel function. The RBF kernel is defined as

$$k(x, x^{'}) = exp(-\gamma \|x - x^{'}\|^2) \qquad (1)$$

where γ is the parameter which determines the spread of the kernel, it decides the region of influence of a single training example. Another hyperparameter of the model is C, which controls the trade-off between misclassification of training examples and model simplicity. The optimal values of these hyperparameters are determined using a grid search approach with k-fold cross-validation.

Feature maps are generated from the images in the test data set using the entropy filter, followed by image flattening and PCA transformation. The transformed examples are fed to the SVM model for classification. Similar to the strategy used by Künster et al.[5] for classification of image volumes, the algorithm labels a volume as motion corrupted when the model detects motion artifacts in at least half of the slices extracted from an image volume.

3   Results

The SVM model's classification performance is illustrated in the confusion matrix in Fig. 3 and Fig. 4 shows examples of model's predictions. The classifier achieved an accuracy of 93.5% in the detection of motion artifacts in individual image slices. The sensitivity and specificity of the classifier were also above

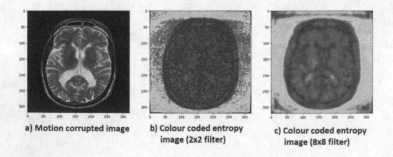

a) Motion corrupted image   b) Colour coded entropy image (2x2 filter)   c) Colour coded entropy image (8x8 filter)

Fig. 2. Entropy image generation from MR image using entropy filter. The motion artifacts caused by patient motion are visible in the entropy images. Local variations in intensity are easier to detect with a smaller filter size.

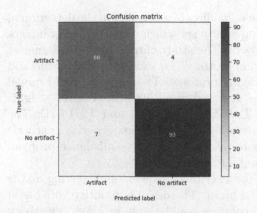

Fig. 3. : Confusion matrix depicting the SVM model's classification performance

90%. In the classification of image volumes, the classifier's sensitivity increased to 100% and a specificity of 90% was achieved. In the instance where the model disagreed with the expert, closer inspection of the image revealed the presence of subtle motion artifact.

4   Discussion and conclusion

In this work, an SVM based method was implemented for the detection of motion artifacts in brain MRI. In the feature extraction stage, we used an entropy filter which could detect even subtle changes in intensity distribution and thereby produce more discriminative features. The proposed model demonstrated classification performance comparable to state-of-the-art deep learning methods. While the CNN based approach investigated by Küstner et al.[5] achieved a sensitivity of 85% and specificity of 91% in the detection of motion artifacts, the SVM model's sensitivity and specificity are 100% and 90% respectively.

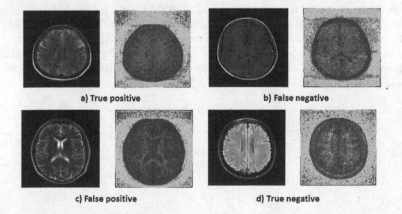

Fig. 4. Examples of MR images and corresponding entropy images for different categories in the confusion matrix

In order to verify the generalization capability of a classifier in the detection of image artifacts, it must be validated on a data set which compromises of images acquired using different imaging protocols.The study carried out by Küstner et al.[5] used images from only two imaging protocols for validation of their method and Oksuz et al. [4] used a single imaging protocol. The proposed SVM model was validated on a data set of images acquired using different contrast weightings and pulse sequences: T1/TSE, T2/TSE, T2/FLAIR and T2/FL2D. The implemented motion simulation framework can generate images with synthetic artifacts of varying severity. It helps to overcome the class-imbalance problem and reduces the dependence on manual data annotation.

The study currently uses a small data set of 17 sequences for testing and it consists of only axial MR images of the brain. The use of a majority vote based approach for classification of image volumes could result in lower sensitivity in the detection of artifacts. Future work will focus on testing the model's performance on a larger data set and extending the model's capability such that it could detect motion artifacts in brain MR images of all orientations.

References

1. Andre JB, Bresnahan BW, Mossa-Basha M, et al. Toward quantifying the prevalence, severity, and cost associated with patient motion During Clinical MR examinations. J Am Coll Radiol. 2015 Jul;12(7):689–695.
2. Juneja M, Bode-Hofmann M, Haong KS, et al. Image quality assessments. In: Informatik aktuell. Springer Fachmedien Wiesbaden; 2019. p. 225–230.
3. Lorch B, Vaillant G, Baumgartner C, et al. Automated detection of motion artefacts in MR imaging using decision forests. J Med Eng. 2017;2017:1–9.
4. Oksuz I, Ruijsink B, Puyol-Antón E, et al. Automatic CNN-based detection of cardiac MR motion artefacts using k-space data augmentation and curriculum learning. Med Image Anal. 2019 Jul;55:136–147.
5. Kustner T, Jandt M, Liebgott A, et al. Automatic motion artifact detection for Whole-Body magnetic resonance imaging. ICASSP. 2018; p. 995–999.
6. Johnson PM, Drangova M. Conditional generative adversarial network for 3d rigid-body motion correction in MRI. Magn Reson Med. 2019 Apr;.
7. Atkinson D, Hill DLG, Stoyle PNR, et al. Automatic correction of motion artifacts in magnetic resonance images using an entropy focus criterion. IEEE Trans Med Imaging. 1997;16(6):903–910.

Tenfold your Photons

A Physically-Sound Approach to Filtering-Based Variance Reduction of Monte-Carlo-Simulated Dose Distributions

Philipp Roser[1,3], Annette Birkhold[2], Alexander Preuhs[1], Markus Kowarschik[2], Rebecca Fahrig[2], Andreas Maier[1,3]

[1]Pattern Recognition Lab, FAU Erlangen-Nürnberg
[2]Siemens Healthcare GmbH, Forchheim Germany
[3]Erlangen Graduate School in Advanced Optical Technologies (SAOT)
philipp.roser@fau.de

Abstract. X-ray dose constantly gains interest in the interventional suite. With dose being generally difficult to monitor reliably, fast computational methods are desirable. A major drawback of the gold standard based on Monte Carlo (MC) methods is its computational complexity. Besides common variance reduction techniques, filter approaches are often applied to achieve conclusive results within a fraction of time. Inspired by these methods, we propose a novel approach. We down-sample the target volume based on the fraction of mass, simulate the imaging situation, and then revert the down-sampling. To this end, the dose is weighted by the mass energy absorption, up-sampled, and distributed using a guided filter. Eventually, the weighting is inverted resulting in accurate high resolution dose distributions. The approach has the potential to considerably speed-up MC simulations since less photons and boundary checks are necessary. First experiments substantiate these assumptions. We achieve a median accuracy of 96.7 % to 97.4 % of the dose estimation with the proposed method and a down-sampling factor of 8 and 4, respectively. While maintaining a high accuracy, the proposed method provides for a tenfold speed-up. The overall findings suggest the conclusion that the proposed method has the potential to allow for further efficiency.

1 Introduction

Over the last years, X-ray dose awareness increased steadily in the interventional environment – also driven by legal regulations requiring evidence of consistent dose application through monitoring tools. Monte Carlo (MC) simulation of particle transport is the de-facto gold standard for computational dose estimation in X-ray imaging. Only its high algorithmic complexity and demand for extensive prior knowledge about the patient anatomy stands in the way of a wider application in the clinical environment outside radiotherapy, especially in the interventional suite.

© Springer Fachmedien Wiesbaden GmbH, ein Teil von Springer Nature 2020
T. Tolxdorff et al. (Hrsg.), *Bildverarbeitung für die Medizin 2020*,
Informatik aktuell, https://doi.org/10.1007/978-3-658-29267-6_24

While the lack of pre-operative computed tomography (CT) scans in general can be overcome by constantly improving patient surface and organ shape modeling algorithms [1], the high arithmetic effort of reliable MC simulations remains a hurdle. Although there exists a variety of GPU-accelerated MC codes applicable to X-ray imaging [2] or radiotherapy [3], their gain in performance mainly depends on the employed hardware, which may vary heavily between different hospitals. Commonly, different variance reduction techniques such as Russian roulette or delta tracking [4] are implemented, which, however, might act contrary to the intention of speeding-up the simulation. For delta tracking e.g., the irradiated volume is assumed to homogeneously consist of the highest-density material during particle tracing to reduce the overall frequency of costly random sampling. This may lead to an undesired slowdown for very dense materials, commonly found in medical applications, e.g., titanium. Recently, convolutional neural networks have been introduced to the problem of dose estimation [5], however, their dependency on diverse training data renders them infeasible for general purpose dose estimation at this point.

To this end, smoothing approaches such as anisotropic diffusion [6] or Savitzky-Golay filtering [7] have been employed successfully, claiming a further reduction of primary particles by a factor of 2 to 20. Based on these concepts, we propose a novel theoretical take on image-processing-based variance reduction. Before simulation, we apply a physically-sound down-sampling strategy on the target volume combined with super-resolving the resulting dose distribution using guided filtering (GF) [8] and the original target volume as guidance. By massively down-sampling the target volume, a further speed-up could possibly be achieved since less boundary checks are necessary.

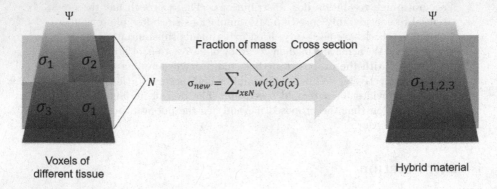

Fig. 1. Basic principle of the proposed method: a hybrid material of the neighborhood $\mathcal{N}$ exposes the same macroscopic properties as its finer counterpart.

2 Methods

2.1 Basic principle

The presented idea depicted in Fig. 1 is based on the assumption that the macroscopic properties, such as the photon fluence $\psi(E)$ with respect to the kinetic energy E, in a neighborhood $\mathcal{N}$ in the voxelized target volume are approximately equal to when its individual voxels are condensed to a mixture material. For instance, the differential cross section $\sigma_\mathcal{N}(E)$ of matter in such a neighborhood is defined by

$$\sigma_\mathcal{N}(E) = \sum_{x \in \mathcal{N}} w(x)\sigma(x, E) \tag{1}$$

where $w(x)$ is the fraction of mass of voxel x, $\sigma(x, E)$ is the differential cross section of its corresponding material, and E is the kinetic energy of the incident particle. Similarly, the mass energy-absorption coefficient $\left(\frac{\mu_{en}(E)}{\rho}\right)_\mathcal{N}$ is defined as

$$\left(\frac{\mu_{en}(E)}{\rho}\right)_\mathcal{N} = \sum_{x \in \mathcal{N}} w(x)\left(\frac{\mu_{en}(x, E)}{\rho}\right) \tag{2}$$

In the following, for the sake of readability, we ignore the energy-dependency in our notation. Bold-typed quantities refer to 3-D tensors $\in \mathbb{R}^3$.

By calculating mixture models for each neighborhood $\mathcal{N}$ in the target volume $\boldsymbol{V}$, we obtain its low resolution representation $\tilde{\boldsymbol{V}}$. Using this down-sampled target volume $\tilde{\boldsymbol{V}}$ in a MC simulation, we obtain the low resolution dose distribution $\tilde{\boldsymbol{D}} = \mathrm{MC}(\tilde{\boldsymbol{V}}) \in \mathbb{R}^3$.

Furthermore, in such large, homogeneous voxels a charged particle equilibrium (CPE) can be assumed. Under CPE, the absorbed dose $\tilde{\boldsymbol{D}}$ in a volume is approximately equal to the respective collision kerma $\tilde{\boldsymbol{K}}_{col}$

$$\tilde{\boldsymbol{D}} = \tilde{\boldsymbol{K}}_{col} + \tilde{\boldsymbol{K}}_{rad} \;,\; \tilde{\boldsymbol{K}}_{rad} \to \boldsymbol{0} \tag{3}$$

given the radiative kerma $\tilde{\boldsymbol{K}}_{rad}$ approaches 0, which is the case for diagnostic X-rays. This allows us to exploit the relationship

$$D_\mathcal{N} = K_{col,\mathcal{N}} = \left(\frac{\mu_{en}}{\rho}\right)_\mathcal{N} \psi_\mathcal{N} \tag{4}$$

to decouple dose or kerma from the absorbance of the irradiated material.

Subsequently, the low resolution fluence $\tilde{\psi}_\mathcal{N}$ is up-sampled to the original resolution $\psi_\mathcal{N}$ using nearest neighbor (NN) interpolation and GF

$$\psi_\mathcal{N} = \mathrm{GF}\left(\frac{\mu_{en}}{\rho}, \mathrm{NN}\left(\tilde{\psi}_\mathcal{N}\right), r\right) \tag{5}$$

where $\frac{\mu_{en}}{\rho}$ functions as guidance and r is the filtering radius. Applying (4), we arrive at the high resolution dose distribution

$$D = \frac{\mu_{en}}{\rho}\psi_\mathcal{N} \tag{6}$$

2.2   Proof of concept

Our MC simulation framework is based on the general purpose MC toolkit Geant4 [9] due to the great flexibility it offers in terms of particle tracking, experiment geometry, and material modeling. Unfortunately, the number of different mixture materials increases exponentially with the down-sampling factor, depending on the degree of distinction of different organs and tissues in the target volume V. This in turn leads to the fact that the calculation of the mixture materials cannot be carried out without further development.

To still provide for a proof of concept, we synthetically create corresponding low resolution dose distributions $\tilde{D}_s$ from high resolution dose distributions D, where s is the sampling factor. The down-sampling is performed by weighting and summing all voxels in the neighborhood $\mathcal{N}(s)$. Again, the weights correspond to the fraction of mass of each individual voxel of the resulting voxel.

3   Results

We investigate our method at four different scales $s \in \{1, 4, 8, 16\}$ of a dose distribution simulated with respect to 10^8 primary photons sampled from a 120 kV peak voltage spectrum using the digital Visible Human dosimetry phantom [10]. As reference, we consider a simulation with 10×10^8 primary photons and otherwise same parameters. Figure 2 shows the initial deviation between these two simulations. Note that both distributions are normalized to a peak dose of 0.5 Gy. We observe an average and median relative error of 34.8 % and 22.3 %, respectively, when no further processing is applied.

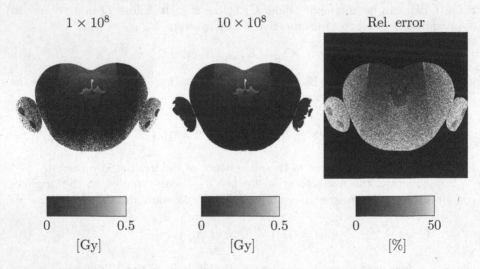

Fig. 2. Baseline error between average dose distributions of 10^8 and 10×10^8 without any processing. Both distributions are scaled to a peak dose of 0.5 Gy.

In comparison, Fig. 3 shows the down-sampled and up-sampled dose distributions using our method, and respective error rates. For the GF operation we set $r = s$. We can see that even for $s = 16$ high resolution dose distributions can be reconstructed with 10.79 % average and 6.36 % median error only. As to be expected, with decreasing sampling factors $s \in \{4, 8\}$, these error rates drop to 4.32 % average and 2.53 % median. Surprisingly, these errors are significantly lower than those arising from smoothing the original dose distribution ($s = 1$) using GF, where no low resolution needs to be compensated. Overall, the highest errors can be observed at the transition of primary X-ray beam to scattered radiation, due to the diffuse border in the low resolution dose distributions.

4 Discussion

We proposed a theoretical framework for accelerated MC simulation based on a down- and up-sampling scheme for the target volume and resulting dose distributions. Since, its implementation is currently not feasible in our MC application, we gave a proof of concept by transferring the basic principle of our method to synthetically down-sampled dose distributions. Promising results could be

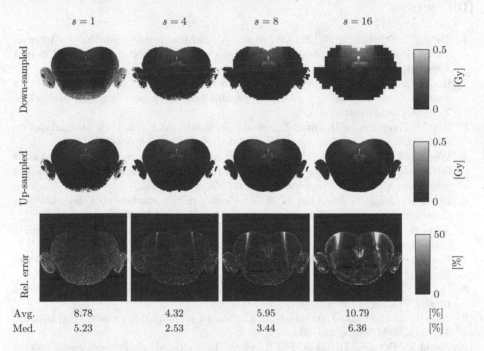

Fig. 3. Exemplary axial slices of dose distributions down-sampled by the factor s (first row) and corresponding reconstructed high resolution distributions (second row). The last row shows the relative error with respect to the reference dose distribution and corresponding averages and medians. Dose distributions are scaled to a peak dose of 0.5 Gy.

reported, which substantiate the assumption of the method being applicable to speed up MC simulations considerably. Future studies will have to focus on a feasible implementation in Geant4 as well as an in-depth analysis of the expected gain in computational performance.

The presented results also suggest the conclusion that the overall method can be used to de-noise MC simulations in general. The down- and up-sampling of the dose distribution could be reformulated to filtering operation.

Inspecting the results visually, it becomes however evident that our method exposes weaknesses at edges and interfaces of different tissues. In addition, for higher down-sampling factors, a systematic error trend in higher density tissues such as bone is observable. These issues could be solved by formulating the GF radius r as function of the tissue densities in the neighborhood $\mathcal{N}$. Furthermore, the inclusion of a voxel-wise distance weighting with respect to the radiation source could be beneficial when applying GF.

Disclaimer. The concepts and information presented in this paper are

based on research and are not commercially available.

References

1. Zhong X, Strobel N, Birkhold A, et al. A machine learning pipeline for internal anatomical landmark embedding based on a patient surface model. Int J Comput Assist Radiol Surg. 2019;14(1):53–61.
2. Badal A, Badano A. Accelerating monte carlo simulations of photon transport in a voxelized geometry using a massively parallel graphics processing unit. Med Phys. 2009;36(11):4878–4880.
3. Bert J, Perez-Ponce H, Bitar ZE, et al. Geant4-based monte carlo simulations on GPU for medical applications. Phys Med Biol. 2013;58(16):5593–5611.
4. Woodcock E, Murphy T, Hemmings P, et al. Techniques used in the GEM code for monte carlo neutronics calculations in reactors and other systems of complex geometry, ANL-7050. Argonne National Laboratory; 1965.
5. Roser P, Zhong X, Birkhold A, et al. Physics-driven learning of x-ray skin dose distribution in interventional procedures. Med Phys. 2019;46(10):4654–4665.
6. Miao B, Jeraj R, Bao S, et al. Adaptive anisotropic diffusion filtering of monte carlo dose distributions. Phys Med and Biol. 2003;48(17):2767–2781.
7. Kawrakow I. On the de-noising of monte carlo calculated dose distributions. Phys Med and Biol. 2002;47(17):3087–3103.
8. He K, Sun J, Tang X. Guided image filtering. IEEE Trans Pattern Anal Mach Intell. 2013;35(6):1397–1409.
9. Agostinelli S, Allison J, Amako K, et al. Geant4–a simulation toolkit. Nucl Instrum Meth A. 2003;506(3):250–303.
10. Zankl M, Petoussi-Henss N, Fill U, et al. Tomographic anthropomorphic models part IV: organ doses for adults due to idealized external photon exposures. Institute of Radiation Medicine (former Institute of Radiation Protection); 2002.

CT-Based Non-Destructive Quantification of 3D-Printed Hydrogel Implants

Jule Steinert[1], Thomas Wittenberg[2,3], Vera Bednarzig[4], Rainer Detsch[4],
Joelle Claussen[1], Stefan Gerth[1]

[1] Fraunhofer Development Center X-Ray Technology EZRT, Fürth
[2] Fraunhofer Institute for Integrated Circuits IIS, Erlangen
[3] Chair of Visual Computing, FAU Erlangen-Nürnberg
[4] Institute of Biomaterials, FAU Erlangen-Nürnberg
stefan.gerth@iis.fraunhofer.de

Abstract. Additive manufacturing of hydrogel-based implants, as e.g
for the human skull are becoming more important as they should allow a modelling of the different natural layers of the skullcap, and support the bone healing process. Nevertheless, the quality, structure and
consistency of such 3D-printed hydrogel implants are important for the
reliable production, quality assurance and further tests of the implant
production. One possibility for non-destructive imaging and quantification of such additive manufactured hydrogels is computed tomography
combined with quantitative image analysis. Hence, the goal of this work
is the quantitative analysis of the hydrogel-air relationship as well as
the automated computation of the hydrogel angles between the different hydrogel layers. This is done by application and evaluation of various classical image analysis methods such as thresholdig, morphological
operators, region growing and Fourier transformation of the CT-slices.
Results show, that the examined quantities (channels in the hydrogel
lattice, angles between the layers) are in the expected ranges, and it can
be concluded that the additive manufacturing process may yield usable
hydrogel meshes for reconstructive medicine.

1 Introduction

Fractures, infections, tumour removal or traumata are clinical incidents where a
hole or crack in the skull has to be covered and filled by an adequate implant
[1, 2]. Such implants have to cover and close the holes or cracks in such a way
that infections, meningitis or pneumocephalus can be avoided. Due to their
complex layer structure, which are quite different from native human bones,
new – additive manufactured – materials are currently under research for the
skullcap, which are biologically, chemically and mechanically compatible to the
surrounding tissue.

Hence, a new generation of additive-manufactured type of *hydrogel-based* implants, as e.g. for the human skull and similar complex bony structures are becoming more important [3, 4]. These 3D-hydrogel mesh prints allow modelling of

© Springer Fachmedien Wiesbaden GmbH, ein Teil von Springer Nature 2020
T. Tolxdorff et al. (Hrsg.), *Bildverarbeitung für die Medizin 2020*,
Informatik aktuell, https://doi.org/10.1007/978-3-658-29267-6_25

the different structural layers of the natural skullcap and are thus of interest for future implant techniques. One such approach of additive-manufactured implant materials consist of a titan mesh layer and different layers of hydrogel, cf. Fig. 1. The porous functional layers are manufactured sequentially on top of each other with varying angles by an extrusion process. The *osseointegration* (meaning the direct structural and functional connection between living bone and the surface of an artificial implant) is decisive for the quality of the implant. Specifically, the channel structures of the *hydrogel grid* are of importance as they relate to the possibility of the osseointegration of the implant.

As the channel structure of the hydrogel-grid as well as the printing quality and consistency of such 3D-printed hydrogel implants is important, an adequate quality assurance of the implant production has to be considered. Thus, computer tomography (CT) as a non-destructive testing method is applied to the 3D-printed hydrogel lattices (Sec. 2.2).

Using a set of classical image analysis approaches the scanned lattices are examined in order to determine the channels in the hydrogel lattice and the angles between the individual layers. Several approaches for angle determination are investigated and the respective results compared with each other. Furthermore, it is checked whether the measured angles agree with the planned angles (Sec. 2.3.)

2   Materials and methods

2.1   Bioprinting

The 3D-printed implants are composite based material manufactured on a titanium mesh. The implant platform is a titanium mesh which is used to mimic the *lamina externa* of the implant, as titanium provides the necessary stability and compensates the weight until the implant is grown into the bone. This layer is pre-manufactured in various sizes. On top of the titan mesh, the hydrogel layers are produced by extrusion (BioScaffolder system, GeSiM Corp.), where the material is liquified by a heated nozzle and fed by compressed air through the extruder [5].

The first hydrogel layer is printed directly onto the titanium mesh and prevents the ingrowth of fibroblasts. The next hydrogel layer has a porous structure and performs the tasks of the *diploe* (the spongiosa layer of the skull bone). The third layer represents the *lamina interna* and is hence similar to the first layer. The *dura mater cranialis* is representing the fourth layer. It provides structures for the functional regeneration and should promote the ingrowth of cells and thus be easily degradable.

The second (diploe) layer, referred to as *hydrogel mesh* consists of a lattice structure with long channels and is intended to promote the ingrowth of blood vessels and bone cells. The grid structure of this mesh is created by additively adding hydrogel sub-layers on top of each other, and rotating them by 60° one to the other, see Fig. 2. Hence the sub-layers result in three different spatial

Fig. 1. CT of an additive manufactured hydrogel mesh of the *diploe* with various functional layers in side (left) and top view (right).

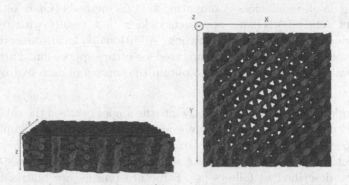

directions, which are repeated several times. $60°$ angles between the individual sub-layers of the grid have been shown to be optimal with respect to space and stability.

2.2 Image data

Four sets of additive manufactured hydrogel structures with changing chemical composites have been scanned using a portable micro-CT system (Fraunhofer CT Portable 160.90). The X-ray consists of a 90 kV tube with 8 Watt (Thermo Scientific PXS5-928 MicroFocus X-Ray), the reconstruction has a voxel size between 2 and 40 μm, and was adjusted to 19.8 μm as compromise between image details and amount of data. Distance between source and detector was 285 mm. Each projection has an integration time of 400 ms and a data size of approximately 11GBytes. Volume reconstructions was obtained from 1200 projections.

2.3 Image analysis

Pre-processing In order to enhance the quality of the volume reconstruction of the mesh-data, a median filter is applied to all projection images for edge-preserving noise-reduction. After the 3D-reconstruction Volumes-of-Interest are

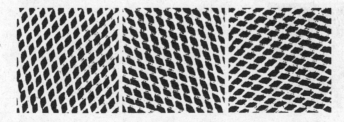

Fig. 2. Axial CT slices of the hydrogel mesh depicting the $60°$ rotations between the additive manufactured hydrogel sub-layers.

manually clipped to focus on the depicted meshes only. This reduces the processing time for subsequent steps. Background noise is eliminated using binary thresholding on all axial slices. Comparing various methods (Otsu [6], Tsai [7], Discriminant Analysis), Otsu's approach yielded best results with respect to noise removal and foreground preservation. Additionally, local connectivity and morphological closing (with $r = 17$) are used for error suppression. Furthermore morphological skeletonizing is used to obtain the centres of each hydrogel line.

2.3.1   Angle measurements To measure the angles between the sub-layers in the hydrogel mesh, two approaches are evaluated. Both have been implemented in ImageJ respectively FIJI, namely *OrientationJ* and *Directionality*.

The mechanics of the *OrientationJ* approach are based on the use of structure tensors, described as follows [8]: Structure tensors are matrix representatives of partial derivatives. To this end the local orientation and isotropic properties (coherency and energy) of every pixel of the image are evaluated. These values are derived from the structure tensor defined for each pixel as the 2×2 symmetric positive matrix $J = \begin{bmatrix} \langle f_x, f_x \rangle_w & \langle f_x, f_y \rangle_w \\ \langle f_x, f_y \rangle_w & \langle f_y, f_y \rangle_w \end{bmatrix}$ where f_x and f_y are partial spatial derivatives of the image $f(x, y)$ along the principal directions X and Y, respectively, and $\langle f, g \rangle_w$ the weighted inner product with a Gaussian weight w. Based on the structure tensor J the local orientation θ, energy E and coherency C can be computed for each pixel. The predominant orientation θ corresponds to the direction of the largest Eigenvector of the tensor: $\theta = \frac{1}{2} \arctan \left(\frac{2\langle f_x, f_y \rangle_w}{\langle f_y, f_y \rangle_w - \langle f_x, f_x \rangle_w} \right)$. The energy is computed from the largest and smallest Eigenvalues $E = \frac{\lambda_{max} - \lambda_{min}}{\lambda_{max} + \lambda_{min}}$ and the coherency $C = trace(J) = \langle f_y, f_y \rangle_w + \langle f_x, f_x \rangle_w$. If the value of C approaches 1, the image depicts highly oriented structures, where as values near 0 relate to isotropic areas. *OrientationJ* provides various methods for the computation of the gradient including cubic-spline-interpolation, finite-differences, Riesz-transform, Gauss-filtering and Hesse-matrix. Fig. 3 gives an example of the colour-coded orientations in a axial mesh slice (left) and the corresponding histogram of detected orientations (right) using the Riesz-transform. The orientation histograms obtained from the other approaches look similar. From the histogram, the dominant angles of the hydro-

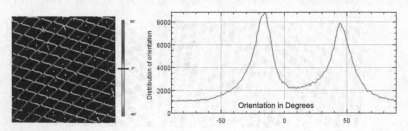

Fig. 3. Example of color coded orientation in the mesh image (left) and corresponding histogram of detected orientations (right) using the Riesz-transform.

gel meshes can be obtained. The *Directionality* approach is based on the classic 2D FFT transform. All images are zero-padded and for weighting the grey-levels the *Blackman* windowing function is applied [9]. The frequencies and directions of the mesh edges are computed using a scale-space-approach [10] from the polar-transformed power spectrum. Fig. 4 gives an example of the colour-coded orientations in a mesh slice (left), the corresponding Fourier-transformed image (center) and the histogram of detected angles (right).

3   Results

To yield space for the ingrowth of cells, ideally, the examined hydrogel mesh should yield a *material-air ratio* r of approximately $1 : 1$. After the pre-processing steps this ratio can be computed. For hydrogel mesh number one (H_1) the material-air ratio was determined as $r = 0.8$ (0.45:0.55) after the binarization-step. After the morphological post-processing correction, the ratio $r_{corr} = 0.92$ (0.48:0.52) was shifted towards the expected value. The difference in the ratio shows, that approx. 3% of air is included within the printed hydrogel material. Similar results were obtained for the other examined meshes, whereas the chemical composition of the printing material influences the determined ratio r. All above described methods for the determination of the *orientation* yield plausible results, but vary within the distribution and frequency of the angles over all examined meshes and data. From the *OrientationJ* approaches the *Riesz-transform* yields the most stable results with respect to angles. In contrast, the 2D-Fourier-Transform shows the most stable results, with angle differences of constantly $60°$ between the examined mesh. These results have also been verified on ideal images with simulated data. Fig. 5 shows the obtained angles of the Riesz- and the Fourier transform.

4   Discussion

Within this work, additive manufactured hydrogel-based implants for the skull-cap are investigated using CT-imaging in order to obtain measures for the material-air relationship, the interconnectivity of the channel and the angles between sub-layers. All values of interest can automatically be extracted and measured

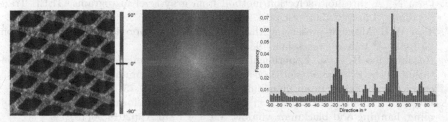

Fig. 4. Example of color coded orientation in the mesh image (left), Fourier transformed slice (center) and resulting histogram of detected angles (right).

Fig. 5. Comparison of angles from Riesz- (yellow) and Fourier transforms (blue).

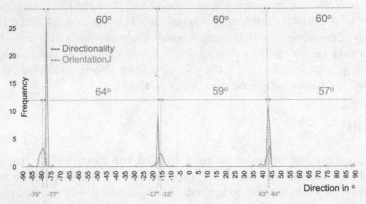

using classical image analysis approaches. Various image analysis approaches have been compared based on real CT-data of 3D-printed implants as well as simulated images and the best combination of methods has been selected for the future non-destructive testing of hydrogel prints.

Acknowledgement. This work was partially supported by the German Federal Ministry of Education and Research (BMBF) with grant number 03XP0097E.

References

1. Diebowski S. Kombination von CT und Hartgewebehistologie bei der Auswertung von in-vivo Untersuchungen an Knochenersatzmaterialien für den Schädelbereich [PhD thesis]; 2014.
2. Rosildo J, Barbara R. Reconstruction of the skull inverting the deformed surface of the bone after exeresis of a frontal arachnoid cyst. Autopsy & case reports. 2017;7(2):69–73.
3. Jang TS, Jung HD, Pan H, et al. 3D printing of hydrogel composite systems: Recent advances in technology for tissue engineering. Int J Bioprinting. 2018;4(01).
4. Detsch R, Sarker B, Grigore A, et al. Alginate and gelatine blending for bone cell printing and biofabrication. In: Proc's Biomed. Eng. 2013. p. 451–455.
5. Žehnder T, Sarker B, Boccaccini A, et al. Evaluation of an alginate-gelatine crosslinked hydrogel for bioplotting. Biofabrication. 2015;7(2).
6. Otsu N. A threshold selection method from gray-level histograms. IEEE Trans Systems, Man & Cybernetics. 1979;9(1):62–66.
7. Tsai WH. Moment-preserving thresolding: A new approach. Computer Vision, Graphics & Image Processing. 1985;2(3):377–93.
8. Rezakhaniha R, et al. Experimental investigation of collagen waviness and orientation in the arterial adventitia using confocal laser scanning microscopy. Biomechanics & modeling in mechanobiology. 2011;11(7):461–73.
9. Podder P, Khan T, Khan MH, et al. Comparative performance analysis of hamming, hanning and blackman window. Int J Comp App 2014;96(18):1–7.
10. Liu Z. Scale space approach to directional analysis of images. Applied Optics. 1991;30(11):1369–73.

Fully-Automatic CT Data Preparation for Interventional X-Ray Skin Dose Simulation

Philipp Roser[1,3], Annette Birkhold[2], Alexander Preuhs[1], Bernhard Stimpel[1], Christopher Syben[1], Norbert Strobel[4], Markus Kowarschik[2], Rebecca Fahrig[2], Andreas Maier[1,3]

[1]Pattern Recognition Lab, FAU Erlangen-Nürnberg
[2]Siemens Healthcare GmbH, Forchheim
[3]Erlangen Graduate School in Advanced Optical Technologies (SAOT)
[4]Fakultät Elektrotechnik, HS für angewandte Wissenschaften Würzburg-Schweinfurt
philipp.roser@fau.de

Abstract. Recently, deep learning (DL) found its way to interventional X-ray skin dose estimation. While its performance was found to be acceptable, even more accurate results could be achieved if more data sets were available for training. One possibility is to turn to computed tomography (CT) data sets. Typically, computed tomography (CT) scans can be mapped to tissue labels and mass densities to obtain training data. However, care has to be taken to make sure that the different clinical settings are properly accounted for. First, the interventional environment is characterized by wide variety of table setups that are significantly different from the typical patient tables used in conventional CT. This cannot be ignored, since tables play a crucial role in sound skin dose estimation in an interventional setup, e. g., when the X-ray source is directly underneath a patient (posterior-anterior view). Second, due to interpolation errors, most CT scans do not facilitate a clean segmentation of the skin border. As a solution to these problems, we applied connected component labeling (CCL) and Canny edge detection to (a) robustly separate the patient from the table and (b) to identify the outermost skin layer. Our results show that these extensions enable fully-automatic, generalized pre-processing of CT scans for further simulation of both skin dose and corresponding X-ray projections.

1 Introduction

Deep learning (DL) is a powerful technique for various applications, with medical X-ray imaging in general and computed tomography (CT) being no exception. Whether for computer-aided diagnosis, semantic segmentation, or 3D reconstruction, DL elevated expected assessment metrics tremendously. As Unberath et al. found, the data situation is excellent for many of these tasks – with the exception of interventional imaging. To exploit the abundance of existing high-quality and open access data libraries, they proposed a DL-fueled framework based on

© Springer Fachmedien Wiesbaden GmbH, ein Teil von Springer Nature 2020
T. Tolxdorff et al. (Hrsg.), *Bildverarbeitung für die Medizin 2020*,
Informatik aktuell, https://doi.org/10.1007/978-3-658-29267-6_26

a poly-chromatic forward projector to generate realistic X-ray projections from CT scans [1]. While challenging tasks in the interventional environment, such as device tracking or learning-based trajectory planning, could be improved or, in some cases, even solved for the first time, skin dose monitoring and optimization does not benefit to the same extent. Besides, DL-based 3D segmentation is often bound to a certain anatomic region and requires top tier hardware.

With increasing dose awareness in the interventional suite, physically-sound real-time tracking of skin dose during interventional procedures is desirable. While being the gold standard, Monte Carlo (MC) simulation of X-ray photon transport typically suffers from high computational complexity. Although hardware acceleration is widely applied for research purposes [2], it may not be available to the same degree in a clinical setting as the available hardware is usually used to support multiple imaging tasks. Recently, DL was used to bypass the hardware bottleneck for dose estimation and promising first results could be reported for both high- and low-end hardware [3]. However, the generation of ground truth data is a tedious task due to (a) the high computational complexity of general purpose MC codes and (b) the lack of open-access digital phantoms. To increase the number of data sets for the generation of ground-truth data using MC simulations, CT scans can be mapped to corresponding tissue types and densities using thresholds. Unfortunately tables, mattresses, and blankets are acquired well in most CT protocols, whereas the skin can not be segmented distinctly. To account for the many different setups (tables, patient preparation) in an interventional environment, a data preparation pipeline capable of removing tables while finding an adequate skin segmentation is needed. To this end, we propose a framework that extends the conventional approach of mapping Hounsfield units (HU) to tissue labels [4] and densities by unsupervised image processing techniques. This ensures smooth tissue distributions, homogeneous skin segmentation, and removes non-patient objects such as tables, blankets, and mattresses. Our framework will be made open source after publication.

2   Methods

The outline of the proposed data preparation pipeline is depicted in Fig. 1. The integer pixel values $I_r \in \mathbb{Z}^3$ are mapped to HU units using the specified rescale intercept $a_r \in \mathbb{Z}$ and slope $b_r \in \mathbb{R}$ according to $I_{HU} = [a_r + b_r I_r] \in \mathbb{Z}^3$. Here '$[\cdot]$' rounds to the next integer number.

2.1   Tissue mapping

To preserve inhomogeneities in the human body that might play a crucial role in realistic data generation, I_{HU} is mapped to mass densities $\rho \in \mathbb{R}^3$ using piecewise linear transforms $\rho(I_{HU}) = a_\rho + b_\rho I_{HU}$, with $a_\rho, b_\rho \in \mathbb{R}$ [4]. To obtain tissue labels $L \in \mathbb{N}^3$, associated HU values are mapped based on a piece-wise constant function. Both transforms are plotted in Fig. 2 a. Note that due to overlapping HU value ranges for certain structures, such as cancellous bone and other organs,

Fig. 1. Flow diagram of the proposed method. Based on the HU values of a CT scan, tissue labels and associated densities are derived. Then a mask of the body is generated using connected component analysis. Finally, the skin is labeled using edge detection on the mask.

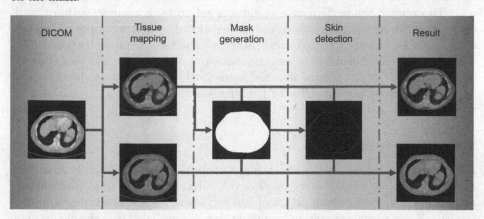

the tissue – and to some extent the density – mapping is not bijective in general. However, in these value ranges, the different tissue types behave similarly. Therefore the tissue label transfer function is defined to provide a meaningful trade-off between all overlapping HU value ranges. In total, we differentiate between lung tissue (1), adipose tissue (2), soft tissue (3), cancellous bone (4), cortical bone (5), and air (0). For convenience, the labels are ordered based on their corresponding nominal mass densities. In addition, outlier pixels in large homogeneoues regions are removed using a median-based hot pixel detection algorithm.

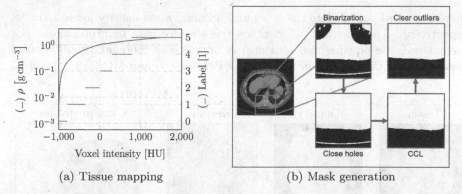

(a) Tissue mapping   (b) Mask generation

Fig. 2. HU values are mapped to mass densities ρ and tissue labels using piece-wise linear and constant transfer functions (a). From the initial tissue labels, a mask is generated. To this end, we apply binarization and close holes found in the lung or esophagus. Afterwards, we separate objects using connected component labeling (CCL). Finally leftover outliers are cleared (b).

2.2 Mask generation

Our approach to generate the patient mask $M \in \{0,1\}^3$ is illustrated in Fig. 2 b. Initially, the tissue labels are binarized, where each non-zero label is assigned to one. To improve the performance of subsequent steps, zero-areas within closed contours, such as the lung or esophagus, are closed. Then we apply connected component labeling (CCL) [5] to separate, e. g., the table from the patient body. The patient is identified by the largest connected cluster, thus all other clusters are assigned to zero. Eventually, the same outlier detection as previously is applied to remove possible leftover hot pixels in the air or near to the patient surface.

2.3 Skin detection

Due to artifacts, interpolation, and tissue ambiguities, the skin is rarely identified as a homogeneous soft tissue region after the initial processing steps. Instead, we rather find a mixture of lung, adipose, and soft tissue. While this is negligible for realistic X-ray image generation, a unique skin surface label is desirable for skin entrance and back-scatter dose estimation. To identify the skin surface, we apply the Canny edge detector [6] with standard deviation $\sigma = 1$ to the binary patient mask yielding a one-voxel thick edge around the patient surface $S \in \{0,1\}^3$.

2.4 Composition

Based on the mask, M, the skin surface, S, the tissue labels, L, and the densities, ρ, the final labeled data set, L', and density distribution, ρ', are computed as

$$L' = (M - S) \odot L + L_{\text{soft}} S \tag{1}$$

$$\rho' = (M - S) \odot \rho + \rho_{\text{soft}} S \tag{2}$$

where L_{soft} and ρ_{soft} denote the label and nominal mass density for soft tissue, respectively. The operator '$\odot$' denotes the element-wise multiplication. For convenience, the pipeline also provides an interface to the penEasy 2008 voxel volume format that is used in the popular Penelope [7] and MC-GPU [2] codes.

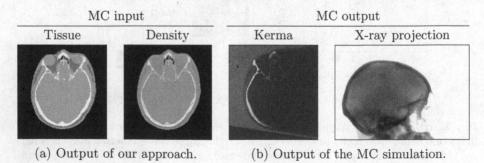

MC input		MC output	
Tissue	Density	Kerma	X-ray projection

(a) Output of our approach.   (b) Output of the MC simulation.

Fig. 3. Sample inputs and outputs of the MC-GPU code of a CT scan pre-processed by the proposed data pre-processing framework.

3   Results

Quantitatively assessing the performance of the proposed data preparation method is inherently difficult as there is currently no ground truth data available. To still obtain some insights into the merits of our work at this point in time, we study how well the anatomical shape is preserved and whether table gets removed without impairing the neighboring patient outline. Figure 3 a shows sample outputs of our proposed approach. We found that the tissue labels obtained were homogeneously distributed. In addition, the estimated tissue densities facilitated the generation of realistic X-ray projection images. This observation is further substantiated by the perceptually realistic kerma distribution and X-ray projection estimated using MC simulation, which are shown in Fig. 3 b. To illustrate the performance of the table removal, Fig. 4 shows average intensity projections of 10 CT scans along the longitudinal axis taken from the HNSCC-3DCT-RT head [8] and the CT Lymph Nodes torso [9] datasets provided in The Cancer Imaging Archive (TCIA) [10]. Evidently, the average shapes are well preserved, while the table and acquisition-induced artifacts were removed completely.

4   Discussion

We presented a fully-automatic, robust, generalized CT scan processing pipeline. It can be used to generate input for MC simulation codes without any need for manual interaction and thus making it attractive for large scale data generation. Thanks to the proposed method, new CT-based digital models can be used to extend our existing training set. Especially the removal of tables as used for conventional spiral CT scans and the inclusion of a distinct skin voxel layer makes it

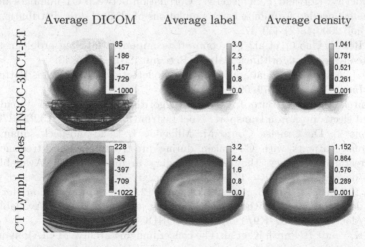

Fig. 4. Average input DICOM, generated labels, densities of 10 volumes from two publicly available datasets. By visual inspection it is evident that table and artifacts get removed completely while the overall correlation is preserved.

possible to transfer the data to interventional setups and use it there for skin dose estimation. We also found that our method produces anatomiccally consistent results for both head and torso scans without adapting any parameters.

Still, the pipeline certainly has limitations. First, overlapping HU value ranges of different tissue types – most prominently soft tissue, brain tissue, and cancellous bone – needs to be addressed in future iterations. This could be achieved using (a) a locally restricted CCL or (b) a DL approach. Second, the skin modelling could be enhanced by differentiating between sub-layers of skin. To this end, a pre-defined skin template could be matched with respect to the normal vector of the patient surface. Third, especially in head CTs, metal artifacts occur and can currently not be dealt with sufficiently well. One way to solve this issue could be an inpainting approach based on template matching or generative adversarial networks.

Disclaimer. The concepts and information presented in this paper are based on research and are not commercially available.

References

1. Unberath M, Zaech JN, Gao C, et al. Enabling machine learning in x-ray-based procedures via realistic simulation of image formation. Int J Comput Assist Radiol Surg. 2019;.
2. Badal A, Badano A. Accelerating monte carlo simulations of photon transport in a voxelized geometry using a massively parallel graphics processing unit. Med Phys. 2009;36(11):4878–4880.
3. Roser P, Zhong X, Birkhold A, et al. Physics-driven learning of x-ray skin dose distribution in interventional procedures. Med Phys. 2019;46(10):4654–4665.
4. Schneider W, Bortfeld T, Schlegel W. Correlation between CT numbers and tissue parameters needed for monte carlo simulations of clinical dose distributions. Phys Med Biol. 2000;45(2):459–478.
5. He L, Ren X, Gao Q, et al. The connected-component labeling problem: a review of state-of-the-art algorithms. Pattern Recognit. 2017;70:25–43.
6. Canny J. A computational approach to edge detection. IEEE Trans Pattern Anal Mach Intell. 1986;8(6):679–698.
7. Sempau J, Acosta E, Baro J, et al. An algorithm for monte carlo simulation of coupled electron-photon transport. Nucl Instrum Meth B. 1997;132(3):377–390.
8. Bejarano T, De Ornelas Couto M, Mihaylov I. Head-and-neck squamous cell carcinoma patients with CT taken during pre-treatment, mid-treatment, and post-treatment dataset. the cancer imaging archive; 2018. Available from: http://doi.org/10.7937/K9/TCIA.2018.13upr2xf.
9. Roth H, Le L, Ari S, et al.. A new 2.5 d representation for lymph node detection in CT. the cancer imaging archive; 2018. Available from: http://doi.org/10.7937/K9/TCIA.2015.AQIIDCNM.
10. Clark K, Vendt B, Smith K, et al. The cancer imaging archive (TCIA): maintaining and operating a public information repository. J Digit Imaging. 2013 07;26:1045–1057.

Prediction of MRI Hardware Failures based on Image Features Using Time Series Classification

Nadine Kuhnert[1], Lea Pflüger[1], Andreas Maier[1]

[1]Pattern Recognition Lab, Friedrich-Alexander University Erlangen-Nuremberg
nadine.kuhnert@fau.de

Abstract. Already before systems malfunction one has to know if hardware components will fail in near future in order to counteract in time. Thus, unplanned downtime is ought to be avoided. In medical imaging, maximizing the system's uptime is crucial for patients' health and healthcare provider's daily business. We aim to predict failures of Head/Neck coils used in Magnetic Resonance Imaging (MRI) by training a statistical model on sequential data collected over time. As image features depend on the coil's condition, their deviations from the normal range already hint to future failure. Thus, we used image features and their variation over time to predict coil damage. After comparison of different time series classification methods we found Long Short Term Memorys (LSTMs) to achieve the highest F-score of 86.43% and to tell with 98.33% accuracy if hardware should be replaced.

1 Introduction

Often it feels like hardware failures occur all of a sudden. However, data contain deviations from the normal range already before breakage and carry hints of future failing parts. In Magnetic Resonance Imaging (MRI), systems are extensively used and unplanned downtimes come with high costs. High image quality and seamless operation are crucial for the diagnostic value. Radiofrequency coils are essential hardware as they receive signals which form the basis of the desired diagnostic image [1]. Thus, the goal is to prevent unplanned coil failure by exchanging or repairing the respective coil before its malfunction. In this work, we predict failures of Head/Neck coils using image-related measurements collected over time. Therefore, we aim to solve a time series classification (TSC) problem.

In literature, time series classification is tackled by a range of traditional Machine Learning (ML) algorithms such as Hidden Markov Models, Neural Networks or Linear Dynamic Systems [2]. Wang et al. [3] are the first who introduced Convolutional Neural Networks (CNN) for the classification of univariate time series where no local pooling layers are included and thus, the length of time series kept the same for all convolutions. They also applied a deep Residual Network (ResNet) for TSC. The main characteristic of a ResNet is the addition of a linear shortcut that connects the output of a residual block to its input. Furthermore,

© Springer Fachmedien Wiesbaden GmbH, ein Teil von Springer Nature 2020
T. Tolxdorff et al. (Hrsg.), *Bildverarbeitung für die Medizin 2020*,
Informatik aktuell, https://doi.org/10.1007/978-3-658-29267-6_27

Recurrent Neural Networks (RNNs) contain loops to allow the network to store previous information which is essential for time series applications. A special kind of RNNs is the Long Short-Term Memory (LSTM) introduced by [4] to specifically incorporate long-term dependencies. Deep neural networks are powerful but often struggle with overfitting and long computation times which one can counteract using the dropout technique [5].

The task of hardware failure prediction using time series data has not been addressed widely in literature. Lipton et al. [6] used LSTMs in order to predict diagnosis based on clinical, time series data. Furthermore, prediction of high performance computing system failures using sequential data was trained using Support Vector Machines [7]. Jain et al. [8] found that hardware failures can be predicted based on image features, but did not examine collections of image features over time.

2 Materials and methods

In order to prevent malfunction, we applied different ML methods to determine broken coils. Firstly, we describe the data and available features. Secondly, we depict preprocessing steps, present the applied models and their configuration.

2.1 Data

We employ classification algorithms on data which was acquired by 238 Siemens MAGNETOM Aera 1.5T MRI systems. Data was collected before every examination using a 20-channel Head/Neck coil since May 1st 2019 all over the world, as well as, from measurements performed at Siemens' research halls specifically generating data sets for various hardware failure cases. This yields 29878 sequences in total which contain 2.2% sequences of defective coils. We derive image features from coil adjustment measurements which are generated before the clinical scan. Thus, reconstruction of any patient-specific features is impossible and guarantees non-clinical, fully anonymized data.

We use image features of coil elements reported by MRI systems which are represented by four continuous numerical measurements per time instance:

- *Channel Signal Noise Level (CNL):* The coil noise is measured every time a new coil configuration is selected or the patient table is moved. This happens at least once per examination. After the noise measurement the noise level is calculated and reported as one value for each channel.
- *Channel Signal to Noise Ratio (CSP):* During coil sensitivity adjustments, both coil noise and sensitivity are measured. Depending on the coil element the signal to noise ratio is estimated.
- *Channel Signal to Signal (SSR):* During the adjustment pre-scanning process also body coil measures are performed. SSR uses the signal measure of the Body coil and the signal around the isocenter of local Head/Neck coil to calculate a signal ratio between Body coil and Head/Neck coil element.

  − *Channel Signal to Noise Ratio at Isocenter (CSI):* CSI combines the channel
    signal to noise ratio (CSP) with the channel signal in the isocenter and
    reports the respective ratio.

2.2 Preprocessing

First, we centered and scaled the data of each individual feature independently
by subtracting the mean and dividing by the standard deviation, respectively.
Furthermore, we artificially produced new defective time series based on training
data set in order to enlarge the number of broken feature sequences used in
training. As the average number of instances per day was found to be 40,
we generated synthetic sequences of length 40 by merging normal and defective
features to mime breaking within one day. We selected one sequence of each class
randomly and filled the new series by fading. During most breakage scenarios
the feature values rose according to a sigmoidal shape. Therefore, fading is
performed using a sigmoid function, which was randomly scaled and shifted
along the y-axis. Equation 1 describes how the synthetic values x for the time
stamps $j \in [0, 40[$ are calculated based on values of randomly chosen normal
($normal[j]$) and broken ($broken[j]$) time series at element j. Equation 2 presents
the used sigmoid function $p[j]$

$$x[j] = (1 - p[j]) \cdot normal[j] + p[j] \cdot broken[j] \qquad (1)$$

$$p[j] = \frac{1}{1 + \exp(-\frac{j-\mu}{\sigma})} \qquad (2)$$

The value for scaling factor σ is randomly chosen out of range $[0.2, 1]$, whereas μ
carries the translation factor which can have values between -13.3 and 13.3. The
allowed ranges were determined experimentally. This is performed for all four
features (CNL, CSP, SSR, CSI) individually using the same sigmoid function.

2.3 Classification

We applied the following four different time series classification methods to the
preprocessed data and compared them. Thus, we determined the best suiting
of the four models in order to predict which coils will change their state from
normal to defective. All parameters were determined using hyper-parameter
tuning. Thus, the model with the lowest validation loss was chosen after random
initialization of weights and optimization following Adam's proposal [9].

  A leave-several-coils-out cross validation was performed, where the respective
non-testing coils were stratified split into 70% training and 30% validation data.
Thus, we can assure that only sequences from distinct coils were used in model
training and testing.

2.3.1   Fully convolutional neural networks Following the approach from Wang et al. [3], we implemented a Fully Convolutional Neural Network (FCN) which is composed of three convolutional blocks. All blocks perform three operations, each. The first block contains a convolution with 128 filters of length eight followed by a batch normalization [10] using 256 filters with a filter length of five in order to speed up convergence. Its result is sent to a ReLu activation function consisting of 128 filters where each has a length equal to three. After the calculation of the third and last convolution block, the average over the complete time is calculated. This step is comparable to a Global Average Pooling (GAP) layer. Finally, the GAP layer's output is fully connected to a traditional softmax classifier. In order to maintain the exact length of the time series throughout the performed convolutions, zero padding and a stride equal to one were used in every convolution step. The FCN does not contain any pooling to prevent overfitting nor a regularization operation.

2.3.2   Residual network Moreover, we set up a ResNet proposed by [3] built out of three residual blocks. Each block is composed of three convolutions. The convolution result of each block is added to the shortcut residual connection (input of each residual block) and is then fed to the following residual block. For all convolutions the number of filters used is set to 64, with the ReLU activation function followed by a batch normalization operation. Within the first block the filter length is set to eight, in the second one to five and in the third to three. The three residual blocks are followed by a GAP layer and a softmax classifier whose number of neurons is equivalent to the number of classes in the data set. The main characteristic of ResNets and the difference to usual convolutions is the linear shortcut between input and residual blocks which allows the flow of the gradient directly through these linear connections. Therefore, training is simplified as the vanishing gradient effect is reduced.

2.3.3   Time convolutional neural networks As an alternative, we implemented a Time Convolutional Neural Network [3](TCNN) constructed of two consecutive convolutional layers with six and twelve filters. A local average pooling operation of length three follows the convolutional layers. Sigmoid is used as the activation function. The network's output results in a fully connected layer, where the number of neurons is in our case two as we focus on two classes in our data set, normal and broken coil.

2.3.4   Long short-term memory The forth method we applied is a LSTM network. It contains two convolutional layers without padding operations. Therefore, the sequence length decreases with every convolution. Each convolutional layer is preceded by local average pooling operation of length three and a dropout operation with a rate equal to 0.2 to prevent overfitting [5]. After the construction of convolutional layers, average pooling and dropout operations, two LSTM layers with 32 units and a tanh activation function follow. A dense

Table 1. Average prediction performance measures and confusion matrix of the applied TSC methods after 10-fold cross-validation.

%	Accuracy	Precision	Recall	F-Score	TN	FP	FN	TP
FCN	97.53	75.54	**85.68**	75.66	97.92	2.08	14.31	85.69
ResNet	97.43	75.73	83.75	73.98	97.72	2.28	16.23	83.77
TCNN	97.72	82.56	68.23	74.16	99.33	0.67	29.35	70.65
LSTM	**98.33**	**90.10**	84.16	**86.43**	98.67	1.33	15.83	84.17

Table 2. Average number of broken instances, prediction performance measures and confusion matrix after 10-fold cross-validation. Different results were achieved with LSTM for different degrees of synthetically increased numbers of broken sequences during model fitting.

Broken instances	Accuracy	Precision	Recall	F-Score	TN	FP	FN	TP
576 (2.2%)	98.33	**90.10**	**84.16**	**86.43**	98.67	1.33	15.83	84.17
641 (2.4%)	97.67	83.32	71.49	76.28	99.18	0.82	28.51	71.49
706 (2.6%)	**98.38**	88.02	82.29	83.59	98.75	1.25	17.71	82.29

layer and a sigmoid classifier whose number of neurons is equivalent to the number of classes in the data set complete the model structure.

3   Results

We applied our algorithms on the given time series data consisting of 97.8% normal and 2.2% broken samples first without adding synthetic sequences. Tab. 1 holds the performance measures accuracy, precision, recall and F-score for the different models where we underlined the best scores. We see that the four models perform very similar in terms of accuracy only ranging from 97.43% for ResNet up to 98.33% reached by LSTM. Furthermore, LSTM classifies coil sequences most precisely with 90.10% and delivers 84.16% recall. This results also in the best F-score for LSTM reporting 86.43%. Next to the performance measures, the confusion matrices are given holding true negative (TN), false positive (FP), false negative (FN), and true positive (TP) rates.

Due to the highly imbalanced class distribution, we generated synthetic data to increase the number of broken samples in the training set. As LSTM achieved the best performances in all four measures, we applied LSTM on three different augmentation degrees. Tab. 2 presents the performance measures and confusion matrices. For comparison, results for the original data set and the augmented datasets containing 2.4% and 2.6% broken instances are listed.

4   Discussion

For the task of predicting normal and broken Head/Neck coils based on collected image features over time, we found the presented LSTM resulting in highest accuracy of 98.33% and F-score of 86.43%. We showed that LSTM, FCN and

ResNet misclassified only few defective coils as normally functioning and thus, received similar recall values. Although ResNet has a deep and flexible architecture, LSTM enabled to classify least sequences within the individual normal coils incorrectly. We explain those results with the mixture of cases in our training data. We observed sequences with very current irregularities as well as features that were collected longer ago. Thus, LSTM considers both cases and combines long and short term instances beneficially. Augmentation of time series data for training by combining normal and defective sequences did not increase the average prediction performance measures significantly. This shows the model did not gain any additional information from the synthetic data which would ease the classification task of the test data. We did not find research applying time series classification methods to image features in order to detect hardware failures. Thus, we consider us to be the first using sequential data for hardware failure prediction while achieving high performance.

We only picked four models for comparison. In a next step, more models should be considered and tested on a larger data set. Moreover, in future work also other augmentation possibilities should be considered. As coils brake because of different reasons reporting different variations in image features, the applied sigmoid function might not reflect real world scenarios, exhaustively. Furthermore, time series classification should be also applied to other MRI hardware in order to determine the generality of our algorithm trained and tested for Head/Neck coils.

References

1. Maier A, Steidl S, Christlein V, et al. Medical imaging systems: an introductory guide. vol. 11111. Springer; 2018.
2. Bishop CM. Pattern recognition and machine learning. springer; 2006.
3. Wang Z, Yan W, Oates T. Time series classification from scratch with deep neural networks: a strong baseline. In: 2017 international joint conference on neural networks (IJCNN). IEEE; 2017. p. 1578–1585.
4. Hochreiter S, Schmidhuber J. Long short-term memory. Neural comput. 1997;9(8):1735–1780.
5. Srivastava N, Hinton G, Krizhevsky A, et al. Dropout: a simple way to prevent neural networks from overfitting. J Mach Learn Res. 2014;15(1):1929–1958.
6. Lipton ZC, Kale DC, Elkan C, et al. Learning to diagnose with LSTM recurrent neural networks. arXiv preprint arXiv:151103677. 2015;.
7. Mohammed B, Awan I, Ugail H, et al. Failure prediction using machine learning in a virtualised HPC system and application. Cluster Computing. 2019;22(2):471–485.
8. Jain B, Kuhnert N, deOliveira A, et al. Image-based detection of MRI hardware failures. In: Bildverarbeitung für die Medizin 2019. Springer; 2019. p. 206–211.
9. Kingma DP, Ba J. Adam: a method for stochastic optimization. arXiv preprint arXiv:14126980. 2014;.
10. Ioffe S, Szegedy C. Batch normalization: accelerating deep network training by reducing internal covariate shift. arXiv preprint arXiv:150203167. 2015;.

Prediction of MRI Hardware Failures Based on Image Features Using Ensemble Learning

Nadine Kuhnert[1], Lea Pflüger[1], Andreas Maier[1]

[1]Pattern Recognition Lab, Friedrich-Alexander University Erlangen-Nuremberg
nadine.kuhnert@fau.de

Abstract. In order to ensure trouble-free operation, prediction of hardware failures is essential. This applies especially to medical systems. Our goal is to determine hardware which needs to be exchanged before failing. In this work, we focus on predicting failures of 20-channel Head/Neck coils using image-related measurements. Thus, we aim to solve a classification problem with two classes, normal and broken coil. To solve this problem, we use data of two different levels. One level refers to one-dimensional features per individual coil channel on which we found a fully connected neural network to perform best. The other data level uses matrices which represent the overall coil condition and feeds a different neural network. We stack the predictions of those two networks and train a Random Forest classifier as the ensemble learner. Thus, combining insights of both trained models improves the prediction results and allows us to determine the coil's condition with an F-score of 94.14% and an accuracy of 99.09%.

1 Introduction

Reliable operation of medical diagnostic imaging systems is crucial for patient's health and healthcare provider's daily business. Thus, the goal is to prevent unplanned system downtimes by exchanging hardware before its malfunction. In Magnetic Resonance Imaging (MRI), one of the crucial hardware components are radiofrequency coils. Those coils can receive and transmit radiofrequency signals which determine the desired, diagnostic image. Coils contain different channels operating as separate, local receivers [1]. In this work, we focus on coils which are specifically used for examinations of the human body's head and neck area. Image features and related measurements depend next to the depicted tissue also on the coil's condition. Before every clinical scanning process, noise and signal measurements are performed from which we derive 1-D features for every coil channel as well as matrix features per coil.

The task of classification is well known in literature, described as assigning an input vector to one out of a set of discrete, predefined classes [2], and applied to various applications [3]. E.g. Kuhnert et al. [4] found Neural Networks to achieve highest accuracy in classifying the examined body parts using MRI

© Springer Fachmedien Wiesbaden GmbH, ein Teil von Springer Nature 2020
T. Tolxdorff et al. (Hrsg.), *Bildverarbeitung für die Medizin 2020*,
Informatik aktuell, https://doi.org/10.1007/978-3-658-29267-6_28

acquisition parameters. Next to Neural Networks, also Random Forest (RF) Classifier is widely used and has been introduced by [5]. Random Forests combine tree predictors where the search space is a randomly chosen subset. Often, several machine learning techniques train an ensemble of models to leverage their results in combination [2]. One form of ensemble learning is stacking which was introduced by Wolpert [6] and refers to a meta learner which is trained on the reliability of base classifiers as inputs.

Several ML techniques have been applied to address the task of hardware failure prediction as described in [7]. For MRI in specific, Jain et al. [8] showed that defective components can be identified using image features.

2   Materials and methods

Our approach classifies image features and consecutively Head/Neck coils of MRI systems as normal or defective. We trained different models on measurements per coil channel and features per coil, individually. In the following, we describe the underlying data, preprocessing, training of our classifiers and the final ensemble learning step in order receive one consolidated prediction per coil.

2.1   Data

All data sets were acquired by 238 Siemens MAGNETOM Aera 1.5T MRI systems using a 20-channel Head/Neck coil. We enrich those data with measurements of normal and broken coils performed at Siemens' research halls. During coil adjustment measurements we collect parameters which represent image features. Thus, we work only on entirely anonymized, non-clinical data.

The collected parameters contain two degrees. On the one hand side, we extract four numerical, one-dimensional features per coil channel. Those features are calculated for all 329338 samples and depict the noise level, signal to noise ratio (CSP), signal ratio of body coil to Head/Neck coil and the ratio of CSP to channel signal in the isocenter. On the other hand side, we use the Noise Covariance Matrix (NCM) as a feature for the entire coil. It holds the covariances of all individual noise values per channel resulting in 19687 matrices.

We perform leave-several-coils-out cross validation to calculate all performance measures on disjoint coil sets for fitting and testing. Furthermore, we apply a stratified split on the fitting data set and use 70% for base model training and 30% for hyper-parameter tuning. On average, one fold contains 29985 one-dimensional features and 1791 matrices.

2.2   Preprocessing

We performed normalization and augmentation. All features were normalized by subtracting the means and scaling to unit variance. To overcome the imbalanced class distribution (6.8% broken coils matrices), we augmented non-testing NCM

Table 1. Configuration details of CNN1 and CNN2 used for training on matrix features.

Layer	1	2	3	4	5	6	7	8	9
CNN1	Conv2D, 6, 'relu', (3,3), padding = 'same'	Average Pooling	Conv2D, 16, 'relu', (3,3), padding = 'same'	Average Pooling	Flatten	Dense, 64, 'relu'	Dense, 2, 'softmax'		
CNN2	Conv2D, 16, 'relu', (3,3), padding = 'same'	Conv2D, 16, 'relu', (3,3), padding = 'same'	Max-Pooling, (2,2)	Conv2D, 32, 'relu', (3,3), padding = 'same'	Conv2D, 32, 'relu', (3,3), padding = 'same'	Max-Pooling, (2,2)	Flatten	Dense, 64, 'relu'	Dense, 2, 'softmax'

instances. Thus, we permuted on-diagonal elements randomly. The off-diagonal elements were placed according to their respective on-diagonal element and thus, the matrices' rows and columns keep their relations. This results in N-1 generated matrices for every NxN matrix entered, where N equals 20 in our case.

2.3 Base learner training

Prediction of coils as normal or defective was achieved using different classification methods on one-dimensional features and matrices, individually.

We applied a Fully Connected Neural Network (FCN) to the numerical features. It consists of four blocks, where each block is composed of one fully connected (FC) layer. This is followed by a batch normalization and a dropout operation to prevent over-fitting. A rectified linear unit (ReLU) activation function is used for all FC layers, only the number of elements is changed within the different FC layers. Parameters and dropout rate were found using hyper-parameter tuning. The result of the four blocks is finally fed to a last FC layer with two elements. As an activation function we used softmax.

Secondly, we trained a Convolutional Neural Network (CNN) on the available NCM input. We tried four different CNN configurations. Please see the exact parameters and structures of CNN1 and CNN2 in Tab. 1. CNN4 is similarly built to CNN2 but has no padding included and contains only one convolutional layer before and after the first MaxPooling layer. CNN3 is comparable to CNN4 but has three dropout layers included. Tab. 2 holds the average prediction performance measures, accordingly. Model CNN1 reached the highest performance with a F-score of 66.00% for all tested cross-validation splits, model CNN3 lowest with 29.29%. CNN4 almost reaches as good results as CNN1.

Table 2. Average prediction performance measures after 10-fold cross-validation for the different CNNs applied to NCMs.

%	Accuracy	Precision	Recall	F-Score
CNN1	94.82	97.99	58.06	66.00
CNN2	92.47	75.92	31.39	36.25
CNN3	92.45	100.00	20.05	29.29
CNN4	93.41	94.62	51.56	60.28

Table 3. Average prediction performance measures and confusion matrix of FCN on coil element level after 10-fold cross-validation.

%	Accuracy	Precision	Recall	F-Score	TN	FP	FN	TP	N	P
FCN	99.74	86.12	82.37	82.43	99.93	0.07	17.61	82.38	97.6	2.4

2.4   Ensemble learner training

Finally, in order to leverage all information and decide for the overall predicted class, we stacked the predictions of two base learners, FCN and CNN2, and applied a RF classifier. We extracted four different features from the two base learners and fed them to the meta learner. We aggregate the FCN prediction results on coil element level, by calculating the minimum, standard deviation and mean prediction values on coil level. Furthermore, we incorporate the CNN2 prediction probability per coil as forth feature. 50% of those extracted feature instances are used for fitting the RF model. We tested the model on the remaining 50% instances. This enables one consolidated prediction result per coil.

3   Results

Main achieved results are presented for the individual models next to the combined model.

3.1   Base learner results 1d

We achieved an average prediction F-score of 82.43% after 10-fold cross-validation by applying the described FCN to our original set of one-dimensional features on coil element level. Tab. 3 shows the respective achieved accuracy of 99.74% next to precision and recall both holding values above 82%. For more details, Tab. 3 also presents the confusion matrix of the FCN showing true negative (TN), false positive (FP), false negative (FN) and true positive (TR) rates and positive (P) and negative (N) samples in percent.

3.2   Base learner results matrix

By augmenting the matrix data set, we achieved the desired ratio of 20% for number of defective vs. normal samples. We gained significant improvement in

Table 4. Average prediction performance measures for CNNs applied to data set with augmentation.

%	Accuracy	Precision	Recall	F-Score	TN	FP	FN	TP
CNN1	98.12	99.13	85.74	91.25	99.85	0.15	14.25	85.75
CNN2	98.27	99.45	86.49	91.86	99.91	0.09	13.50	86.50
CNN3	97.61	99.90	82.33	88.83	99.91	0.09	17.66	82.34
CNN4	98.09	99.52	85.30	91.05	99.92	0.08	14.69	85.31

prediction performance after augmentation. Thus, all further results shown in this section are based on training with artificial instances added during preprocessing. Tab. 4 presents the performances of the four CNNs applied to our data set including artificial instances next to the respective confusion matrix.

3.3 Ensemble learner results

Through aggregating the FCN results and only using their minimal prediction probability per coil, we observe an increase in performance from an average F-score of 82.43% to 91.04%. The average F-score for the best NCM classification lies at 91.86%. By combining the predictions of those two base learners and training a Decision Tree on these predicted instances we reach a final F-score of 94.14% and accuracy of 99.09%. The individual model performances are visualized in Fig. 1.

4   Discussion

We achieve satisfying results by training a FCN on features per coil element and aggregating the individual decision to a prediction per entire coil. The aggregation is necessary to overcome correlations of broken and normal elements within one coil affecting normal channels and their measurements such that they lead to false positives. In case of training a model on our matrix features, augmentation of data allowed to improve the classification result drastically due to avoiding overfitting to specific coil elements. As the prediction should not be affected by the location of the highest on-diagonal element value, augmentation was necessary to overcome unrealistic correlation of broken coil to specific coil elements. By combining the learnings of the two trained models in a final ensemble learning step, we could leverage the two different view points and information degrees of our data. Thus, stacking improved the resulting performance measures even more.

To our knowledge, we are the first ones to combine coil features with coil channel specific information using ensemble learning for the application of hardware failure prediction. For further research, the method should be expanded to different coil types and even larger data sets. As this approach is planned to be integrated into the Quality Assurance procedure, a next step is to also incorporate a feedback loop from technicians validating the model's prediction for self-learning improvement.

Fig. 1. Average prediction scores for the two base classifiers FCN and CNN2 next to FCN aggregated per coil and the stacked meta learner.

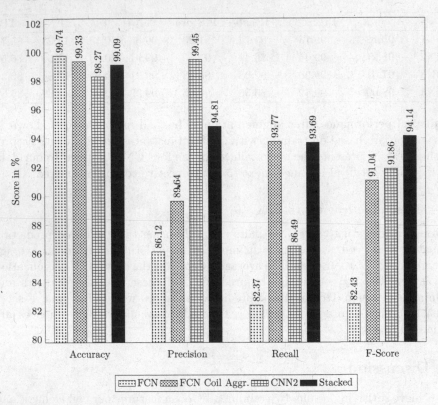

References

1. Maier A, Steidl S, Christlein V, et al. Medical imaging systems: an introductory guide. vol. 11111. Springer; 2018.
2. Witten IH, Frank E, Hall MA, et al. Data mining, fourth edition: practical machine learning tools and techniques. 4th ed. San Francisco, CA, USA: Morgan Kaufmann Publishers Inc.; 2016.
3. Maier A, Syben C, Lasser T, et al. A gentle introduction to deep learning in medical image processing. Zeitschrift für Medizinische Physik. 2019;29(2):86–101.
4. Kuhnert N, Lindenmayr O, Maier A. Classification of body regions based on MRI log files. In: Proc ICCRS. Springer; 2017. p. 102–109.
5. Breiman L. Random forests. Mach Learn. 2001;45(1):5–32.
6. Wolpert DH. Stacked generalization. Neural Netw. 1992;5:241–259.
7. Chigurupati A, Thibaux R, Lassar N. Predicting hardware failure using machine learning. In: Proc RAMS; 2016. p. 1–6.
8. Jain B, Kuhnert N, deOliveira A, et al. Image-based detection of MRI hardware failures. In: Proc BVM. Springer; 2019. p. 206–211.

Abstract: Estimation of the Principal Ischaemic Stroke Growth Directions for Predicting Tissue Outcomes

Christian Lucas[1], Linda F. Aulmann[2], André Kemmling[3],
Amir Madany Mamlouk[4], Mattias P. Heinrich[1]

[1]Institute of Medical Informatics, University of Lübeck, Lübeck
[2]Department of Neuroradiology, University Hospital UKSH, Lübeck
[3]Department of Neuroradiology, Westpfalz Hospital, Kaiserslautern
[4]Institute for Neuro- and Bioinformatics, University of Lübeck, Lübeck
lucas@imi.uni-luebeck.de

The estimates of traditional segmentation CNNs for the prediction of the follow-up tissue outcome in strokes are not yet accurate enough or capable of properly modeling the growth mechanisms of ischaemic stroke [1]. In our previous shape space interpolation approach [2], the prediction of the follow-up lesion shape has been bounded using core and penumbra segmentation estimates as priors. One of the challenges is to define well-suited growth constraints, as the transition from one to another shape may still result in a very unrealistic spatial evolution of the stroke. In this work, we address this shortcoming by explicitly incorporating vector fields for the spatial growth of the infarcted area. Since the anatomy of the cerebrovascular system defines the blood flow along brain arteries, we hypothesise that we can reasonably regularise the direction and strength of growth using a lesion deformation model. We show that a Principal Component Analysis (PCA) model computed from the diffeomorphic displacements between a core lesion approximation and the entire tissue-at-risk can be used to estimate follow-up lesions (0.74 F1 score) for a well-defined growth problem with accurate input data better than with the shape model (0.62 F1 score) by predicting the PCA coefficients through a CNN [3].

References

1. Winzeck S, Hakim A, McKinley R, et al. ISLES 2016 and 2017-benchmarking ischemic stroke lesion outcome prediction based on multispectral MRI. Front Neurol. 2018;9:679.
2. Lucas C, Kemmling A, Bouteldja N, et al. Learning to predict ischemic stroke growth on acute CT perfusion data by interpolating low-dimensional shape representations. Front Neurol. 2018;9:989.
3. Lucas C, Aulmann LF, Kemmling A, et al. Estimation of the principal ischaemic stroke growth directions for predicting tissue outcomes. MICCAI BrainLes. 2019;.

© Springer Fachmedien Wiesbaden GmbH, ein Teil von Springer Nature 2020
T. Tolxdorff et al. (Hrsg.), *Bildverarbeitung für die Medizin 2020*,
Informatik aktuell, https://doi.org/10.1007/978-3-658-29267-6_29

Assistive Diagnosis in Opthalmology Using Deep Learning-Based Image Retrieval

Azeem Bootwala[1], Katharina Breininger[1], Andreas Maier[1], Vincent Christlein[1]

[1]Pattern Recognition Lab, Friedrich-Alexander-Universität Erlangen-Nürnberg
azeem.bootwala@fau.de

Abstract. Image-based diagnosis of the human eye is crucial for the early detection of several diseases in ophthalmology. In this work, we investigate the possibility to use image retrieval to support the diagnosis of diabetic retinopathy. To this end, we evaluate different feature learning techniques. In particular, we evaluate the performance of cost functions specialized for metric learning, namely, contrastive loss, triplet loss and histogram loss, and compare them with the classification cross-entropy loss. Additionally, we train the network on images graded by diabetic retinopathy severity and transfer the knowledge learned, to retrieve images that are graded by diabetic macular edema severity and evaluate our algorithm on three different datasets. For the task of detecting referable/non-referable diabetic retinopathy, we achieve a sensitivity of 0.84 and specificity of 0.88 on the Kaggle dataset using histogram loss. On the Messidor dataset, we achieve a sensitivity and specificity score of 0.79 and 0.84, respectively.

1 Introduction

About 422 million people worldwide suffered from diabetes mellitus in 2014 [1]. As one of its side effect, diabetes mellitus can damage blood vessels in the retina and cause diabetic retinopathy (DR), one of the leading causes of blindness. Seven percent of people suffering from diabetes also suffer from vision-threatening retinopathy [1]. Early detection of changes in retinal vessels can help to reduce such severe consequences. For a medical expert, grading of diabetic retinopathy is time-consuming and strenuous. The accurate interpretation of fundus images depends on experience and meticulousness of the rater.

Lately, deep learning has been successfully incorporated into facial recognition and verification tasks [2]. A similar system has been used to obtain similarity rankings and allows for content-based image retrieval [3]. To this end, a convolutional neural network is employed that acts as a hierarchical feature extractor. An appropriate cost function forces the network to extract features that are close to each other for images from the same category, but further apart for images from different categories. While the performance of such cost functions [4, 2, 5] is well evaluated on common multimedia benchmark datasets, their outcomes on

© Springer Fachmedien Wiesbaden GmbH, ein Teil von Springer Nature 2020

T. Tolxdorff et al. (Hrsg.), *Bildverarbeitung für die Medizin 2020*,
Informatik aktuell, https://doi.org/10.1007/978-3-658-29267-6_30

Fig. 1. Example images from the Kaggle diabetic retinopathy dataset.

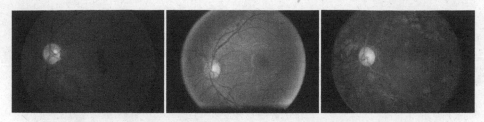

medical image data require further investigation. To reduce the variability and workload of human interpretation, image analysis systems have been developed that can support medical experts in diagnosis and grading of DR [6], where deep learning is used for classification.

In contrast, we propose a method for image retrieval for retinal images that can both support training of medical experts and diagnosis. A system that provides labeled references with similar appearance for an unclassified image may help in case of difficult pathologies. The main contributions are as follows: (1) We perform a comparative evaluation of different loss functions. In particular, we evaluate contrastive [4], triplet [2] and histogram [5] loss, when training a feature extraction network (VGG-19) from scratch. (2) We show how these loss functions compare to the classical softmax cross-entropy loss for the task of image retrieval. (3) We demonstrate that the learned network parameters can be adapted to other disease types without retraining. To achieve this, we evaluate the performance of the network on images graded by the severity of diabetic macular edema (DME).

2   Materials and methods

2.1   Datasets

We use three datasets in our evaluation where each dataset represents a different population. The kaggle diabetic retinopathy dataset [7] consists of 88,702 high-resolution retinal images. Each image is graded depending on the severity of diabetic retinopathy on a scale from 0 (no DR) to 4 (proliferative DR). Fig. 1 shows examples from this dataset. The dataset contains a variety of images with different illuminations, color characteristics, and pathologies.

Two additional datasets are taken as a basis for evaluation, the Messidor database [8][1], which consists of 1200 color fundus eye images, and the Indian diabetic retinopathy dataset [9] with 516 images. Both datasets provide DR labels with the same 5-step grading. Additionally, they provide labels for diabetic macular edema severity, with three grading steps.

---

[1] Kindly provided by the Messidor program partners (http://www.adcis.net/en/third-party/messidor/).

2.2 Preprocessing

The original images are preprocessed using border removal, local average color subtraction, and hue normalization by setting the background to gray. We then resize the original images to 400×400 pixels. We normalize the images to zero mean and unit variance based on the training set.

2.3 Network architecture and training

We use VGG-19 [10] as base architecture, but replace the last fully-connected layer after the final convolutional layer with an additional layer with 128 nodes.

Networks trained with contrastive, triplet, and histogram loss use multiple samples at a time according to the loss functions (see definitions below) to maximize the difference between embeddings extracted from images of different classes and minimize the difference of embeddings of the same class. For the standard cross-entropy loss, a fully-connected layer with softmax activation is added to differentiate between the five different classes during training. During inference, this layer is removed and the output of the 128-dimensional layer is used to obtain the embedding used for image retrieval. For all losses, the final layer is normalized by its ℓ^2 norm before training with the respective loss. In order to counter the class imbalance of the datasets, we oversample the minority class by applying data augmentation using random image transformations, such as rotation, horizontal and vertical flipping, and Gaussian blurring.

During inference, the 128-dimensional activation vector of the final layer serves as the image representation. Given a query representation, we conduct a nearest neighbor search using the Euclidean distance to find the K closest images in the dataset.

2.4 Loss functions

2.4.1 Contrastive loss The contrastive loss function [4] only requires neighbourhood relationships between images and is defined as

$$L(\boldsymbol{\theta}, \mathcal{D}) = \sum_{\{\boldsymbol{x}_i, \boldsymbol{x}_j\} \in \mathcal{D}} (1 - y_{i,j}) \frac{1}{2} d(\boldsymbol{x}_i, \boldsymbol{x}_j)^2 + y_{i,j} \frac{1}{2} \{\max\left(0, m - d(\boldsymbol{x}_i, \boldsymbol{x}_j)\right)\}^2 \quad (1)$$

where $\mathcal{D}$ denotes the set of all embedding tuples, i.e., all possible combinations of image embeddings; $d(\boldsymbol{x}_i, \boldsymbol{x}_j)$ is the Euclidean distance between the pair of inputs, while $y_{i,j}$ is 1 if they belong to the same class and 0 otherwise. Dissimilar pairs can only have a maximum distance of m (the margin) to contribute to the loss.

2.4.2 Triplet loss The triplet loss [2] requires triplets of three images to learn for the loss computation. A triplet consists of the embedding of an anchor image $\boldsymbol{x}_a$, a positive image $\boldsymbol{x}_p$, i.e., from the same class, and a negative image

Table 1. Sensitivity, Specificity, κ for binary retrieval, and MP and MRR for multi-class retrieval.

Dataset	Loss	Sens.	Spec.	κ	MP	MRR
Kaggle	Cross-entropy	0.62	0.83	0.46	-	-
	Contrastive	**0.86**	0.85	0.72	**0.51**	**0.66**
	Triplet	0.84	0.83	0.68	0.49	0.64
	Histogram	0.84	**0.88**	**0.74**	0.50	0.65
Messidor	Cross-entropy	0.54	0.76	0.31	-	-
	Contrastive	**0.82**	0.81	**0.63**	**0.56**	0.70
	Triplet	0.80	0.79	0.60	0.55	**0.72**
	Histogram	0.79	**0.84**	**0.63**	0.52	0.69
IDRiD	Cross-entropy	0.78	0.77	0.54	-	-
	Contrastive	**0.91**	0.82	0.75	0.57	**0.72**
	Triplet	0.90	0.82	0.71	0.58	0.71
	Histogram	**0.91**	**0.85**	**0.76**	**0.59**	0.71

x_n comming from a different class. Then the triplet loss over the set of possible triplets $\mathcal{T}$ of the training set is defined as

$$L(\boldsymbol{\theta}, \mathcal{T}) = \sum_{\{\boldsymbol{x}_a, \boldsymbol{x}_b, \boldsymbol{x}_p\} \in \mathcal{T}} \max\left(0, d(\boldsymbol{x}_a, \boldsymbol{x}_p) + m - d(\boldsymbol{x}_a, \boldsymbol{x}_n)\right) \qquad (2)$$

2.4.3 Histogram loss In contrast to contrastive and triplet loss, histogram loss [5] does not rely on any margin value. It computes two distributions of similarities of positive (matching) and negative (non-matching) pairs and computes the probability of a positive pair to have lower similarity score than a negative pair [5]. The final loss is given by

$$L_{\text{histogram}}(\boldsymbol{\theta}, \mathcal{X}) = \sum_{r=1}^{R} h_r^- \Phi_r^+ \qquad (3)$$

where $L(\boldsymbol{\theta})$ is the loss function computed on a batch of images $\mathcal{X}$, R is the number of histogram bins, h_r^- is the histogram of negative distances. Φ^+ is the cumulative density function computed from the histogram of positive distances h^+.

3 Results

Assessment of diabetic retinopathy can be done as a binary classification problem, i. e., non-referable (healthy and mild) and referable (moderate, severe, proliferative). During inference, the class frequency was set to 50 % for referable and non-referable DR in the binary retrieval problem. Balancing the datasets during evaluation is important as image retrieval favours the class with more instances

Table 2. Multi-class retrieval performance on the kaggle dataset.

Metric	Loss	Healthy	Mild	Moderate	Severe	Proliferative
	Contrastive	**0.67**	0.40	0.32	**0.55**	0.60
MP	Triplet	0.60	**0.44**	0.34	0.51	0.55
	Histogram	0.57	0.38	**0.36**	0.53	**0.63**
	Contrastive	**0.81**	0.57	0.50	**0.69**	0.70
MRR	Triplet	0.72	**0.59**	0.55	0.66	0.65
	Histogram	0.70	0.57	**0.56**	**0.69**	**0.73**

Table 3. Performance of image retrieval for DME on Messidor and IDRiD datasets, network trained with contrastive loss.

Metric	Messidor			IDRiD		
	Grade 0	Grade 1	Grade 2	Grade 0	Grade 1	Grade 2
MP	0.70	0.46	0.54	0.70	0.46	0.62
MRR	0.78	0.69	0.76	0.80	0.78	0.83

in the dataset. We also assess our model by their average retrieval capacity on a 5-point scale, since there are five classes (healthy, mild, moderate, severe, proliferative). For multi-class retrieval assessment the class frequency is set to 20 % per class. We use sensitivity, specificity and Cohen's kappa (κ) metric for binary retrieval while mean precision (MP) and mean reciprocal rank (MRR) were used for multi-class retrieval. MRR is defined as the average reciprocal rank of the first relevant image. All metrics are computed on the first ten retrieved images. We divide the kaggle dataset into 80 % training, 10 % validation and 10 % test set. Messidor and IDRiD datasets are used entirely for evaluation. The results for the binary and multi-class retrieval task are presented in Tab. 1 and Tab. 2. In Fig. 2, we show an image overlaid with a class activation map.

An important advantage of training a few-shot learning algorithm is that the training is not specific to a particular disease type. Instead, the network learns a similarity mapping that applies to all pathologies and data that share similar features. Without retraining the network for this task, we evaluate the

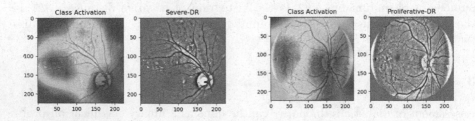

Fig. 2. Class activation maps: The class activation map is overlaid on the input image on Messidor dataset as a heat map. Red areas indicate parts of the image the network considers essential for retrieval.

performance of image retrieval for DME severity on the Messidor and IDRiD datasets. The class frequency of each class was set to 33 %. Tab. 3 presents the evaluation of image retrieval on Messidor and IDRiD DME datasets.

4   Discussion

Our results show that loss functions specialized for metric learning perform better than cross-entropy loss and retrieve more relevant images. Out of these three, there is no clear winner, however, contrastive and histogram loss perform slightly better compared to triplet loss. When looking at the multi-class task, we observe a higher performance for grade 0 and grade 4 compared to the in-between classes. This may be due to the gradual changes that occur in these diseases and hinder a clear discrimination. The heat maps indicate that the network focuses on disease relevant regions with microaneurysms and hemoraging. The performance on the DME task demonstrates that the networks trained with contrastive, triplet and histogram loss are task agnostic and can be easily applied to similar tasks without the need of retraining. Our results indicate significant potential of image retrieval for diagnosis of eye diseases, and future work will focus on investigating the clinical applicability.

References

1. World Health Organization. Global report on diabetes; 2016.
2. Schroff F, Kalenichenko D, Philbin J. FaceNet: a unified embedding for face recognition and clustering. In: Proc CVPR; 2015. p. 815–823.
3. Zhang X, Felix XY, Kumar S, et al. Learning spread-out local feature descriptors. In: Proc ICCV; 2017. p. 4605–4613.
4. Hadsell R, Chopra S, LeCun Y. Dimensionality reduction by learning an invariant mapping. In: Proc CVPR. vol. 2; 2006. p. 1735–1742.
5. Ustinova E, Lempitsky V. Learning deep embeddings with histogram loss. In: Proc NIPS; 2016. p. 4170–4178.
6. Krause J, Gulshan V, Rahimy E, et al. Grader variability and the importance of reference standards for evaluating machine learning models for diabetic retinopathy. Ophthalmology. 2018 Aug;125(8):1264–1272.
7. EyePACS. Diabetic retinopathy detection;. Accessed: 2019-11-1. https://www.kaggle.com/c/diabetic-retinopathy-detection.
8. Decencière E, Zhang X, Cazuguel G, et al. Feedback on a publicly distributed database: the messidor database. Image Anal & Stereology. 2014 Aug;33(3):231–234.
9. Porwal P, Pachade S, Kamble R, et al. Indian diabetic retinopathy image dataset (IDRiD): a database for diabetic retinopathy screening research. Data. 2018;3(3).
10. Simonyan K, Zisserman A. Very deep convolutional networks for large-scale image recognition. arXiv e-prints. 2014; p. arXiv:1409.1556.

Multitask-Learning for the Extraction of Avascular Necrosis of the Femoral Head in MRI

Duc Duy Pham[1], Gurbandurdy Dovletov[1], Sebastian Serong[2],
Stefan Landgraeber[2], Marcus Jäger[3,4], Josef Pauli[1]

[1]Intelligent Systems, Faculty of Engineering, University of Duisburg-Essen, Germany
[2]Department of Orthopedics and Orthopedic Surgery,
Saarland University Medical Center, Germany
[3] Department of Orthopedics, Trauma and Recontructive Surgery, St. Marien Hospital Mülheim
[4] Chair of Orthopaedics and Trauma Surgery, University Hospital Essen, Germany
duc.duy.pham@uni-due.de

Abstract. In this paper, we present a 2D deep multitask learning approach for the segmentation of small structures on the example of avascular necrosis of the femoral head (AVNFH) in MRI. It consists of one joint encoder and three separate decoder branches, each assigned to its own objective. We propose using a reconstruction task to initially pre-train the encoder and shift the objective towards a second necrosis segmentation task in a reconstruction-dependent loss adaptation manner. The third branch deals with the rough localization of the topographical neighborhood of possible femoral necrosis areas. Its output is used to emphasize the roughly approximated location of the segmentation branch's output. The evaluation of the segmentation performance of our architecture on coronal T1-weighted MRI volumes shows promising improvements compared to a standard U-Net implementation.

1 Introduction

Necrosis is a disease process of non-programmed premature cell death. In case of the hip joint, various causes can lead to avascular necrosis of the femoral head (AVNFH), such as a disruption of the blood supply by means of traumatic injuries, physical obstructions or metabolic issues. A collapse of the femoral head can lead to functional damage of the hip joint [1]. A precise assessment of the necrotic area helps in operative planning and may prevent unnecessary total endoprosthesis (TEP). Since manual segmentation is expensive and time consuming, there is a high demand for computerized fully automated methods. AVNFH presents large variability in its shape and appearance, which makes the segmentation a challenging problem. Zoroofi et al. [2] present a semi-automated necrosis segmentation pipeline of traditional image processing methods, using histogram based thresholding in a region of interest (ROI) and ellipse fitting in

© Springer Fachmedien Wiesbaden GmbH, ein Teil von Springer Nature 2020
T. Tolxdorff et al. (Hrsg.), *Bildverarbeitung für die Medizin 2020*,
Informatik aktuell, https://doi.org/10.1007/978-3-658-29267-6_31

oblique slices, which are set to be perpendicular to the femoral collum. Similar approaches, that also estimate the ROI beforehand, can be observed for other segmentation tasks, which deal with the extraction of small structures. For the segmentation of brain lesions Song et al. [3] use a two-stage strategy in first approximating the ROI by means of thresholding and GrowCut, in order to use a random forest classifier afterwards for pixelwise classification. As deep learning methods have become a preferred strategy for segmentation, the use of multi-stage approaches can also be observed in these techniques. For the extraction of liver lesions both Christ et al. [4] and Vorontsov et al.[5] essentially segment the liver first, in order to find the lesions afterwards. Hatamizadeh et al. [6] combine the output of a Convolutional Neural Network with an extended Level Set method for the refinement of the initial lesion segmentation. In this paper, we investigate, how well Ronneberger et al.'s widely used U-Net [7] deals in segmenting rather small structures in large MRI volumes, and propose an alternative deep 3-branch multitask fully convolutional architecture.

2   Materials and methods

2.1   Deep 3-branch multitask fully convolutional architecture

In multitask learning several tasks are addressed simultaneously in order to leverage common properties across related tasks. In our deep learning setting, we use a joint convolutional encoder, followed by three task-specific convolutional decoder branches. The main objective is represented by the segmenter branch, that aims at segmenting the femoral necrotic area. We denote y_{seg} as the output of the segmenter branch. We define an auxiliary task of reconstructing the input from a latent representation by means of an autoencoder branch. The idea is to particularly enforce a compact latent representation of the necrotic area, from which the autoencoder branch can reconstruct it. Motivated by Erhan et al's [8]

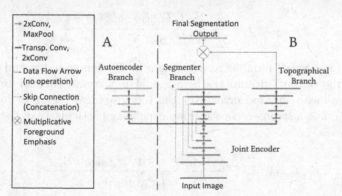

Fig. 1. Multitask architecture consisting of joint encoder and 3 different decoder branches. For the final segmentation the segmenter branch is fused with the topographical branch (side B). The autoencoder output is omitted for inference (side A).

work on unsupervised pre-training, we aim at regularizing the learning process by this auxiliary task on the fly. In contrast to Wiehman et al.'s [9] approach, the branching point of our method is in latent space, whereas Wiehman et al. add their reconstruction task in their final layer. The result of this branch is depicted as y_{auto}. We introduce an additional task of approximating the location of the topographical neighborhood of the femoral necrosis. The idea is to learn features that are activated by inter-patient consistent anatomical structures within that location, e.g. the femoral head. The output of this topographical branch is denoted as y_{topo}. As shown in Fig. 1, we use skip connections between the joint encoder and the segmenter branch to improve the fine pixel localization capabilities of this decoder. We do not use any skip connections for the topographical branch, since the rough topographical approximation of the surroundings does not need any high-resolution information. The autoencoder branch does not receive any skip connections, either, as these would allow the decoder to copy the relevant information for the image reconstruction task from the high-resolution encoder layers. In both cases we intend to enforce the necessity to compress the input image into a compact representation in latent space. For the final segmentation, the foreground output of the topographical branch is multiplied with the segmenter branch output to emphasize on this topographical neighborhood, i.e. $y_{final}^{fg} := y_{topo}^{fg} \otimes y_{seg}^{fg}$, where $\otimes$ denotes the Hadamard product and $y_{(\cdot)}^{fg}$ the foreground (necrosis) channel(s) of the output $y_{(\cdot)}$. The background channel of the final output is adjusted to $y_{final}^{bg} := 1 - y_{final}^{fg}$, such that $y_{final}^{bg}, y_{final}^{fg} \in [0,1]$. Leaving out any superscript annotation denotes using all channels.

2.2 Training

Since the necrotic area only consists of a small fraction of the whole image, it is essential to only consider the foreground channel of the segmentation output for the DSC loss of the segmenter branch, i.e.

$$\mathcal{L}_{\text{seg}} := 1 - \frac{2 \cdot \sum_p GT_{seg}^{fg}(p) \cdot y_{\text{seg}}^{fg}(p) + \epsilon}{\sum_p GT_{seg}^{fg}(p) + \sum_p y_{\text{seg}}^{fg}(p) + \epsilon} \tag{1}$$

where $\epsilon > 0$ is a small number to avoid zero in the denominator and p depicts a point in the output/ground truth image. For the autoencoder branch, we calculate the mean squared error over the topographical region of interest, as we aim to enforce a strong reconstruction capability particularly in the probable area of necrosis, i.e.

$$\mathcal{L}_{\text{auto}} := \frac{\sum_p GT_{topo}^{fg}(p) \cdot (x(p) - y_{auto}(p))^2}{\sum_p GT_{topo}^{fg}(p) + \epsilon} \tag{2}$$

where x denotes the input image. The autoencoder and segmenter branches' loss functions are combined to a reconstruction-dependent loss function

$$\mathcal{L}_{\text{seg,auto}} := \alpha \mathcal{L}_{\text{auto}} + (1 - \alpha)\mathcal{L}_{\text{seg}} \tag{3}$$

where $\alpha \in [0,1]$ is a weighing factor, set to $\alpha := \mathcal{L}_{\text{auto}}$, as proposed by our previous work [10]. It should be noted that when taking the gradient of $\mathcal{L}_{\text{seg,auto}}$ during training, the autoencoder branch within α is not considered in our implementation. The adaptive weighting scheme encourages the joint encoder to pre-generate features and a latent representation for image reconstruction before focusing on the segmentation task.

To train the topographical branch, we need to generate a ground truth for the desired neighborhood. For this, we relax the original ground truth necrosis segmentation (GT_{seg}) to squared environments around the necrotic area with an empirical width of a third of the input image. Since we desire a necrosis-independent localization, we mirror each box along the vertical axis, as can be seen in Fig. 2(e). The overlay of ground truths from both sides is particularly visible in the stepped upper and lower bounding lines. We use this relaxed ground truth (GT_{topo}) to train the topographical branch by means of a DSC loss function $\mathcal{L}_{\text{topo}}$. The topographical branch is trained separately with its own optimizer. Therefore, we propose using two optimizers in an alternating fashion, starting with the topographical branch. In both cases we use an Adam optimizer with initial learning rate of 10^{-3}. It should be noted, that we only need the autoencoder branch for training, leaving its result out during inference, as indicated in Fig.1 by the separation line between side A and B.

2.3 Evaluation

We evaluated the proposed architecture on our inhouse T1-weighted coronal MRI data sets, consisting of twelve patients, each comprising 19 to 30 slices. We compared our results to a standard U-Net implementation. For training and inference we resized the MRI slices to an input size of 512×512 and normalized the intensity range to $[-1,1]$. In a leave-one-out cross validation manner, we kept one patient volume for testing and trained the networks with the remaining patient volumes. The coronal slices of an arbitrary patient volume were used as validation data to monitor the training process. We applied data augmentation by means of flipping, rotation and translation. For the evaluation, our 2D segmentation outputs are stacked to 3D segmentations and compared to the desired 3D ground truths. We choose Dice Similarity Coefficient (DSC), Precision, and Recall as quality metrics. In our experiments we differentiate between AVNFH on the right and left femur.

3 Results

The achieved mean DSC, precision and recall values are depicted in table 1. The standard U-Net achieves a mean DSC of 32.5% on the right and 34.1% on the left femur. Our proposed 3-Branch Multitask Fully Convolutional Network (3B-MT-FCN) on the other hand results in higher mean DSCs of 37.1% and 38.9%, respectively. This is reflected in the average precision values, i.e. 47.4% and 21.4% by the U-Net compared to 56.8% and 21.4%, achieved by

Table 1. Mean DSC, precision and recall from a standard U-Net compared to the proposed architecture.

mean DSC [%]	Necrosis on right femur	Necrosis on left femur
U-Net	0.325 ± 0.253	0.341 ± 0.396
3B-MT-FCN	0.371 ± 0.268	0.389 ± 0.442
mean Precision [%]		
U-Net	0.474 ± 0.337	0.214 ± 0.309
3B-MT-FCN	0.568 ± 0.375	0.214 ± 0.330
mean Recall [%]		
U-Net	0.347 ± 0.282	0.151 ± 0.234
3B-MT-FCN	0.335 ± 0.237	0.119 ± 0.230

3B-MT-FCN. Regarding mean recall the U-Net implementation yields slightly higher values with 34.7% and 15.1% for the U-Net and 33.5% and 11.9% for 3B-MT-FCN.

4   Discussion

From the results we can conclude that our proposed 3B-MT-FCN yields better segmentation results than the U-Net baseline. While its mean recall values for AVNFH are slightly lower, its higher mean precision is an indicator for fewer false positive predictions. Therefore U-Net appears to be more prone to dilated segmentations. This can be observed in the exemplary comparison of segmentation outputs in Fig. 2(b) and (d). It is noticable that the segmenter branch output (Fig. 2(c)) yields contours, that are closer to the boundaries of the necrotic area, but it also contains some outlier segmentations. This may be due to the spatial restriction of the reconstruction loss to the surrounding neighborhood in Eq.2, which leads to arbitrarily high values in irrelevant locations at the image boundaries. This is corrected in the final segmentation (Fig. 2(d)) by the multiplicative foreground emphasis by means of the topographical branch's output. This yields a segmentation result for small structures, that is less prone to di-

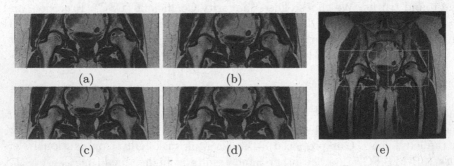

Fig. 2. Exemplary (cropped) coronal MRI slice with overlayed (a) ground truth, (b) U-Net output, (c) segmenter branch output, (d) final output, (e) relaxed ground truth

lated convolutions than a standard U-Net implementation. Although we make use of this property, a drawback is, however, the assumption, that the necrotic area is surrounded by inter-patient consistent anatomical structures, such as the femoral head. It is also noticeable that the DSC scores are rather low for all approaches. This may be due to the fact, that the foreground area of the ground truth is very small compared to the whole volume. Therefore, the higher risk of false positives in all approaches may negatively impact the dice scores.

4.1 Conclusion

In this work we present a 2D multitask deep learning architecture for the segmentation of small structures, such as AVNFH. We leverage the reconstruction property of autoencoders and define a topographical localization objective to improve the main task of segmenting AVNFH, and during training we apply a reconstruction-dependent adaptation scheme. In our evaluation we observe promising improvements compared to U-Net.

References

1. Baig SA, Baig M. Osteonecrosis of the femoral head: etiology, investigations, and management. Cureus. 2018;10(8).
2. Zoroofi RA, Nishii T, Sato Y, et al. Segmentation of avascular necrosis of the femoral head using 3-d MR images. Comput Med Imaging Graph. 2001;25(6):511–521.
3. Song B, Chou CR, Chen X, et al. Anatomy-guided brain tumor segmentation and classification. In: Brainlesion: Glioma, Multiple Sclerosis, Stroke and Traumatic Brain Injuries. Springer International Publishing; 2016. p. 162–170.
4. Christ PF, Elshaer MEA, Ettlinger F, et al. Automatic liver and lesion segmentation in CT using cascaded fully convolutional neural networks and 3d conditional random fields. In: Proc MICCAI. Springer; 2016. p. 415–423.
5. Vorontsov E, Tang A, Pal C, et al. Liver lesion segmentation informed by joint liver segmentation. In: Proc IEEE ISBI; 2018. p. 1332–1335.
6. Hatamizadeh A, Hoogi A, Sengupta D, et al. Deep active lesion segmentation. In: Suk HI, Liu M, Yan P, et al., editors. Machine Learning in Medical Imaging. Cham: Springer International Publishing; 2019. p. 98–105.
7. Ronneberger O, Fischer P, Brox T. U-net: convolutional networks for biomedical image segmentation. In: International Conference on Medical Image Computing and Computer-Assisted Intervention. Springer; 2015. p. 234–241.
8. Erhan D, Bengio Y, Courville A, et al. Why does unsupervised pre-training help deep learning? J Mach Learn Res. 2010;11(Feb):625–660.
9. Wiehman S, Kroon S, De Villiers H. Unsupervised pre-training for fully convolutional neural networks. In: 2016 Pattern Recognition Association of South Africa and Robotics and Mechatronics International Conference (PRASA-RobMech). IEEE; 2016. p. 1–6.
10. Pham DD, Dovletov G, Warwas S, et al. Deep segmentation refinement with result-dependent learning. In: Bildverarbeitung für die Medizin 2019. Wiesbaden: Springer Fachmedien Wiesbaden; 2019. p. 49–54.

Investigation of Feature-Based Nonrigid Image Registration Using Gaussian Process

Siming Bayer[1,*], Ute Spiske[1,*], Jie Luo[2], Tobias Geimer[1],
William M. Wells III[2], Martin Ostermeier[3], Rebecca Fahrig[3], Arya Nabavi[4],
Christoph Bert[5], Ilker Eyüpoglo[6], Andreas Maier[1]

[1]Pattern Recognition Lab, FAU Erlangen-Nürnberg
[2]Brigham and Women's Hospital, Harvard Medical School
[3]Advanced Therapies, Siemens Healthare GmbH, Forchheim
[4]Department of Neurosurgery, KRH Klinikum Nordstadt, Hannover
[5]Department of Radiation Therapy, Universität Klinikum Erlangen, Erlangen
[6]Department of Neurosurgery, Univerisät Klinikum Erlangen, Erlangen
*These authors contributed equally and are listed in alphabetical order
siming.bayer@fau.de

Abstract. For a wide range of clinical applications, such as adaptive treatment planning or intraoperative image update, feature-based deformable registration (FDR) approaches are widely employed because of their simplicity and low computational complexity. FDR algorithms estimate a dense displacement field by interpolating a sparse field, which is given by the established correspondence between selected features. In this paper, we consider the deformation field as a Gaussian Process (GP), whereas the selected features are regarded as prior information on the valid deformations. Using GP, we are able to estimate the both dense displacement field and a corresponding uncertainty map at once. Furthermore, we evaluated the performance of different hyperparameter settings for squared exponential kernels with synthetic, phantom and clinical data respectively. The quantitative comparison shows, GP-based interpolation has performance on par with state-of-the-art B-spline interpolation. The greatest clinical benefit of GP-based interpolation is that it gives a reliable estimate of the mathematical uncertainty of the calculated dense displacement map.

1 Introduction

For many clinical applications, nonrigid image registration is a key enabling technique. Compared to intensity-based deformable registration approaches, feature-based methods are intuitive and have low computational cost. Furthermore, human interactions, such as manual adjustment of landmarks, can be integrated easily. Basically, feature-based deformable registration methods estimate the suitable dense deformation field between two images by interpolating

© Springer Fachmedien Wiesbaden GmbH, ein Teil von Springer Nature 2020
T. Tolxdorff et al. (Hrsg.), *Bildverarbeitung für die Medizin 2020*,
Informatik aktuell, https://doi.org/10.1007/978-3-658-29267-6_32

the correspondence of sparse feature sets.An explicit interpolation step is therefore necessary to propagate the information from the control points to the whole image space. Hence, the choice of the interpolation technique and its underlying deformation model affects the overall performance of the registration method greatly.

One of the state-of-the-art interpolation technique is B-Spline interpolation [1]. It has been widely employed for various clinical applications such as registration of breast MR images [1] or intraoperative brain shift compensation [2]. Thin-Plate-Splines (TPS) proposed in [3] are another common choice for deformable image warping, and has been applied e. g. for 3D-3D [4] registration of vasculature.

Gaussian Process (GP) introduced in [5] is a powerful tool to resolve regression, classification, and interpolation problems. The major advantage of Gaussian Process is the capability to estimate the result and its own uncertainty at once. Therefore, it has been applied in a wide variety of disciplines. However, in medical image processing its applications to date are limited. Recently, [6] presented a generative model for intensity-based rigid registration with Gaussian processes, dealing with the interpolation uncertainty of the resampling step. A feature-based semi-automatic registration framework using Gaussian Process interpolation for the estimation of the dense displacement field has been proposed in [7]. Although those works indicate the general applicability of GP for medical image registration, a comparison between GP and state-of-the-art image interpolation techniques and a comprehensive performance analysis is still missing.

We present a first investigation of the performance of GP for feature-based deformable registration, including comparison with B-Spline interpolation and analysis of hyperparameter setting. To this end, correspondence of selected features are established using the method proposed in [2] and [8]. Subsequently, GP with squared exponential kernel is employed to interpolate the sparse deformation field to a dense one and to estimate an associated uncertainty map. Furthermore, we compare three different approaches for the hyperparameter tuning. Finally, experiments with synthetic, phantom and clinical data for two clinical applications, namely intraoperative brain shift compensation and adaptive treatment planning for multi-catheter brachytherapy [8] are conducted for the performance analysis.

2   Materials and method

The goal of image registration is to find a optimal transformation $\mathcal{T}$ maps the source image $\mathbf{I}_s$ to the target image $\mathbf{I}_t$. For the sake of simplicity, we only consider the case where $\mathbf{I}_s$ and $\mathbf{I}_t$ have the same dimensionality $\mathbb{R}^d$. The transformation $\mathcal{T}_{deformable}$ that maps $\mathbf{I}_s$ and $\mathbf{I}_t$ in a nonrigid fashion is a dense displacement field $\mathbf{V} = \{\mathbf{v}_i \in \mathbb{R}^d, i = 1 : N\}$ with N denotes the size of $\mathbf{I}_s$.

2.1   Feature extraction and feature matching

Prior to the estimation of the dense deformation field, two sets of sparse features $\mathbf{P} = \{\mathbf{x}_i^s \in \mathbb{R}^d, i = 1 : N_s\}$ and $\mathbf{Q} = \{\mathbf{y}_i \in \mathbb{R}^d, i = 1 : N_t\}$ with N_s and N_t features are selected from $\mathbf{I}_s$ and the target $\mathbf{I}_t$, respectively. In the feature matching step, the source feature set $\mathbf{P}$ is updated to a corresponding set $\tilde{\mathbf{P}} = \{\tilde{\mathbf{x}}_i \in \mathbb{R}^d, i = 1 : N_s\}$, which is aligned with $\mathbf{Q}$. Consequently, a sparse displacement field maps the sparse feature sets $\mathbf{P}$ to $\mathbf{Q}$ is straightforwardly obtained as $\mathbf{D} = \{\mathbf{d}_i = \tilde{\mathbf{x}}_i - \mathbf{x}_i, i = 1 : N_s\}$.

2.2   Estimation of dense deformation field and uncertainty map

In order to interpolate $\mathbf{V}$ from $\mathbf{D}$, we consider the location of each voxel $\mathbf{x}_i$ in $\mathbf{V}$ as a multivariate Gaussian random variable. Each vector of the sparse displacement field $\mathbf{d}_i = \mathbf{d}(\mathbf{x}_i)$ for the voxel at the location $\mathbf{x}_i$ is treated as an observation of $\mathbf{V}$. According to the definition of GP provided in [5], the prior distribution of the spatial position $\mathbf{x}_i$ is given as $\mathbf{d}(\mathbf{x}_i) \sim \mathrm{GP}(\mathrm{m}(\mathbf{x}_i), \mathrm{k}(\mathbf{x}_i, \mathbf{x}_j))$. Hereby, $\mathrm{m}(\mathbf{x}_i) = 0$ is the mean function. The spatial correlation of the displacement vectors at the positions $\mathbf{x}_i$ and $\mathbf{x}_j$ is represented by the GP kernel $\mathrm{k}(\mathbf{x}_i, \mathbf{x}_j)$.

Following the GP modeling assumption, that the functions of all $\mathbf{x}_i$ in a set of random variables $\mathbf{X}$ are jointly Gaussian distributed, the dense displacement field can be formulated as a normal distribution $\mathrm{p}(\mathbf{V} \mid \mathbf{X}) = \mathcal{N}(\mathbf{V} \mid \boldsymbol{\mu}, \mathbf{K})$, with mean $\boldsymbol{\mu} = (\mathrm{m}(\mathbf{x}_1), \ldots, \mathrm{m}(\mathbf{x}_N))$, and covariance $\mathbf{K} = \{K_{ij} = \mathrm{k}(\mathbf{x}_i, \mathbf{x}_j)\}$. Consequently, the relationship between the $N_* = N - N_s$ unknown displacements $\mathbf{d}_*$ at the positions $\mathbf{X}_*$ and the N_s known deformation vectors $\mathbf{d}$ at the locations $\mathbf{X}$ can be expressed as the Equation. 1, where $\mathbf{K} = \mathrm{k}(\mathbf{X}, \mathbf{X})$, $\mathbf{K}_* = \mathrm{k}(\mathbf{X}, \mathbf{X}_*)$, and $\mathbf{K}_{**} = \mathrm{k}(\mathbf{X}_*, \mathbf{X}_*)$ are covariance matrices with the size $N_s \times N_s$, $N_s \times N_*$ and $N_* \times N_*$ respectively

$$\begin{pmatrix} \mathbf{d} \\ \mathbf{d}_* \end{pmatrix} \sim \mathcal{N}\left(0, \begin{pmatrix} \mathbf{K} & \mathbf{K}_* \\ \mathbf{K}_*^T & \mathbf{K}_{**} \end{pmatrix}\right) \tag{1}$$

Having the observations $\mathbf{d}$, the prior GP assumption can be converted into GP posterior $p(\mathbf{d}_* \mid \mathbf{X}_*, \mathbf{X}, \mathbf{d}) = \mathcal{N}(\mathbf{d}_* \mid \boldsymbol{\mu}_*, \boldsymbol{\Sigma}_*)$ via bayesian inference, where $\boldsymbol{\mu}_* = \mathbf{K}_*^T \mathbf{K}^{-1} \mathbf{d}$. Simultaneously, an uncertainty map indicates the mathematical confidence of the estimated displacement vectors can be obtained from the diagonal entries of the covariance matrix $\boldsymbol{\Sigma}_*$, defined in Equation. 2)

$$\boldsymbol{\Sigma}_* = \mathbf{K}_{**} - \mathbf{K}_*^T \mathbf{K}^{-1} \mathbf{K}_* \tag{2}$$

2.2.1   GP kernel estimation
The zero mean assumption of GP implies, that GP is completely defined by its second-order statistics [9]. Hence, the choice of the kernel and its parameter setting are the key factors defining the behavior of the GP model. In order to preserve the smoothness of the resulting dense displacement field, we use a Squared Exponential kernel, $\mathrm{k}(x, x') =$

Table 1. Summary of the conducted quantitative experiments with synthetic, phantom, and clinical data. Clinical data has different size in the axial direction, but has the same resolution as the phantom data.

Data	Voxels	Features	Used	Image pairs	Metric
Synthetic	256^3	$[1000, 2000]$	20%	6	$\frac{No.(I_{warp} \neq I_{target})}{No.\,Voxel}$
Phantom	512^3	$[3000, 4000]$	20%	4	MHD[2]
Clinical	$512 \times 512 \times n$	$[200, 400]$	100%	6	$\frac{|\Delta HU|}{No.\,Voxel}$

$\sigma^2 exp(-\frac{\|x-x'\|^2}{2l^2})$ (also known as Gaussian kernel). The characteristic of the Squared Exponential (SE) kernel is defined by l and σ. The former is the length-scale of the random variable that controls the smoothness of the kernel, and the latter represents the relationship between output displacement vectors.

In this work, we use three different method for automatic calculation of the hyperparameters l and σ:

MEAN Initially, the standard deviation of the kernel is computed as the mean standard deviation of the sparse displacement vectors used to train the GP model. It can be expressed as $\sigma_{mean} = \text{mean}\{\sigma_{disp} := \sigma(\mathbf{D}_x), \sigma(\mathbf{D}_y), \sigma(\mathbf{D}_z)\}$. The length-scale is initialized as $l_{mean} = \{\text{mean}(\|\mathbf{x}_i - \mathbf{x}_j\|^2), i \neq j \wedge i, j = 1 : N_s, \mathbf{x} \in \mathbb{R}^d\}$.

NML Negative log marginal likelihood minimization proposed by [8]. The start parameters are estimated using the MEAN method.

DGS Use discrete grid search to optimize the hyperparamter σ and l in the following discrete space:
- $\sigma_{dgs} \in \{\min(\sigma_{disp}), \sigma_{mean}, \max(\sigma_{disp})\}$,
- $l_{dgs} \in \{\min(\|\mathbf{x}_i - \mathbf{x}_j\|^2), l_{mean}, \max(\|\mathbf{x}_i - \mathbf{x}_j\|^2), i \neq j \wedge i, j = 1 : N_s\}$

The objective function of the grid search optimization is the root mean squared error (RMSE) between the updated image I_{warp} and the target image I_{target}.

3 Results

In order to evaluate the accuracy and applicability of GP for different medical applications, we conduct quantitative experiments with synthetic data [10] and anthropomorphic phantom data [11] for intraoperative brain shift compensation. For the adaptive treatment planning for multi-catheter HDR Brachytherapy, a retrospective clinical study is conducted.

A summary of the conducted quantitative experiments is presented in Tab. 1. The vessel centerline of the synthetic data and phantom data are extracted and aligned using the framework proposed in [2]. The catheters in the clinical data are registered as described in [8]. Since the number of the homologous features differs in the three categories of experiments greatly, we randomly select 20% features from the registered vessel centerlines from the synthetic and phantom data

Fig. 1. Quantitative results of all experiments conducted. MEAN, NML and DGS are compared with B-Spline interpolation. For phantom data b), MHD of the vessel centerline extracted from the warped and target image is calculated. Average intensity difference is used as metrics for synthetic a) and clinical c) data.

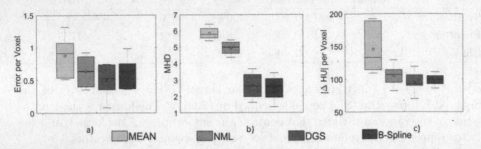

for a fair comparison. Considering the image properties [1], number of homologous features and the availability of the ground truth, we calculated modified hausdorff distance (MHD) between the extracted vessel centerlines from the warped and target image for the evaluation of phantom experiments. For the synthetic and clinical data, pro voxel intensity difference are estimated.

The performance of MEAN, NML and DGS are compared with the state-of-the-art B-Spline interpolation technique [1]. The quantitative results are presented in Fig. 1. For the qualitative inspection, overlays of the warped clinical images and their corresponding uncertainty maps are presented in Fig. 2.

4   Discussion

The quantitative results of all experiments conducted show the same trend, namely DGS and B-Spline interpolation outperforming MEAN and NML. Moreover, DGS outperforms B-Spline slightly both for synthetic and clinical data. For phantom data, DGS and B-spline show comparable results. These results indicate, that modeling nonrigid deformation as a GP with Squared Exponential kernel presents a reliable alternative to B-Spline interpolation in terms of accuracy. Additionally, the qualitative results of the cinical data presented in Fig. 2 underline our quantitative findings, namely, the result of DGS and B-Spline being comparable. The uncertainty map on Fig. 2 a), b), and c) visualize the mathematical confidence of the estimated voxel-wise displacement. Hereby, MEAN and NML tend to be overconfident about its own estimation of dense displacement, whereas DGS produces a uncertainty map with more credability. Considering both quantitative and qualitative results, a conclusion about the self-confidence of GP interpolation with Squared Exponential kernel can be drawn: with the suitable choice of hyperparameter, GP-based interpolation is comparable with B-Spline interpolation, in term of accuracy. More importantly, it produce a con-

---

[1] Synthetic data are binarized (background: 0; brain parenchyma: 255) [10], phantom data have unrealistic Hounsfield Unit (HU) value [11]

Fig. 2. Overlay of the warped clinical images and their corresponding uncertainty map (color map). The dense displacement fields are interpolated from the sparse field (established with the corresponding catheter points, i.e. the black dots on the images) using a) MEAN, b), DGS c) NML, and d) B-Spline respectively.

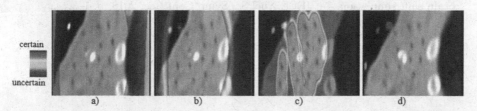

certain

uncertain

a)   b)   c)   d)

fidence map about its own estimation with high credability, which could be used as a guidance for clinicians.

In general, GP belongs to the family of non-parametric methods. For the interpolation of each unknown displacement vector, the entire set of training data is taken into account. Hence, the run time of GP depends on the size of the sparse displacement vectors and the size of the image. In contrast, B-Spline interpolation is locally controlled, which means only the number of the homologous points on a predefined mesh grid affects its computational cost. Consequently, B-Spline interpolation is suitable for time critical applications such as intraoperative brain shift compensation, whereas GP-based interpolation is an excellent candidate for applications with lower real-time requirement, such as treatment planning in radiation therapy. In the subsequent studies, a detailed run time analysis of the GP-based interpolation technique will be performed. Furthermore, qualitative studies with clinicians are planned, where the clinician will ask to give scores for different interpolation methods.

References

1. Rueckert D, Sonoda LI, Hayes C, et al. Nonrigid registration using free-form deformations: application to breast MR images. IEEE Trans Med Imaging. 1999 Aug;18(8):712-721.
2. Bayer S, Zhai Z, Strumia M, et al. Registration of vascular structures using a hybrid mixture model. Int J Comput Assist Radiol Surg. 2019 June;14.
3. Bookstein FL. Principal warps: thin-plate splines and the decomposition of deformations. IEEE Trans Pattern Anal Mach Intell. 1989 Jun;11(6):567-585.
4. Reinertsen I, Descoteaux M, Siddiqi K, et al. Validation of vessel-based registration for correction of brain shift. Med Img Anal. 2007;11(4):374 – 388.
5. Rasmussen CE, Williams CKI. Gaussian processes for machine learning. MIT Press; 2006.
6. Wachinger C, Golland P, Reuter M, et al. Gaussian process interpolation for uncertainty estimation in image registration. In: Proc MICCAI; 2014. p. 267–274.
7. Luo J, Toews M, Machado I, et al. A Feature-Driven active framework for Ultrasound-Based brain shift compensation. In: Proc MICCAI; 2018. p. 30–38.
8. Kallis K, Kreppner S, Lotter M, et al. Introduction of a hybrid treatment delivery system used for quality assurance in multi-catheter interstitial brachytherapy. Phys Med Biol. 2018 may;63(9).

9. Bishop CM. Pattern recognition and machine learning. Berlin: Springer; 2006.
10. Bayer S, Maier A, Ostermeier M, et al. Generation of synthetic image data for the evaluation of brain shift compensation methods. In: Proc CIGI; 2017. p. 10.
11. Bayer S, Wydra A, Zhong X, et al. An anthropomorphic deformable phantom for brain shift simulation. In: IEEE Nucl Sci Symp Conf Rec; 2018. p. 1–3.

Intensity-Based 2D-3D Registration Using Normalized Gradient Fields

Annkristin Lange, Stefan Heldmann

Fraunhofer MEVIS, Lübeck
annkristin.lange@mevis.fraunhofer.de

Abstract. 2D-3D registration is central to image guided minimal invasive endovascular therapies such as the treatment of aneurysms. We propose a novel intensity-based 2D-3D registration method based on digitally reconstructed radiographs and the so-called Normalized Gradient Fields (NGF) as a distance measure. We evaluate our method on publicly available clinical data and compare it to five other state-of-the-art 2D-3D registration methods. The results show that our method achieves better accuracy with comparable results in terms of the number of successful registrations and robustness.

1 Introduction

2D-3D image registration is the process of finding the spatial orientation between a 3D volume and a 2D projection of that volume. In the medical context, the treatment of vascular diseases, e.g. abdominal aneurysms, is a possible field of application. Minimally invasive image-guided therapies are often used for this treatment. During the intervention, live X-ray (fluoroscopic) images are taken by a C-arm system. These are used e.g. to track catheters. Therefore the 2D images should be aligned with the 3D planning image to determine the correct 3D position of the catheter in the 3D vascular system.

Over the years different 2D-3D registration methods have been developed. A good overview and classification of methods can be found in [1]. The 2D-3D registration methods can roughly be divided into feature-based and intensity-based methods. Feature-based methods attempt to align features extracted directly from the images. Intensity-based methods are based on synthetic 2D projections that are computed from given 3D images. These projections mimic the real 2D physical projection process and are referred to as digitally reconstructed radiographs (DRRs) [2, 3]. They are explained in more detail in Section 2.1. However, the alignment is then computed by comparing the DRR to a measured projection.

In our target application, we aim for the alignment of 2D vascular X-ray (fluoroscopic) images. These images do not contain large structures with textures, but a lot of local gradient information from projected vessels. Therefore, a suitable intensity-based method should be based on image gradients. This

© Springer Fachmedien Wiesbaden GmbH, ein Teil von Springer Nature 2020
T. Tolxdorff et al. (Hrsg.), *Bildverarbeitung für die Medizin 2020*,
Informatik aktuell, https://doi.org/10.1007/978-3-658-29267-6_33

conclusion is not new, and there exist related work that builds on gradients such as Gradient Information [4] or Gradient Correlation [1].

Here we propose an novel approach that, to the best of our knowledge for the first time in 2D-3D registration, uses the so-called Normalized Gradient Fields (NGF) image similarity measure [5, 6]. NGF is based on orientation of gradients and well-suited for local edge/gradient-based alignment. It is simple to compute (function values and derivatives) and has been proven being very efficient for CT registration [6, 7]. In Section 2.2 it will be explained in more detail. The proposed method is therefore intensity-based but also based on the gradients and can thus be seen as an intermediate between pure intensity-based and feature-based methods, which directly measure the similarity between the 3D gradients and the 2D gradients without calculating DRRs.

We evaluate our method on public available data and compare it to five other intensity- and feature-based methods [8, 9].

2   Materials and methods

2.1   Digitally reconstructed radiographs

An X-ray image is the result of attenuation and detected radiation, respectively, that is emitted by a radiation source q with an initial energy I_0. We model this process with a projection operator $\mathcal{P}$ that maps a 3D attenuation map $\mu : \mathbb{R}^3 \to \mathbb{R}$ to a 2D image. Let $x \in \mathbb{R}^2$ be a location in the 2D projection image and let $d(x) \in \mathbb{R}^3$ be the location of the corresponding detector element in 3D-space. Then the projection is given by

$$\mathcal{P}[\mu](x) := I_0 \exp\left(-\int_{L(q,d(x))} \mu \, d\ell\right) \tag{1}$$

where $L(q, d(x)) := \{q + t(d(x) - q) \mid t \in [0,1]\}$ is the line from the radiation source q to the detector element $d(x)$.

In the following we aim to simulate 2D X-ray images from attenuation maps μ that are estimated from 3D images. In case of CT, the image values are given in Hounsfield units, i.e., $\mathrm{CT}(x) := \frac{\mu(x) - \mu_{\mathrm{water}}}{\mu_{\mathrm{water}}} \cdot 1000$, such that the attenuation is given by $\mu(x) = \alpha \, \mathrm{CT}(x) + \beta$ with $\alpha = \frac{\mu_{\mathrm{water}}}{1000}$ and $\beta = \mu_{\mathrm{water}}$. Practical experiments show, that these values are not optimal and only valid in a simplified theoretical setting. However, we generally assume an affine relationship of a 3D image T and attenuation μ with parameters α and β that are determined experimentally. In the following, we simply write $\mathcal{P}[T]$ with the implicit understanding that we first convert from image intensity to attenuation by affine scaling with fixed parameters for α, β, i.e., we set $\mathcal{P}[T] \equiv \mathcal{P}[\alpha T + \beta]$. This synthetic projection from an given 3D image is called digitally reconstructed radiograph (DRR). As the calculation of the DRRs is computationally expensive, we implemented a GPU-version.

2.2   2D-3D image registration

In general, the image registration can be described as follows: Given a so-called reference image R and a so-called template image T, the goal is finding a plausible spatial transformation y such that the transformation applied to the template image $T(y)$ is as similar to the reference R as possible. To this end, image similarity is measured by a suitable cost-function a so-called called distance or similarity measure $\mathcal{D}$, and the registration problem is in finding y such that $\mathcal{D}(R, T(y)) = \min$. We model d-dimensional images as intensity mappings, i.e. an image $I : \mathbb{R}^d \to \mathbb{R}$ maps position $x \in \mathbb{R}^d$ to an intensity $I(x)$. In our case of 2D-3D registration, reference and template are of different dimensionality. That is, the reference $R : \mathbb{R}^2 \to \mathbb{R}$ is a 2D measured projection image and the template $T : \mathbb{R}^3 \to \mathbb{R}$ is a 3D image. We seek a 3D transformation $y : \mathbb{R}^3 \to \mathbb{R}^3$ such that the 2D reference R and the 2D projection $P[T(y)]$ of the 3D deformed template $T(y) := T \circ y$ are similar, i.e., $\mathcal{D}(R, P[T(y)]) = \min$ where $\mathcal{D}$ is a 2D distance measure. In this work we propose using the 2D version of the normalized gradient field NGF distance measure [5, 6]. For 2D images $R, \widetilde{T} : \mathbb{R}^2 \to \mathbb{R}$, it is given by

$$\mathrm{NGF}(R, \widetilde{T}) = \int_\Omega 1 - \left(\frac{\langle \nabla R(x), \nabla \widetilde{T}(x) \rangle_{\varepsilon_R \varepsilon_T}}{\|\nabla R(x)\|_{\varepsilon_R} \|\nabla \widetilde{T}(x)\|_{\varepsilon_T}} \right)^2 dx \qquad (2)$$

with $\langle x, y \rangle_\varepsilon := x^\top y + \varepsilon^2$, $\|x\|_\varepsilon = \sqrt{\langle x, x \rangle_\varepsilon}$, domain $\Omega \subset \mathbb{R}^2$, that models the 2D field-of-view of the detector and so-called edge parameters $\varepsilon_R, \varepsilon_T > 0$.

Here, we are particularly interested in rigid transformations $y(x) = Qx + b$ with 3-by-3 rotation matrix $Q \in \mathrm{SO}(3)$ and translation vector $b \in \mathbb{R}^3$. The rotation matrix can be parameterized by three rotation angles, such that we end up with a six parameter deformation model $y \equiv y_\theta$ with parameters $\theta \in \mathbb{R}^6$. Summarizing, our 2D-3D rigid registration approach is

$$\min_{\theta \in \mathbb{R}^6} \mathrm{NGF}\left(R, \mathcal{P}[T(y_\theta)]\right) \qquad (3)$$

To compute a solution, we tried a Gauss-Newton type and a L-BFGS optimization scheme with backtracking Armijo linesearch. The Gauss-Newton scheme led to better results and is therefore used. Furthermore, to avoid local minima, for better robustness and large capture range and to speed-up run-times, optimization is embedded into a multi-level and multi-resolution strategy.

2.3   Clinical database

Our evaluation is based on the public available clinical data and the results presented in [8]. The data consists of image from 10 patients with cerebral vascular diseases such as aneurysms. Each data set contains a 3D digitally subtracted rotational angiogram (3D-DSA) volume, two 2D digitally subtracted angiograms (2D-DSA) from lateral (LAT) and anterior-posterior (AP) views (Fig. 1) and a rigid gold-standard transformation for the 3D volume. The gold-standard transformation was derived from fiducial markers. In addition, landmarks and initial transformations are provided for comparative evaluation.

2.4   Evaluation parameters

Common measures for assessing the quality of the resulting registration depend
on landmarks. One of the most popular measures is the so-called target registration error (TRE) [10]. Given N landmarks $\ell_1, ..., \ell_N \in \mathbb{R}^3$, the mean TRE
(mTRE) between transformation y_{reg} and gold-standard y_{gold} is given by

$$\text{mTRE} = \frac{1}{N} \sum_{i=1}^{N} \|y_{\text{reg}}(\ell_i) - y_{\text{gold}}(\ell_i)\| \tag{4}$$

Another measure, particularly designed for 2D-3D registration, is the mean
re-projection distance (mRPD) [10]. It measures the distance of the ray passing
through source q and transformed landmark to gold-standard. It is defined as

$$\text{mRPD} = \frac{1}{N} \sum_{i=1}^{N} \min_{x \in L(q, y_{\text{reg}}(\ell_i))} \|x - y_{\text{gold}}(\ell_i)\| \tag{5}$$

where $L(q, y_{\text{reg}}(\ell_i))$ is the line passing through the source q and the registered
landmark $y_{\text{reg}}(\ell_i)$. Together with the data a set of 400 initial displacements
was specified for each dataset. The displacements were created by randomly
translating about (-20 mm, 20 mm) and rotating around (-10°, 10°) all three
axes. The mTRE of all displacements was calculated and then sorted in a way,
that 20 displacements were in each 1 mm interval from 0-20 mm.

The workflow is as follows: First, the volume of the gold-standard registration
is transformed with the specified initial transformations. Then the parametric
registration is performed and the mRPD & mTRE values are calculated.

Validation criteria are the percentage of successful registration (SR), the
mean and standard deviation of all successful registrations and the capture range
(CR). A registration is viewed as successful, if the mTRE respectively the mRPD
is less then 2 mm, which is approximately the radius of the larger cerebral vessels.
The capture range is defined as the first interval in which less than 95 % of the
registrations are successful.

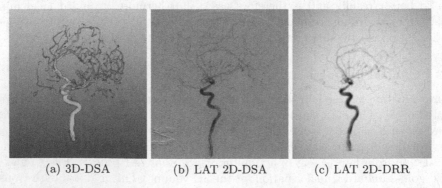

(a) 3D-DSA   (b) LAT 2D-DSA   (c) LAT 2D-DRR

Fig. 1. Example dataset with 3D-DSA, 2D-DSA from lateral (LAT) view and calculated DRR from the same view.

Table 1. Results for the registering of a 3D-DSA to a 2D-DSA from LAT or AP view averaged over all 10 datasets of the proposed *DRR-NGF* method compared to the results of 5 other state-of-the-art methods reported in [8].

View	Method	Success rate (%)	Mean ± Std (mm)	Capture Range (mm)	Time (s)
LAT	MIP-MI	77.43	0.30 ± 0.29	5	84.3
	ICP	45.05	0.41 ± 0.34	0	0.5
	BGB	52.38	0.40 ± 0.37	3	11.6
	MGP	73.23	0.61 ± 0.37	5	0.5
	MGP+BGB	79.45	0.28 ± 0.21	6	15.3
	DRR-NGF	78.60	0.16 ± 0.004	5	3.1
AP	MIP-MI	92.43	0.26 ± 0.29	11	52.3
	ICP	72.48	0.32 ± 0.25	1	0.4
	BGB	58.18	0.39 ± 0.35	3	10.8
	MGP	92.23	0.55 ± 0.29	11	0.5
	MGP+BGB	95.45	0.28 ± 0.19	12	11.5
	DRR-NGF	86.70	0.12 ± 0.003	10	1.7

3 Results

The results of the evaluation of our proposed method (DRR-NGF) with the clinical database averaged over all 10 datasets are given in (Tab. 1) for the LAT and AP images. For comparison the results for several state-of-the-art methods from [8] are listed as well. With the exception of MIP-MI, which uses maximum intensity projections instead of DRRs and mutual information as distance measure, are all other methods feature- or gradient-based. The DRR-NGF achieves in 78.60% a successful registration with a mean mRPD of 0.16 mm ± 0.004 mm in successful cases for the LAT images. The capture range is 5 mm for the LAT images and 10 mm for the AP images. There the registration is in 86.70% successful with a mean mRPD of 0.12 mm ± 0.003 mm. The mean execution time for one registration is 3.1 seconds for LAT and 1.7 seconds for AP images. The mTRE values are not listed in (Tab. 1) because the comparison results are missing. Our proposed method achieves in successful cases a mTRE averaged over all datasets of 1.05 mm ± 0.140 mm for the LAT images and 0.64 mm ± 0.114 mm for the AP images.

4 Discussion

Compared to the other state-of-the-art methods our method achieves significantly higher accuracy while being comparable in terms of success rate and capture range, especially for the LAT 2D-DSA. The mean execution times are not directly comparable, as different hardware is used. However, our experiments show, that run-times for intensity-based 2D-3D NGF registration are fast on of-the-shelf hardware.

We conclude that NGF is very well suited for 2D-3D registration as it provides very accurate results.

One aim of further investigation is to transfer the results to the specific use-case of abdominal aneurysms, using abdominal vascular structures and different systems for acquiring the 3D image and the 2D images. Furthermore we are planning to add an initialisation strategy, to cope with larger initial displacements.

Acknowledgement. This work was funded by the German Federal Ministry of Education and Research (BMBF, project NavEVAR, funding code: 13GW0228C).

References

1. Markelj P, Tomaževič D, Likar B, et al. A review of 3D/2D registration methods for image-guided interventions. Med Image Anal. 2012;16(3):642–61.
2. Goitein M, Abrams M, Rowell D, et al. Multi-dimensional treatment planning: II. Beam's eye-view, back projection, and projection through CT sections. Int J Radiat Oncol Biol Phys. 1983;9(6):789 – 97.
3. Russakoff DB, Rohlfing T, Mori K, et al. Fast generation of digitally reconstructed radiographs using attenuation fields with application to 2D-3D image registration. IEEE Trans Med Imaging. 2005;24(11):1441–54.
4. Otake Y, Armand M, Armiger RS, et al. IEEE Trans Med Imaging. 2011;31(4):948–62.
5. Haber E, Modersitzki J. Intensity gradient based registration and fusion of multi-modal images. In: Proc MiCCAI; 2006. p. 726–33.
6. Rühaak J, Heldmann S, Kipshagen T, et al. Highly accurate fast lung CT registration. In: SPIE Medical Imaging 2013: Image Processing; 2013. .
7. Rühaak J, Polzin T, Heldmann S, et al. Estimation of large motion in lung CT by integrating regularized keypoint correspondences into dense deformable registration. IEEE Trans Med Imaging. 2017;36(8):1746–57.
8. Mitrović U, Pernuš F, Špiclin Ž, et al. 3D-2D registration of cerebral angiograms: a method and evaluation on clinical images. IEEE Trans Med Imaging. 2013;32(8):1550–63.
9. Mitrović U, Likar B, Pernuš F, et al. 3D–2D registration in endovascular image-guided surgery: evaluation of state-of-the-art methods on cerebral angiograms. Int J Comput Assist Radiol Surg. 2018;13(2):193–202.
10. Van de Kraats EB, Penney GP, Tomazevic D, et al. Standardized evaluation methodology for 2-D-3-D registration. IEEE Trans Med Imaging. 2005;24(9):1177–89.

Deep Autofocus with Cone-Beam CT Consistency Constraint

Alexander Preuhs[1], Michael Manhart[2], Philipp Roser[1], Bernhard Stimpel[1], Christopher Syben[1], Marios Psychogios[3], Markus Kowarschik[2], and Andreas Maier[1]

[1]Pattern Recognition Lab, Friedrich-Alexander-Universität Erlangen-Nürnberg
[2]Siemens Healthcare GmbH, Forchheim, Germany
[3]Department of Neuroradiology, University Hospital Basel, Switzerland
alexander.preuhs@fau.de

Abstract. High quality reconstruction with interventional C-arm cone-beam computed tomography (CBCT) requires exact geometry information. If the geometry information is corrupted, e.g., by unexpected patient or system movement, the measured signal is misplaced in the back-projection operation. With prolonged acquisition times of interventional C-arm CBCT the likelihood of rigid patient motion increases. To adapt the backprojection operation accordingly, a motion estimation strategy is necessary. Recently, a novel learning-based approach was proposed, capable of compensating motions within the acquisition plane. We extend this method by a CBCT consistency constraint, which was proven to be efficient for motions perpendicular to the acquisition plane. By the synergistic combination of these two measures, in and out-plane motion is well detectable, achieving an average artifact suppression of 93 %. This outperforms the entropy-based state-of-the-art autofocus measure which achieves on average an artifact suppression of 54 %.

1 Introduction

Cone-beam computed tomography (CBCT) using interventional C-arm systems has gained strong interest since an update of the guidelines of the American Stroke Association favoring mechanical thrombectomy [1, 2]. The procedure needs to be guided by an interventional C-arm system capable of 3-D imaging with soft tissue image quality comparable to helical CT [3]. This allows to perform diagnostic stroke imaging before therapy directly on the C-arm system without prior patient transfers to CT or MRI. This one-stop procedure improves the time-to-therapy [4], but 3-D image acquisition is challenging due to the prolonged acquisition time compared to helical CT. Rigid patient head motion is more likely to occur, which leads to motion artifacts in the reconstructed slice images. Thus, a robust patient motion compensation technique is highly demanded.

© Springer Fachmedien Wiesbaden GmbH, ein Teil von Springer Nature 2020
T. Tolxdorff et al. (Hrsg.), *Bildverarbeitung für die Medizin 2020*,
Informatik aktuell, https://doi.org/10.1007/978-3-658-29267-6_34

Rigid patient motion in CBCT can be compensated by adapting the projection matrices, which represent the acquisition trajectory. This compensated trajectory is denoted as the motion free trajectory. Multiple methods for rigid motion estimation in transmission imaging have been proposed, which can be clustered in three categories: (1) image-based autofocus [5, 6], (2) registration-based [7] and (3) consistency-based [8, 9]. Within those categories, learning-based approaches have been presented that detect anatomical landmarks for registration [10, 11] or assess the reconstruction quality to guide an image-based autofocus [12]. The latter approach demonstrates promising initial results, capable of competing with the state of the art, but the motion estimation is restricted to in-plane motion [12].

As a counterpart, consistency-based methods are merely sensitive to in-plane motion, as they evaluate their consistency by the comparison of epipolar lines. For circular trajectories, epipolar lines are dominantly parallel to the acquisition plane allowing precise detection of out-plane motion. This pose consistency conditions a synergetic constraint for the deep autofocus approach presented in Preuhs et al. [12].

We propose an extension of this learning-based autofocus approach which is constrained by the epipolar consistency conditions (ECC) derived from Grangeat's theorem [13].

2   Motion estimation and compensation framework

2.1   Autofocus

Autofocus frameworks iteratively find a motion trajectory $\mathcal{M}$ by optimizing an image-quality metric (IQM) evaluated on intermediate reconstructions which are updated according to the current estimated motion trajectory. The motion trajectory defines a transformation for each acquired projection i representing the view-dependent patient orientation $M_i \in \mathbb{SE}(3)$. $\mathcal{M}$ is used, together with the offline-calibrated trajectory $\mathcal{T}$, for the backprojection operation in the Feldkamp-Davis-Kress (FDK) reconstruction algorithm [14]. If the image-quality metric saturates, the method outputs a motion compensated reconstruction as illustrated in Fig. 1.

We use a data driven IQM which is computed by a convolutional neural network (CNN) trained to regress the reprojection error (RPE) from the observable motion artifacts within a reconstructed slice image. To account for out-plane motion, the autofocus framework is further constrained using the ECC based on Grangeat's theorem [13, 15]. Thus, in inference, we estimate the motion free trajectory $\hat{\mathcal{M}}$ by iteratively minimizing

$$\hat{\mathcal{M}} = \underset{\mathcal{M}}{\operatorname{argmin}} \; \text{CNN}(\text{FDK}(\mathcal{M})) + \lambda \cdot \text{ECC}(\mathcal{M}) \tag{1}$$

with $\text{CNN}(\text{FDK}(\mathcal{M}))$ denoting the network output (Sec. 2.2) for an intermediate reconstruction and $\text{ECC}(\mathcal{M})$ the consistency constraint (Sec. 2.3), both for a current motion estimate $\mathcal{M}$. The regularization weight λ is choosen such that both metrics are within the same range.

Fig. 1. Flowchart describing the proposed autofocus framework. First, in the initialization, all necessary inputs for the respective methods are computed, then in an iterative compensation-estimation step the motion trajectory is derived. After convergence, the method provides the motion compensated reconstruction.

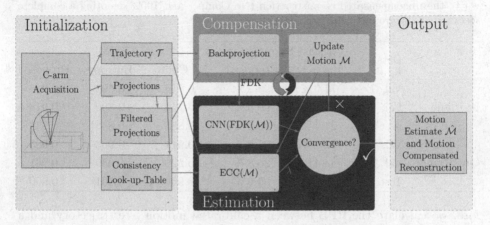

2.2   Reprojection error regression

A highly accurate method for geometry alignment is the minimization of the RPE which is computed as

$$\text{RPE} = ||\boldsymbol{T}'\boldsymbol{x} - \boldsymbol{T}\boldsymbol{x}|| = ||\boldsymbol{T}\boldsymbol{M}\boldsymbol{x} - \boldsymbol{T}\boldsymbol{x}|| \tag{2}$$

This measure evaluates the reconstruction relevant deviations of projection $\boldsymbol{T}'$ and $\boldsymbol{T}$. When applying this measure in practice, the 3-D position of the marker $\boldsymbol{x}$ must be determined, which is a non-trivial task, especially in the presence of geometry misalignment. However, the measure has nice properties, e.g., it increases linearly for translational motion in $\boldsymbol{M}$. To this end, we train a network to regress the RPE based on a reconstructed slice as depicted in Fig. 2. There-

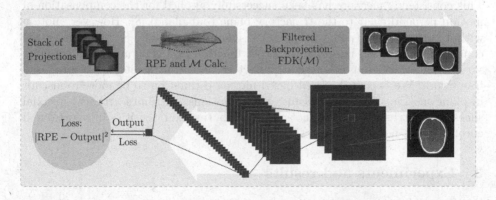

Fig. 2. Schematic description of the training process for the regression network.

Table 1. Motion compensation results for the proposed autofocus method (Proposed) and a state-of-the-art autofocus method employing entropy as an IQM (Entropy) using in-plane and out-plane motion applied to the validation and test patients. Artifact suppression describes the improvement of the RMSE, with 0% being no improvement w.r.t. the uncompensated reconstruction (No Comp.) and 100% denoting a complete recovery of the ground truth reconstruction.

| | Dataset | Artifact Suppression | | SSIM | | |
		Entropy	Proposed	No Comp.	Entropy	Proposed
	Val. 1	77.0 %	94.2 %	0.814	0.892	0.944
In-Plane	Val. 2	89.3 %	96.5 %	0.742	0.890	0.918
	Test 1	21.4 %	90.1 %	0.835	0.855	0.931
	Val. 1	92.1 %	96.8 %	0.911	0.963	0.983
Out-Plane	Val. 2	44.4 %	86.8 %	0.926	0.939	0.981
	Test 1	2.0 %	94.0 %	0.904	0.901	0.990

fore, we calculate the RPE between a calibrated motion free trajectory and a simulated motion trajectory using virtual marker positions x.

We use the same ResNet-like regression network as presented in Preuhs et al. [16] using the same training strategy based on 16 different patients. This results in 7200 reconstructions with random motion and corresponding RPE, differing in their shape and amplitude.

2.3   Cone-beam consistency constraint

Grangeat described a connection of the derivative in the line-integral space — the 2-D Radon domain — of a cone-beam projection to the derivative in the plane-integral space — the 3-D Radon domain [13, 15]. As a result, this measure can be used to judge the consistency of any two epipolar lines in a pair of projection images. The summed pairwise consistency of all sampled epipolar lines defines the consistency of a whole trajectory which we have denoted in (1) as ECC. This consistency measure has been successfully applied for the compensation of motion perpendicular to the trajectory plane (out-plane) [8]. However, motion within the trajectory plane (in-plane) is merely detectable [8]. This poses the consistency condition improper as a cost function in a general motion compensation framework, but makes it a perfect fit as a constraint for the proposed framework. We expect the IQM-based motion estimation to be more robust for in-plane motion detection, because these motions distribute artifacts in axial slices. In contrast, out-plane motion redistributes the intensities in sagittal and coronal slices, not available to the network.

3   Experiments and results

We generate motion trajectories using Akima splines. To prevent an inverse crime scenario we use a Piecewise Cubic Hermite Interpolating Polynomial

(PCHIP) for the estimate of the motion trajectory. By modeling the motion with a spline, we achieve a lower computational complexity in the optimization, as only the spline nodes need to be estimated instead of every motion matrix and additionally we implicitly regularize the motion to be smooth. The motion compensation is performed by optimizing (1) using the Nelder-Mead simplex method. We initialize the simplex corresponding to the initial estimated RPE. If the initial RPE is close to zero, we expect only a small motion, whereas a high initial RPE is expected for greater motion amplitudes. We use a block-based motion estimation strategy, where within each block we only optimize a subset of neighboring spline nodes, while keeping the other nodes fixed. To enforce $M_i \in \mathbb{SE}(3)$ we construct the motion matrices as a function of rotation and translation parameters.

Using the motion affected trajectory we perform an initial reconstruction and apply the proposed motion compensation algorithm (Fig. 1). In addition, we use the best performing IQM from [6] as a baseline compensation. Quantitative results for the test patient and the two validation patients are described in Tab. 1 and visual results for the test patient are depicted in Fig. 3.

4   Conclusion and discussion

We present a novel combination of synergistic motion estimation strategies: a consistency-based method for out-plane motion estimation and a novel data-driven image quality metric for the estimation of in-plane motion. The presented

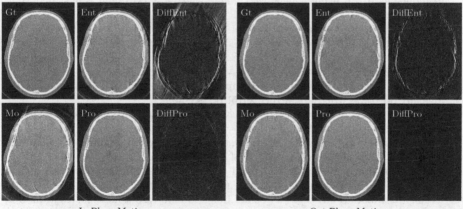

In-Plane Motion   Out-Plane Motion

Fig. 3. Reconstructions of the test patient visualized using a bone-window. For in-plane and out-plane motion, the ground truth (Gt) together with the motion affected reconstruction (Mo) is depicted in the respective leftmost columns. Next to it, the motion compensation result using the state-of-the-art entropy-based autofocus (Ent) and the result using our proposed method (Pro) are depicted. The respective rightmost column shows the difference image of the compensated images to the ground truth using entropy (DiffEnt) or the proposed method (DiffPro), respectively.

metric is computed fast, as the network relies only on an axial slice, reducing the computational burden of the FDK to that of a fan-beam reconstruction. In addition, the consistency-based metric is inherently fast, because the consistency look-up-table can be pre-computed (Fig. 1) and remains constant during the motion compensation. The final motion compensated reconstruction is solely based on the projection raw-data and the estimated motion trajectory. This allows us to use a learning-based approach while ensuring data integrity, as we are not manipulating any of the raw data.

Disclaimer: The concepts and presented in this paper are based on research and are not commercially available.

References

1. Powers WJ, et al. 2015 AHA/ASA focused update of the 2013 guidelines for the early management of patients with acute ischemic stroke regarding endovascular treatment. Stroke. 2015;46(10):3020–3035.
2. Berkhemer ea. A randomized trial of intraarterial treatment for acute ischemic stroke. NEJM. 2015;372(1):11–20.
3. Leyhe JR, Tsogkas I, Hesse AC, et al. Latest generation of flat detector CT as a peri-interventional diagnostic tool: a comparative study with multidetector CT. JNIS. 2017;9(12):1253–1257.
4. Psychogios M, Behme D, Schregel K, et al. One-Stop management of acute stroke patients: minimizing door-to-reperfusion times. Stroke. 2017;.
5. Sisniega A, Stayman JW, Yorkston J, et al. Motion compensation in extremity cone-beam CT using a penalized image sharpness criterion. Phys Med Biol. 2017;62(9):3712.
6. Wicklein J, Kunze H, Kalender WA, et al. Image features for misalignment correction in medical flat-detector CT. Med Phys. 2012;39(8):4918–4931.
7. Ouadah S, Stayman W, Gang J, et al. Self-Calibration of cone-beam CT geometry using 3D–2D image registration. Phys Med Biol. 2016;61(7):2613.
8. Frysch R, Rose G. Rigid motion compensation in c-arm CT using consistency measure on projection data. Proc. 2015; p. 298–306.
9. Preuhs A, Maier A, Manhart M, et al. Symmetry prior for epipolar consistency. IJCARS. 2019;14(9):1541–1551.
10. Bier B, Aschoff K, Syben C, et al. Detecting anatomical landmarks for motion estimation in weight-bearing imaging of knees. MLMIR. 2018; p. 83–90.
11. Bier B, Unberath M, Zaech JN, et al. X-Ray-Transform invariant anatomical landmark detection for pelvic trauma surgery. Proc. 2018; p. 55–63.
12. Preuhs A, Manhart M, Roser P, et al. Image quality assessment for rigid motion compensation. MedNeurIPS. 2019;.
13. Aichert A, Berger M, Wang J, et al. Epipolar consistency in transmission imaging. TMI. 2015;34(11):2205–19.
14. Feldkamp L, Davis L, Kress J. Practical cone-beam algorithm. J Opt Soc Am A. 1984;1(6):612–619.
15. Defrise M, Clack R. A cone-beam reconstruction algorithm using shift-variant filtering and cone-beam backprojection. TMI. 1994;13(1):186–195.
16. Preuhs A, Manhart M, Maier A. Fast epipolar consistency without the need for pseudo matrix inverses. CT-Meeting. 2018; p. 202–205.

Abstract: mlVIRNET

Improved Deep Learning Registration Using a Coarse to Fine Approach to Capture all Levels of Motion

Alessa Hering[1,2], Stefan Heldmann[1]

[1]Fraunhofer MEVIS, Lübeck, Germany
[2]Diagnostic Image Analysis Group, Radboudumc, Nijmegen, Netherlands
alessa.hering@mevis.fraunhofer.de

While deep learning has become a methodology of choice in many areas, relatively few deep-learning-based image registration algorithms have been proposed. One reason for this is lack of ground-truth and the large variability of plausible deformations that can align corresponding anatomies. Therefore, the problem is much less constrained than for example image classification or segmentation. Nevertheless, several methods have been presented in the last years which aim to mimic iterative image registration methods by training a convolutional network which predicts the non-linear deformation function given two new unseen images. However, these algorithms are still limited to relatively small deformations.

To overcome this shortcoming, in our work [1] we present mlVIRNET - a multilevel variational image registration network. We proposed to compute deformation fields on different scales, similar to iterative methods. Starting on a coarse grid with smoothed and down-sampled versions of the input images a deformation field is computed which is subsequently prolongated on the next finer level as a initial guess. Hereby, a coarse level alignment is obtained first that typically captures the large motion components and which is later improved on finer levels for the alignment of more local details.

We validated our framework on the challenging task of large motion inspiration to expiration lung registration using large image data of the multi-center COPDGene study. We have shown that our proposed method archives better results than the comparable single level variant. In particular with regard to the alignment of inner lung structures and the presence of foldings. Moreover, we demonstrated the transferability of our approach to new datasets by evaluating our learned method on the publicly available DIRLAB dataset and showing a lower landmark error than other deep learning based registration methods.

References

1. Hering A, van Ginneken B, Heldmann S. MIVIRNET: multilevel variational image registration network. In: International Conference on Medical Image Computing and Computer-Assisted Intervention. Springer; 2019. p. 257–265.

© Springer Fachmedien Wiesbaden GmbH, ein Teil von Springer Nature 2020
T. Tolxdorff et al. (Hrsg.), *Bildverarbeitung für die Medizin 2020*,
Informatik aktuell, https://doi.org/10.1007/978-3-658-29267-6_35

Font Augmentation

Implant and Surgical Tool Simulation for X-Ray Image Processing

Florian Kordon[1,2,3], Andreas Maier[1], Benedict Swartman[4], Holger Kunze[3]

[1]Pattern Recognition Lab, Department of Computer Science,
Friedrich-Alexander-Universität Erlangen-Nürnberg, Erlangen, Germany
[2]Erlangen Graduate School in Advanced Optical Technologies (SAOT),
Friedrich-Alexander-Universität Erlangen-Nürnberg, Erlangen, Germany
[3]Advanced Therapies, Siemens Healthcare GmbH, Forchheim, Germany
[4]Department for Trauma and Orthopaedic Surgery, BG Trauma Center
Ludwigshafen, Ludwigshafen, Germany
florian.kordon@fau.de

Abstract. This study investigates a novel data augmentation approach for simulating surgical instruments, tools, and implants by image composition with transformed characters, numerals, and abstract symbols from open-source fonts. We analyse its suitability for the common spatial learning tasks of multi-label segmentation and anatomical landmark detection. The proposed technique is evaluated on 38 clinical intra-operative X-ray images with a high occurrence of objects overlaying the target anatomy. We demonstrate increased robustness towards superimposed surgical objects by incorporating our technique and provide an empirical rationale about the neglectable influence of realistic object shape and intensity information.

1 Introduction

To ensure the success of orthopedic and trauma surgery, it is often mandatory to verify key steps of an operation by analysing and assessing intra-operative X-ray images [1]. Recently, such image guidance is frequently facilitated by computer-aided learning algorithms which select and process the relevant semantic information for a given intervention step, e.g. by segmentation of the target structure or by detection of anatomical landmarks [2]. The performance of those algorithms however is limited by both the overall image quality as well as the visibility of the relevant objects. Particularly in intra-operative settings, this visibility is frequently impaired by superimposed surgical tools and instruments or by implants and screws inserted into the patient [1] (Fig. 1). These can partially or completely occlude important anatomical structures, so that additional manual steps such as repositioning of the patient, re-acquisition of the X-ray image under potentially suboptimal orientation, or temporary removal of those objects might be needed.

© Springer Fachmedien Wiesbaden GmbH, ein Teil von Springer Nature 2020
T. Tolxdorff et al. (Hrsg.), *Bildverarbeitung für die Medizin 2020*,
Informatik aktuell, https://doi.org/10.1007/978-3-658-29267-6_36

Fig. 1. Intra-operative X-ray images with various kinds of occluding objects.

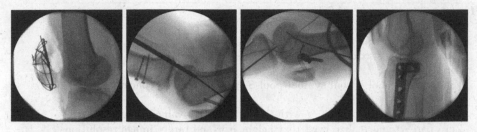

This raises the question how learning algorithms could be designed so that they can reliably interpolate occluded structures and encode spatial and structural relationships to infer meaningful and clinically accepted predictions. A straight-forward strategy is to provide the algorithm a large enough and representative training set from which it can learn an abstract representation model of the underlying anatomy. However, such extensive acquisition of clinical data and annotations is often infeasible as it typically requires costly and time-consuming manual labor of medical experts [2]. Although techniques like domain adaptation and re-training aid to tackle these shortcomings, their successful outcome strongly depends on the relatedness between the source and problem domains. Another strategy is limiting the space of plausible solutions by explicitly incorporating knowledge-driven priors or shape regularization techniques [3]. Designing these however is task-dependent and cannot be applied without rephrasing or adapting the implemented constraints. More recently, Unberath et al. proposed a different approach by extending their work on realistic simulation of X-ray images from 3D-CT data by incorporating 3D models of tools and implants [4, 5]. The computed forward projection of the anatomy is augmented by combining it with density and material samples at the respective object positions. Such data augmentation is an attractive solution as it can be integrated in any algorithm pipeline with little to none computational overhead and effort for the user.

Building upon this motivation and principle idea of [6], this study investigates a novel type of data augmentation for simulating implants and surgical tools on 2D X-ray images. We seek to supply a generalized technique which can be used for a variety of different object types. This technique utilizes a broad set of characters, numerals, and abstract symbols from different open-source fonts, transforms their appearance, and subsequently overlays it on the original anatomy image. We call this approach "Font Augmentation" [1].

2   Materials and methods

2.1   Font augmentation

Font augmentation is a simple technique which tries to approximate characteristic shape and intensity distributions of real implants and surgical tools by using

---

[1] Code available at https://github.com/FlorianKordon/FontAugmentation.

Algorithmus 2 Font augmentation

Input: x {input image}, S {hyper-parameters}
    Sample string length l with $l \sim S.stringLength$
    Sample font f from font pool $S.fontPool$
    Initialize empty sequence of symbols: $t \leftarrow$ ""
    for $i \leftarrow 0; i < l; i + +$ **do**
        Sample symbol c from symbol pool $S.symbolPool$ and concatenate: $t \leftarrow t \oplus c$
    end for
    Binarized render r of string t with font f onto zero-valued envelope
    Zero-pad r to normalize w.r.t text height in r and target image resolution
    Perform affine transformations and intensity scaling (configured in S) on r
    Image blending: $x_{aug} \leftarrow x * (1 - r)$
Output: x_{aug} {augmented image}

---

and composing symbols from a large pool of different fonts. In general, a set of symbols (e.g. latin alphabet, arabic numerals, etc.) is selected, rendered to a binary mask, transformed (rotation, scaling, intensity shifts, etc.), and subsequently composed by image blending with the original anatomy image (Fig. 2). Both parametrization of this technique and selection of fonts and symbols might be adapted to the target task. Note that we intentionally omit exact positioning of the overlaid object since we want the algorithm to be generally invariant to objects at any location. The algorithm is summarized in Algorithm 2 and can be repeated several times for a single image to simulate multiple occluding objects.

2.2 Experiments

To evaluate the suitability of the font augmentation technique, the experiments target two common spatial tasks. First, its behaviour is investigated for multi-label bone segmentation (femur, patella, tibia, and fibula at the knee joint [7]). The successful outcome and clinical applicability of such task largely depends on a contiguous and consistent segmentation outline and hence is prone to ambiguous structure boundaries. Secondly, anatomical landmark detection is considered. We predict spatial heat-maps of two auxiliary landmarks for automatic planning of a drilling point in medial patellofemoral ligament reconstruction surgery [7]. Such point-like anatomical features and structures are often small, which means that typically overlaid objects could suppress low-level visual cues for its actual position.

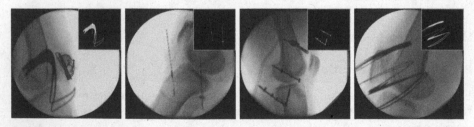

Fig. 2. Examples of images processed with the proposed font augmentation.

For both these tasks the effect of different data augmentation techniques on the algorithm's capability to interpolate the missing information is analysed. To aid the experiment setup, two auxiliary questions are posed: 1) What influence has the intensity of the overlaid object on the performance of learning algorithms on such spatial tasks? 2) Is it important to approximate or mimic the shape of real and task-related surgical tools and implants? To tackle these questions, five augmentation levels with varying amount of retained shape and intensity information are compared to a baseline without additional augmentation.

1. Building upon [4, 5], images are composed with 2D projections of proprietary 3D-CAD data (Fig. 2.2). An image blending is computed between the image and a projection with randomized rotation, translation, and intensity scaling [6]. In total, 9955 projections with task-related objects are used.
2. To suppress any residual information of the superimposed anatomy, the image blending of 1. is binarized so that every pixel belonging to the overlaid object is set to zero intensity.
3. The images are processed with the proposed font augmentation. For every image composition, a pool of 15 open-source fonts is sampled, one to two string-instances with a length up to two are rendered under randomized transformations (rotation, translation, intensity scaling, piece-wise drop-out and Gaussian blur to simulate screw structure).
4. In analogous fashion, all pixels of the rendered font samples described in 3. are truncated to zero intensity.
5. For comparison with a variant without shape and intensity information, coarse dropout of image pixels similar to DropBlock [8] is performed (Fig. 2.2). The pixel dropout mask is calculated on a down-sampled spatial resolution (factor $f \in [0.01, 0.075]$ w.r.t. the image resolution) so that larger contiguous regions are dropped. The probability of one pixel in the down-sampled mask being suppressed is set to $p \in [0.01, 0.1]$.

2.3   Dataset and training protocol

Training for each experiment was performed on 246 lateral X-ray images of the knee anatomy. Of these, 223 are conventional radiographs acquired prior to

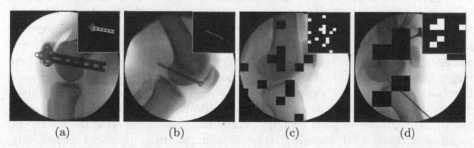

| (a) | (b) | (c) | (d) |

Fig. 3. (a) and (b) show superimpositions of images with 3D-CAD projections. (c) and (d) depict images with a dropout of coarse pixel regions.

surgery while the remaining 23 are intra-operative images from image intensifier systems. The evaluation data consists of 38 intra-operative images, which suffer from large-scale spatial occlusions caused by a variety of different tools and instruments. The training ground truth of the anatomical landmarks was provided by one orthopedic surgeon. Both landmark annotation on the evaluation data as well as the segmentation masks for the femur, patella, tibia, and fibula on both splits were created by the first author under medical supervision.

Upon training, online-augmentation with random affine transformations (rotation, scaling, horizontal flipping) and linear contrast scaling for each image pixel were used [6]. To obtain a common spatial resolution, all images were down-sampled maintaining their aspect-ratio and subsequently zero-padded to square image dimensions of 256 x 256 pixels. For both experiments, a default U-Net neural network architecture with a feature root of 64 and ReLU nonlinearities was implemented in PyTorch (v1.3) [9]. In addition, instance normalization was used for a smoothed optimization landscape [6]. For the segmentation task, separate output channels per target label were appended and evaluated with binary cross-entropy terms and subsequent linear summation. Similar to [7], the localization loss was derived by evaluating the linear sum of mean-squared errors on every output channel, each corresponding to a heat-map representation of a single landmark (centered Gaussian with standard deviation $\sigma = 6$).

Each augmentation technique as well as the baseline with no additional augmentation were evaluated for ten different random seeds, while the sampled augmentation parameters were conditioned to that random seed for valid comparison. All network parameters were optimized over 300 epochs with stochastic gradient descent with Nesterov momentum. A batch size of 6, learning rate of 0.07, momentum term of 0.86, and learning rate decay of 0.89 upon reaching a plateau (no reduction of the loss for 4 consecutive epochs) were used. Those values were acquired by a prior hyper-parameter optimization on a subset of the training data via 150-step random search.

3   Results

Evaluating the performance of the different augmentation techniques on the segmentation task shows a substantial performance gain when using any kind of object overlay or information dropout (Fig. 3). Especially for the patella and fibula which mark smaller anatomies, using font augmentation with intensity scaling boosts the average symmetric surface distance (ASD) from $7.6 \pm 1.9\,\mathrm{px}$ (mean $\pm$ std) to $3.6 \pm 0.9\,\mathrm{px}$ and $9.0 \pm 1.5\,\mathrm{px}$ to $6.0 \pm 1.6\,\mathrm{px}$ respectively. The two larger bones (femur and tibia) exhibit a noticeably lower performance increase. For both the ASD and mean intersection over union (mean IOU) the difference between shape and intensity-informed variants, their binarized version, and the model with coarse pixel dropout is only marginal. Observing the landmark localization task, both binarized versions and the dropout model consistently outperform the baseline and the intensity-informed versions of font-augmentation and 3D render overlay (Fig. 3). Where landmark 1) shows only a minimal improvement w.r.t. the Euclidean distance (ED) metric upon binary font-augmentation, the ED for landmark 2) considerably improves from 17.7 ± 7.2 px to 7.9 ± 2.1 px.

4 Discussion

We proposed a novel data augmentation strategy for simulating surgical tools and implants on 2D X-ray images. We evaluated this technique on clinical data for multi-label segmentation and landmark localization tasks and demonstrated its usefulness for boosting the learning algorithm's performance in ambiguous image regions. Interestingly, the benefit of using realistic shape and intensity information is generally rather small. This indicates that a partial dropout of precise spatial information does not necessarily lead to anatomically aberrant solutions but rather promotes the network to learn the often relatively static relationships between anatomical structures. This finding is backed by a generally good performance of coarse pixel dropout, where neither information about

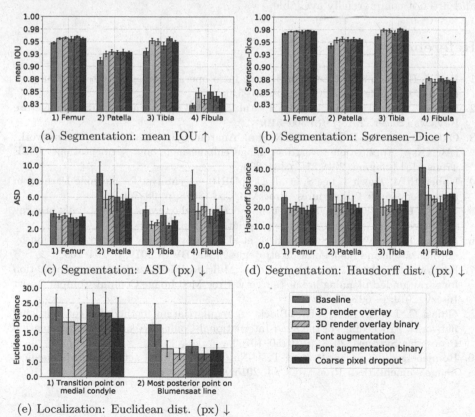

(a) Segmentation: mean IOU ↑   (b) Segmentation: Sørensen–Dice ↑

(c) Segmentation: ASD (px) ↓   (d) Segmentation: Hausdorff dist. (px) ↓

(e) Localization: Euclidean dist. (px) ↓

Fig. 4. Results for the devised augmentation strategies for multi-label bone segmentation and anatomical landmark detection on the femur (refer to [7] for a thorough description). ↑ marks a metric to maximize, ↓ marks a metric to minimize.

shape nor intensity are retained. This further translates to the task domain of reconstructing missing or incomplete parts in an image, which is known as image inpainting. Instead of phrasing such reconstruction task explicitly as an auxiliary task prior, font augmentation presumably enables the learning algorithm to perform semantic reconstruction implicitly and aids to refine its learned representation. We see limitations in our study in that we evaluated the technique only on proprietary data with a single algorithm. We therefor seek to extend this study to multiple anatomies and evaluate the font augmentation technique on public data with similar occlusion problems.

Acknowledgement. The authors gratefully acknowledge funding of the Erlangen Graduate School in Advanced Optical Technologies (SAOT) by the German Research Foundation (DFG) in the framework of the German excellence initiative.

Disclaimer. The methods and information presented here are based on research and are not commercially available.

References

1. Keil H, Beisemann N, Swartman B, et al. Intra-operative imaging in trauma surgery. EFORT Open Reviews. 2018;3(10):541–549.
2. Hosny A, Parmar C, Quackenbush J, et al. Artificial intelligence in radiology. Nature Reviews Cancer. 2018;18(8):500–510.
3. Oktay O, Ferrante E, Kamnitsas K, et al. Anatomically constrained neural networks (ACNNs): Application to cardiac image enhancement and segmentation. IEEE Trans Med Imaging. 2018;37(2):384–395.
4. Unberath M, Zaech J, Lee S, et al. DeepDRR – A catalyst for machine learning in fluoroscopy-guided procedures. Proc MICCAI. 2018; p. 98–106.
5. Gao C, Unberath M, Taylor R, et al. Localizing dexterous surgical tools in x-ray for image-based navigation. arXiv preprint. 2019; p. 98–106.
6. Kordon F, Lasowski R, Swartman B, et al. Improved x-ray bone segmentation by normalization and augmentation strategies. Proc BVM. 2019; p. 104–109.
7. Kordon F, Fischer P, Privalov M, et al. Multi-task localization and segmentation for x-ray guided planning in knee surgery. Proc Med Image Comput Comput Assist Interv. 2019; p. 622–630.
8. Ghiasi G, Lin T, Le Q. DropBlock: A regularization method for convolutional networks. Proceedings of the 32nd International Conference on Neural Information Processing Systems. 2018; p. 10750–10760.
9. Ronneberger O, Fischer P, Brox T. U-Net: Convolutional networks for biomedical image segmentation. Proc MICCAI. 2015;9351:234–241.

Abstract: Segmentation of Retinal Low-Cost Optical Coherence Tomography Images Using Deep Learning

Timo Kepp[1], Helge Sudkamp[2], Claus von der Burchard[3], Hendrik Schenke[3], Peter Koch[2], Gereon Hüttmann[2,4], Johann Roider[2], Mattias P. Heinrich[1], Heinz Handels[1]

[1]Institut für Medizinische Informatik, Universität zu Lübeck
[2]Medizinisches Laserzentrum Lübeck GmbH
[3]Klinik für Ophthalmologie, Universität zu Kiel
[4]Institut für Biomedizinische Optik, Universität zu Lübeck
kepp@imi.uni-luebeck.de

The treatment of age-related macular degeneration (AMD) requires continuous eye examinations using optical coherence tomography (OCT). The need for treatment is indicated by the presence or change of disease-specific OCT-based biomarkers. Therapeutic response and recurrence patterns of patients, however, vary widely between individuals and represent a major challenge for physicians. Therefore, the monitoring frequency plays an important role in the success of AMD therapy. While a higher monitoring frequency would have a positive effect on the success of the treatment, it can only be achieved with a home monitoring solution in practice. One of the most important requirements of an OCT system for home monitoring is computer-aided quantification of pathological changes using specific OCT-based biomarkers. In this work, retinal scans of a novel self-examination low-cost full-field OCT (SELF-OCT) system are segmented for the first time using a deep learning approach [1]. A convolutional neural network (CNN) is used to segment the entire retina as well as pigment epithelial detachments (PED) as biomarkers. Due to the special acquisition technique of the SELF-OCT system, densely sampled volumes are generated, making a 3D CNN architecture a natural choice for OCT segmentation. In contrast to current state of the art methods, the 3D CNN receives a complete OCT volume as input instead of individual 2D-B scans. It is shown that our approach can segment the retina with high accuracy, while segmenting the PED remains difficult because of the low contrast of these structures in the OCT images. In addition, it is shown that the use of a convolutional denoising autoencoder as refinement step corrects segmentation errors caused by artifacts in the OCT image.

References

1. Kepp T, Sudkamp H, von der Burchard C, et al. Segmentation of retinal low-cost optical coherence tomography images using deep learning. In: Proc. SPIE Med Imaging; 2020. Accepted.

© Springer Fachmedien Wiesbaden GmbH, ein Teil von Springer Nature 2020
T. Tolxdorff et al. (Hrsg.), *Bildverarbeitung für die Medizin 2020*,
Informatik aktuell, https://doi.org/10.1007/978-3-658-29267-6_37

Abstract: RinQ Fingerprinting

Recurrence-Informed Quantile Networks for Magnetic Resonance Fingerprinting

Elisabeth Hoppe[1,*], Florian Thamm[1,*], Gregor Körzdörfer[2],
Christopher Syben[1], Franziska Schirrmacher[1], Mathias Nittka[2], Josef Pfeuffer[2],
Heiko Meyer[2], Andreas Maier[1]

[1]Pattern Recognition Lab, Department of Computer Science,
Friedrich-Alexander-Universität Erlangen-Nürnberg, Erlangen, Germany
[2]MR Application Development, Siemens Healthcare, Erlangen, Germany
*These authors contributed equally and are listed in alphabetical order.
elisabeth.hoppe@fau.de, florian.thamm@fau.de

Recently, Magnetic Resonance Fingerprinting (MRF) was proposed as a quantitative imaging technique for the simultaneous acquisition of tissue parameters such as relaxation times T_1 and T_2. Although the acquisition is highly accelerated, the state-of-the-art reconstruction suffers from long computation times: Template matching methods are used to find the most similar signal to the measured one by comparing it to pre-simulated signals of possible parameter combinations in a discretized dictionary. Deep learning approaches can overcome this limitation, by providing the direct mapping from the measured signal to the underlying parameters by one forward pass through a network. In this work, we propose a Recurrent Neural Network (RNN) architecture in combination with a novel quantile layer [1]. RNNs are well suited for the processing of time-dependent signals and the quantile layer helps to overcome the noisy outliers by considering the spatial neighbors of the signal. We evaluate our approach using in-vivo data from multiple brain slices and several volunteers, running various experiments. We show that the RNN approach with small patches of complex-valued input signals in combination with a quantile layer outperforms other architectures, e.g. previously proposed CNNs for the MRF reconstruction reducing the error in T_1 and T_2 by more than 80 %.

References

1. Hoppe E, Thamm F, Körzdörfer G, et al. RinQ fingerprinting: recurrence-informed quantile networks for magnetic resonance fingerprinting. In: Proc MIC-CAI. Springer; 2019. p. 92–100.

© Springer Fachmedien Wiesbaden GmbH, ein Teil von Springer Nature 2020
T. Tolxdorff et al. (Hrsg.), *Bildverarbeitung für die Medizin 2020*,
Informatik aktuell, https://doi.org/10.1007/978-3-658-29267-6_38

Abstract: Learning to Avoid Poor Images
Towards Task-Aware C-Arm Cone-Beam CT Trajectories

Jan-Nico Zaech[1,2,3], Cong Gao[1], Bastian Bier[1,2], Russell Taylor[1],
Andreas Maier[2], Nassir Navab[1], Mathias Unberath[1]

[1]Laboratory for Computational Sensing and Robotics, Johns Hopkins University
[2]Pattern Recognition Lab, Friedrich-Alexander-Universität Erlangen-Nürnberg
[3]Computer Vision Laboratory, Eidgenössische Technische Hochschule Zürich
unberath@jhu.edu

Metal artifacts in computed tomography (CT) arise from a mismatch between physics of image formation and idealized assumptions during tomographic reconstruction. These artifacts are particularly strong around metal implants, inhibiting widespread adoption of 3D cone-beam CT (CBCT) despite clear opportunity for intra-operative verification of implant positioning, e.g. in spinal fusion surgery. On synthetic and real data, we demonstrate that much of the artifact can be avoided by acquiring better data for reconstruction in a task-aware and patient-specific manner, and describe the first step towards the envisioned task-aware CBCT protocol. The traditional short-scan CBCT trajectory is planar, with little room for scene-specific adjustment. We extend this trajectory by autonomously adjusting out-of-plane angulation. This enables C-arm source trajectories that are scene-specific in that they avoid acquiring "poor images", characterized by beam hardening, photon starvation, and noise. The recommendation of ideal out-of-plane angulation is performed on-the-fly using a deep convolutional neural network that regresses a detectability-rank derived from imaging physics. This work was first presented at MICCAI 2019 [1].

References

1. Zaech JN, Gao C, Bier B, et al. Learning to avoid poor images: towards task-aware c-arm cone-beam CT trajectories. In: Proc – MICCAI 2019. Cham: Springer International Publishing; 2019. p. 11–19.

© Springer Fachmedien Wiesbaden GmbH, ein Teil von Springer Nature 2020
T. Tolxdorff et al. (Hrsg.), *Bildverarbeitung für die Medizin 2020*,
Informatik aktuell, https://doi.org/10.1007/978-3-658-29267-6_39

Field of View Extension in Computed Tomography Using Deep Learning Prior

Yixing Huang[1], Lei Gao[1], Alexander Preuhs[1], Andreas Maier[1,2]

[1]Pattern Recognition Lab, Friedrich-Alexander-University Erlangen-Nuremberg
[2]Erlangen Graduate School in Advanced Optical Technologies (SAOT)
yixing.yh.huang@fau.de

Abstract. In computed tomography (CT), data truncation is a common problem. Images reconstructed by the standard filtered back-projection algorithm from truncated data suffer from cupping artifacts inside the field-of-view (FOV), while anatomical structures are severely distorted or missing outside the FOV. Deep learning, particularly the U-Net, has been applied to extend the FOV as a post-processing method. Since image-to-image prediction neglects the data fidelity to measured projection data, incorrect structures, even inside the FOV, might be reconstructed by such an approach. Therefore, generating reconstructed images directly from a post-processing neural network is inadequate. In this work, we propose a data consistent reconstruction method, which utilizes deep learning reconstruction as prior for extrapolating truncated projections and a conventional iterative reconstruction to constrain the reconstruction consistent to measured raw data. Its efficacy is demonstrated in our study, achieving small average root-mean-square error of 24 HU inside the FOV and a high structure similarity index of 0.993 for the whole body area on a test patient's CT data.

1 Introduction

In computed tomography (CT), image reconstruction from truncated data occurs in various situations. In region-of-interest (ROI) imaging, also known as interior tomography, collimators are inserted between the X-ray source and the detector of a CT scanner for low dose considerations. In addition, due to the limited detector size, large patients cannot be positioned entirely inside the field-of-view (FOV) of a CT scanner. In both scenarios, acquired projections are laterally truncated. Images reconstructed by the standard filtered back-projection (FBP) algorithm from such truncated data suffer from cupping artifacts inside the FOV, while anatomical structures are severely distorted or missing outside the FOV.

So far, many approaches have been investigated for truncation correction. Among them, a major category of methods are based on heuristic extrapolation, including symmetric mirroring, cosine or Gaussian functions, and water cylinder

© Springer Fachmedien Wiesbaden GmbH, ein Teil von Springer Nature 2020
T. Tolxdorff et al. (Hrsg.), *Bildverarbeitung für die Medizin 2020*,
Informatik aktuell, https://doi.org/10.1007/978-3-658-29267-6_40

extrapolation (WCE) [1]. Such extrapolation methods seek for a smooth transition between measured and truncated areas to alleviate cupping artifacts. Another category of methods seek for an alternative to the standard FBP method, where the high-pass ramp filter is the main cause of cupping artifacts. Decomposing the ramp filter into a local Laplace filter and a nonlocal low-pass filter [2] is one of such methods. Another strategy is the differentiate back-projection (DBP) [3] approach, one milestone for interior tomography. With DBP, theoretically exact solutions have been developed based on *a priori* knowledge [4]. With the development of compressed sensing technologies, iterative reconstruction with total variation (TV) regularization [5] is a promising approach for interior tomography, despite its high computation.

Recently, deep learning has achieved impressive results in various CT reconstruction fields, including low-dose denoising, sparse-view reconstruction, limited angle tomography, and metal artifact reduction. In the field of interior tomography, Han and Ye applied the U-Net to remove null space artifacts [6] from FBP reconstruction. Observing its instability, they propose to use DBP reconstruction instead of the FBP reconstruction as the input of the U-Net for various types of ROI reconstruction tasks [7]. Except for learning-based post-processing methods, interior tomography images can be directly learned from truncated data by the iCT-Net [8] based on known operators [9]. For FOV extension, Fournié et al. [10] have demonstrated the efficacy of the U-Net in this application. However, no thorough evaluation is provided in their preliminary results.

Although deep learning surpasses conventional methods in many CT reconstruction fields, its robustness remains a concern for clinical applications [11]. Since post-processing neural networks have no direct connections to measured projection data, incorrect structures, even inside the FOV, might be reconstructed. Therefore, generating reconstructed images directly from a post-processing neural network is inadequate. In this work, we propose a data consistent reconstruction (DCR) method to improve the image quality of deep learning reconstruction for FOV extension. It utilizes deep learning reconstruction as prior for data extrapolation and a conventional iterative reconstruction method to constrain the reconstruction consistent to measured projection data.

2   Materials and methods

Our proposed DCR method consists of three main steps: deep learning artifact reduction, data extrapolation using deep learning prior, and iterative reconstruction with TV regularization.

2.1   Deep learning artifact reduction

As displayed in Fig. 1, the state-of-the-art U-Net is used for truncation artifact reduction. Images reconstructed by FBP directly from truncated projections suffer from severe cupping artifacts, especially at the FOV boundary. It is difficult for the U-Net to learn the corresponding artifacts accurately, according to our experiments. Instead, FBP reconstruction from extrapolated projections contains much fewer cupping artifacts. Therefore, in this work, an image reconstructed from WCE [1] processed projections, denoted by f_{WCE}, is chosen as the input of the U-Net. The output of the U-Net is its corresponding artifact image, denoted by f_{artifact}. Then an estimation of the artifact-free image, denoted by $f_{\mathrm{U\text{-}Net}}$, is obtained by $f_{\mathrm{U\text{-}Net}} = f_{\mathrm{WCE}} - f_{\mathrm{artifact}}$.

2.2 Data extrapolation using deep learning prior

For data consistent reconstruction, we propose to preserve measured projections entirely and use the deep learning reconstruction as prior for extrapolating missing (truncated) data. We denote measured projections by p_{m} and their corresponding system matrix by A_{m}. We further denote truncated projections by p_{t} and their corresponding system matrix by A_{t}. The deep learning reconstruction $f_{\mathrm{U\text{-}Net}}$ provides prior information for the truncated projections p_{t}. Therefore, an estimation of p_{t}, denoted by $\hat{p}_{\mathrm{t}}$, is achieved by forward projection of $f_{\mathrm{U\text{-}Net}}$,

$$\hat{p}_{\mathrm{t}} = A_{\mathrm{t}} f_{\mathrm{U\text{-}Net}} \tag{1}$$

Combining $\hat{p}_{\mathrm{t}}$ with p_{m}, a complete projection set is obtained for extended FOV reconstruction.

2.3 Iterative reconstruction with TV regularization

Due to intensity discontinuity between $\hat{p}_{\mathrm{t}}$ and p_{m} at the transition area, artifacts occur at the boundary of the original FOV in the image reconstructed directly by FBP. Therefore, iterative reconstruction with reweighted total variation (wTV) regularization is utilized

$$\min \|f\|_{\mathrm{wTV}}, \text{subject to} \begin{cases} \|A_{\mathrm{m}} f - p_{\mathrm{m}}\| < e_1 \\ \|A_{\mathrm{t}} f - \hat{p}_{\mathrm{t}}\| < e_2 \end{cases} \tag{2}$$

Here e_1 is a noise tolerance parameter for the data fidelity term of the measured projections and the other tolerance parameter e_2 accounts for the inaccuracy of the deep learning prior $f_{\mathrm{U\text{-}Net}}$. $\|f\|_{\mathrm{wTV}}$ is an iterative reweighted total

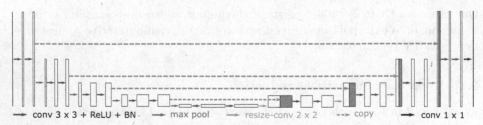

conv 3 x 3 + ReLU + BN   max pool   resize-conv 2 x 2   copy   conv 1 x 1

Fig. 1. The U-Net architecture for truncation artifact reduction.

Table 1. The system configuration of cone-beam CT to validate the proposed DCR method for FOV extension.

Parameter	Value
Scan angular range	$360°$
Angular step	$1°$
Source-to-detector distance	$1200.0\,\mathrm{mm}$
Source-to-isocenter distance	$600.0\,\mathrm{mm}$
Detector size	500×960
Extended virtual detector size	1000×960
Detector pixel size	$1.0\,\mathrm{mm} \times 1.0\,\mathrm{mm}$
Volume size	$256 \times 256 \times 256$
Voxel size	$1.25\,\mathrm{mm} \times 1.25\,\mathrm{mm} \times 1.0\,\mathrm{mm}$

variation (wTV) term defined as the following [12]

$$||\boldsymbol{f}^{(n)}||_{\mathrm{wTV}} = \sum_{x,y,z} \boldsymbol{w}^{(n)}_{x,y,z}||\mathcal{D}\boldsymbol{f}^{(n)}_{x,y,z}||$$
$$\boldsymbol{w}^{(n)}_{x,y,z} = \frac{1}{||\mathcal{D}\boldsymbol{f}^{(n-1)}_{x,y,z}|| + \epsilon}$$

(3)

where $\boldsymbol{f}^{(n)}$ is the image at the nth iteration, $\boldsymbol{w}^{(n)}$ is the weight vector for the nth iteration which is computed from the previous iteration, and ϵ is a small positive value added to avoid division by zero.

To solve the above objective function, simultaneous algebraic reconstruction technique (SART) + wTV is applied [12]. To save computation, the iterative reconstruction is initialized by $\boldsymbol{f}_{\mathrm{U\text{-}Net}}$.

2.4   Experimental setup

We validate the proposed DCR method using 18 patients' data from the AAPM Low-Dose CT Grand Challenge in cone-beam CT with Poisson noise. For each patient's data, truncated projections are simulated in a cone-beam CT system with parameters listed in Tab. 1. Poisson noise is simulated considering an initial exposure of 10^5 photons at each detector pixel before attenuation.

For training, 425 2-D slices are chosen from 17 patients' 3-D volumes, i.e., picking 1 slice among every 10 slices for each patient. For test, all the 256 slices from the WCE reconstruction $\boldsymbol{f}_{\mathrm{WCE}}$ are fed to the U-Net for evaluation. Both the training data and test data contain Poisson noise. The Hounsfield scaled images are normalized to [-1, 1] for stable training. The U-Net is trained on the above data using the Adam optimizer for 500 epochs. An ℓ_2 loss function is used.

For reconstruction, the parameter e_1 is set to 0.01 for Poisson noise tolerance. A relatively large tolerance value of 0.5 is chosen empirically for e_2. For the wTV regularization, the parameter ϵ is set to 5 HU for weight update. With the initialization of $f_{\text{U-Net}}$, 10 iterations of SART + wTV only are applied to get the final reconstruction.

3 Results

The reconstruction results of two example slices from the test patient are displayed in Fig. 3. In the FBP reconstruction f_{FBP} (Figs. 3(b) and (h)), the original FOV is observed. The anatomical structures outside this FOV are missing, while the structures inside the FOV suffer from cupping artifacts. WCE reconstructs certain structures outside the FOV and alleviates the cupping artifacts, according to f_{WCE} in Figs. 3(c) and (i). However, the reconstructed structures outside the FOV is not accurate and shadow artifacts remain near the FOV boundary. In the wTV reconstruction f_{wTV} (Figs. 3(d) and (j)), the cupping artifacts are mitigated. Moreover, Poisson noise is reduced as well. It achieves small root-mean-square error (RMSE) values of 32 HU and 42 HU for Fig. 2(d) and Fig. 2(j) inside the FOV, respectively. Nevertheless, the structures outside the FOV are still missing. Figs. 3(e) and (k) demonstrate that the U-Net is able to reduce the cupping artifacts and to reconstruct the anatomical structures outside the FOV as well. However, Poisson noise remains. The relative high RMSE inside the FOV indicates incorrect structures reconstructed by the U-Net. The proposed DCR method combines the advantages of wTV and U-Net. It reconstructs the anatomical structures outside the FOV well. Meanwhile, it reduces both the cupping artifacts and the Poisson noise, as demonstrated in Figs. 3(f) and (l). Among all the algorithms, it achieves the smallest RMSE value of 21 HU inside the FOV.

The average RMSE and structure similarity (SSIM) values of all the 256 slices in the test patient for different methods are displayed in Tab. 2. DCR achieves the smallest value of 24 HU and 66 HU for RMSE inside the FOV and for the whole patient body, respectively. It also reaches the highest SSIM index of 0.993, which highlights the efficacy of the proposed DCR method.

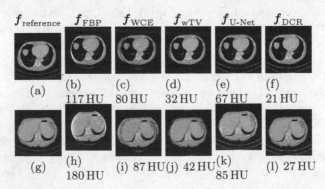

Fig. 2. Reconstruction results of two example slices from the test patient, window: [-600, 500] HU. The RMSE value inside the FOV for each method is displayed.

Table 2. The quantitative evaluation results of different methods using the RMSE and SSIM metrics.

Method	FBP	WCE	wTV	U-Net	DCR
RMSE in FOV	162 HU	85 HU	41 HU	77 HU	24 HU
RMSE	353 HU	179 HU	137 HU	127 HU	66 HU
SSIM	0.834	0.948	0.968	0.975	0.993

4 Discussion

With deep learning prior for initialization, only a small number of iterations, e. g. 10 iterations in this work, are required. Therefore, it is more efficient than conventional iterative reconstruction methods. Meanwhile, the deep learning provides information for structures outside the FOV. Therefore, it is more effective than conventional iterative reconstruction methods in the regard of FOV extension. With the integration of iterative reconstruction, it is more effective in reducing Poisson noise and more robust as well than deep learning. All in all, the proposed DCR method is a hybrid method combining the advantages of deep learning and iterative reconstruction while overcoming their shortcomings.

References

1. Hsieh J, Chao E, Thibault J, et al. A novel reconstruction algorithm to extend the CT scan field-of-view. Med Phys. 2004;31(9):2385–2391.
2. Xia Y, Hofmann H, Dennerlein F, et al. Towards clinical application of a Laplace operator-based region of interest reconstruction algorithm in C-arm CT. IEEE Trans Med Imaging. 2013;33(3):593–606.
3. Noo F, Clackdoyle R, Pack JD. A two-step Hilbert transform method for 2D image reconstruction. Phys Med Biol. 2004;49(17):3903–3923.
4. Kudo H, Courdurier M, Noo F, et al. Tiny a priori knowledge solves the interior problem in computed tomography. Phys Med Biol. 2008;53(9):2207.
5. Yu H, Wang G. Compressed sensing based interior tomography. Phys Med Biol. 2009;54(9):2791.
6. Schwab J, Antholzer S, Haltmeier M. Deep null space learning for inverse problems: convergence analysis and rates. Inverse Probl. 2019;.
7. Han Y, Ye JC. One network to solve all ROIs: Deep learning CT for any ROI using differentiated backprojection. arXiv. 2018;.
8. Li Y, Li K, Zhang C, et al. Learning to reconstruct computed tomography (CT) images directly from sinogram data under a variety of data acquisition conditions. IEEE Trans Med Imaging. 2019;8:2469–2481.
9. Maier AK, Syben C, Stimpel B, et al. Learning with known operators reduces maximum training error bounds. Nat Mach Intell. 2019;.
10. Fournié É, Baer-Beck M, Stierstorfer K. CT Field of View Extension Using Combined Channels Extension and Deep Learning Methods. Proc MIDL. 2019;.
11. Huang Y, Würfl T, Breininger K, et al. Some investigations on robustness of deep learning in limited angle tomography. Proc MICCAI. 2018; p. 145–153.
12. Huang Y, Taubmann O, Huang X, et al. Scale-space anisotropic total variation for limited angle tomography. IEEE Trans Radiat Plasma Med Sci. 2018;2(4):307–314.

Abstract: Self-Supervised 3D Context Feature Learning on Unlabeled Volume Data

Maximilian Blendowski, Mattias P. Heinrich

Institut für Medizinische Informatik, Universität zu Lübeck
blendowski@imi.uni-luebeck.de

Deep learning with convolutional networks (DCNN) has established itself as a powerful tool for a variety of medical imaging tasks. However, DCNNs in particular require strong monitoring by expert annotations, which cannot be generated cost-effectively by laymen. In contrast to manual annotations, the mere availability of medical volume data is not a problem. In our MICCAI 2019 conference paper [1], we present a fully self-supervised method to learn 3D context features by exploiting data-inherent patterns and leveraging anatomical information freely available from medical images themselves.

Closely related to the context prediction of neighboring patches as classification task (e.g. top/bottom, left/right) by Doersch et al. [2], we alter this self-supervised pretext loss to a more flexible regression task. We propose to appropriately leverage spatial information in 3D scans by predicting orthogonal offsets of two planar patches that are extracted with a small intermediate gap. In addition, we use an auxiliary decoder network for 2D heatmap regression that increases the robustness of this offset regression.

Using our Vantage Point Forest method [3] for an approximate k-Nearest Neighbor search in an atlas database, we predict labels without any subsequent finetuning strategies for a multi-organ segmentation task. Compared to a naive 3D extenstion of [2], we obtain a large increase in mean Dice scores from 55.2% to 65.5%. While we only trained with spatial relations, we also achieve state-of-the-art results for one-shot-segmentation on a public abdominal CT dataset.

Acknowledgement. This work was supported by the German Research Foundation (DFG) under grant number 320997906 (HE 7364/2-1) and by the NVIDIA Corporation with their GPU donations. Find our code here:
https://github.com/multimodallearning/miccai19_self_supervision

References

1. Blendowski M, Nickisch H, Heinrich MP. How to learn from unlabeled volume data: self-supervised 3d context feature learning. In: MICCAI. Springer; 2019. p. 649–657.
2. Doersch C, Gupta A, Efros AA. Unsupervised visual representation learning by context prediction. In: Proc IEEE Int Conf Comput Vis; 2015. .
3. Heinrich MP, Blendowski M. Multi-organ segmentation using vantage point forests and binary context features. In: MICCAI. Springer; 2016. p. 598–606.

© Springer Fachmedien Wiesbaden GmbH, ein Teil von Springer Nature 2020
T. Tolxdorff et al. (Hrsg.), *Bildverarbeitung für die Medizin 2020*,
Informatik aktuell, https://doi.org/10.1007/978-3-658-29267-6_41

Deep Learning Algorithms for Coronary Artery Plaque Characterisation from CCTA Scans

Felix Denzinger[1,2], Michael Wels[2], Katharina Breininger[1], Anika Reidelshöfer[3], Joachim Eckert[4], Michael Sühling[2], Axel Schmermund[4], Andreas Maier[1]

[1]Pattern Recognition Lab, Friedrich-Alexander-University Erlangen-Nuremberg, Erlangen, Germany
[2]Computed Tomography, Siemens Healthineers, Forchheim, Germany
[3]University Clinic Frankfurt, Frankfurt am Main, Germany
[4]Cardioangiological Centrum Bethanien, Frankfurt am Main, Germany
`felix.denzinger@fau.de`

Abstract. Analysing coronary artery plaque segments with respect to their functional significance and therefore their influence to patient management in a non-invasive setup is an important subject of current research. In this work we compare and improve three deep learning algorithms for this task: A 3D recurrent convolutional neural network (RCNN), a 2D multi-view ensemble approach based on texture analysis, and a newly proposed 2.5D approach. Current state of the art methods utilising fluid dynamics based fractional flow reserve (FFR) simulation reach an AUC of up to 0.93 for the task of predicting an abnormal invasive FFR value. For the comparable task of predicting revascularisation decision, we are able to improve the performance in terms of AUC of both existing approaches with the proposed modifications, specifically from 0.80 to 0.90 for the 3D-RCNN, and from 0.85 to 0.90 for the multi-view texture-based ensemble. The newly proposed 2.5D approach achieves comparable results with an AUC of 0.90.

1 Introduction

Cardiovascular diseases (CVDs) remain the leading cause of natural death [1]. In diagnosis and treatment of CVDs, the identification of functionally significant atherosclerotic plaques that narrow the coronary vessels and cause malperfusion of the heart muscle plays an important role. In clinical practice, this is typically assessed using fractional flow reserve (FFR) measurements.

This measurement is performed minimally invasively and therefore induces a small but existing risk to the patient. A non-invasive modality capable of visualising and assessing coronary artery plaque segments is coronary computed tomography angiography (CCTA). Current research tries to simulate the FFR value from CCTA scans [2]. Approaches based on this mostly rely on a prior segmentation of the whole coronary tree which is computationally intensive, prone to errors and may need manual corrections [3].

© Springer Fachmedien Wiesbaden GmbH, ein Teil von Springer Nature 2020
T. Tolxdorff et al. (Hrsg.), *Bildverarbeitung für die Medizin 2020*,
Informatik aktuell, https://doi.org/10.1007/978-3-658-29267-6_42

In this work, we investigate three lumen-extraction independent deep learning algorithms for the task of predicting the revascularisation decision and the significance of a stenosis on a lesion-level. We propose a multi-view 2.5D approach, which we compare with two previously published methods, a 3D-RCNN approach [4] and a multi-view texture-based ensemble approach [5]. Additionally, we introduce adaptions to improve the performance of all approaches on our task. These include resizing lesions to an intermediate length instead of padding them and the usage of test-time augmentations. Also, we propose to use a different feature extraction backbone than described in [5] for the respective approach. Note that both reference approaches were originally used to detect lesions and characterise them. Contrary to this we characterise annotated lesions with a defined start and end point.

2   Material and methods

2.1   Data

The data collection used contains CCTA scans from 95 patients with suspected coronary artery disease taken within 2 years at the same clinical site. For each patient, the resulting clinical decision regarding revascularisation was made by trained cardiologists, based on different clinical indications. This decision was monitored on a branch level. Lesions were annotated using their start and end point on the centerline, which was extracted automatically using the method described in [6]. We binarise the stenosis grade, which is estimated based on the lumen segmentation and defined as the ratio between the actual lumen and an estimated healthy lumen, using a threshold of 50 %. The branch-wise revascularisation decision is propagated only to the lesion with the highest stenosis grade in branches known to be revascularised. Of the total of 345 lesions in our data set, 85 lesions exhibit a significant stenosis grade, and 93 require revascularisation.

2.2   Methods

2.2.1   3D-RCNN The first network we use is identical to the method described in [4]. In this approach, after extracting the coronary centerlines, a multi-planar reformatted (MPR) image stack is created by interpolating an orthogonal plane for each centerline point. Next, the MPR image stack is cut into a sequence of 25 overlapping cubes with size 25x25x25 and a stride of 5. During training, data augmentation using random rotations around the centerline and random shifts in all directions is used. Moreover, the data set is resampled for batch creation to achieve class balance during training. Since detection instead of sole characterisation is performed in [4], padding the inputs to the same length was not needed in their work.

2.2.2   Texture-based multi-view 2D-CNN The second baseline approach is described in reference [5]. A VGG-M network backbone pretrained on the

ImageNet challenge dataset is used as a texture-based feature extractor. The extracted features are encoded as Fisher vectors and used for classification using a linear support vector machine. As inputs for this classification pipeline, different 2D views of the MPR image stack are combined for a final vote.

2.2.3   2.5D-CNN Both aforementioned methods utilize a sliced 3D representation of the lesion or a multitude of 2D representations, which is computationally expensive to obtain and to process by the subsequent machine learning pipeline. To mitigate this, we propose a 2.5D multi-view approach as shown in Figure 1. From the MPR image stack, only two orthogonal slices are selected, concatenated and forwarded to a 2D-CNN.

2.2.4   Modifications In this work, we examine the effect of three different padding strategies for all three approaches: zero-padding, stretching the volume stack to the longest lesion and resizing all lesions to an intermediate size. Stretching and squeezing of the image stacks along the centerline is performed with linear interpolation. Each MPR image stack for each lesion has a resolution of 64x32x32 and 170x32x32 after padding depending on the method used. For the 3D-RCNN approach, we downscale the y and x dimension further to 25x25 to match the original algorithm described in [4]. For augmentation of the data set all single volumes are rotated around the centerline in steps of 20°, which leads to an 18 times larger data collection. In order to create valid rotational augmentations of the image stack without cropping artefacts, we cut out a cylindrical ROI and set all values around it to zero. We confirmed in preliminary experiments that this computationally cheaper procedure does not to impact the results compared to cutting out a rotated view from the original data. In contrast to [4, 5], no class resampling was necessary during training, since the class imbalance is not as severe for classification given the start and end point of a lesion compared to detecting lesions as well. Instead of the originally proposed VGG-M backbone used in [5], we use the VGG-16 network architecture as a backbone since it was already shown to yield better performance in the original paper on texture-based filter banks [7]. The data set was normalised to fit ImageNet statistics. We also evaluate the performance of this approach using a pretrained Resnet50 architecture [8] as backbone.

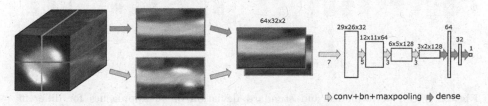

Fig. 1. Algorithm overview: Extraction of two orthogonal views of the lesion of interest. These are concatenated and then used as an input for a 2D-CNN (conv = convolutional layer, bn = batch normalisation layer, dense = fully connected layer).

Table 1. Results for predicting stenosis degree prediction on a lesion-level (18 and 8 correspond to the amount of views considered for data augmentation during training and test time, + = single view classification, * = combined view classification, | | = resizing to intermediate size, | → | = resizing to the longest sequence).

Model/Metric	AUC	Accuracy	F1-score	Sensitivity	Specificity	MCC
3D-RCNN[4, 9]	0.89	0.85	0.67	*0.79*	0.86	0.59
3D-RCNN[4]$^{18|}$ $^|$	*0.92±0.03*	0.88±0.02	0.69±0.06	0.68±0.11	0.93±0.03	0.62±0.06
2D[5]$^{8*|→|VGG}$	0.85±0.07	0.86±0.04	0.62±0.10	0.56±0.15	0.94±0.02	0.54±0.12
2D[5]$^{18+|}$ $^{|RES}$	0.78±0.04	0.82±0.03	0.61±0.05	0.70±0.08	0.85±0.03	0.50±0.06
2D[5]$^{18*|}$ $^{|RES}$	0.90±0.04	0.87±0.03	0.68±0.08	0.71±0.13	0.91±0.03	0.60±0.09
2.5D$^{18+|}$ $^|$	*0.92±0.03*	0.89±0.02	0.70±0.06	0.64±0.10	0.95±0.03	0.64±0.06
2.5D$^{18*|}$ $^|$	*0.92±0.03*	*0.90±0.02*	*0.71±0.07*	0.64±0.10	*0.96±0.03*	*0.66±0.08*

2.2.5 Evaluation No hyperparameter optimisation is performed. Parameters are either taken from the references or default values are used. To reduce the influence of random weight initialisation and other random effects on the results, we repeat a 5-fold cross validation with five different initialisations, leaving a total of 25 splits. All splits are performed patient-wise. We also use the aforementioned rotational augmentation during test-time, and compare how the mean prediction over all rotations performs in comparison to a single input.

3 Results

The most important results are provided in Table 1, Table 2 and Figure 2. The results for the 3D-RCNN approach are also compared to the results of our previous work [9], where similar experiments are performed on the same data set as here but with the workflow described in [4], zero-padding and a different

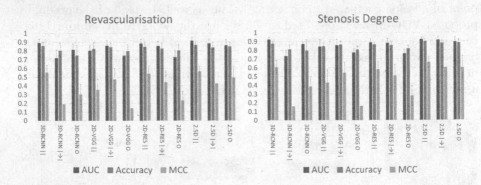

Fig. 2. Mean performance and standard deviation of all approaches for different padding strategies. These experiments are performed using only 8 instead of the 18 views (| | = resizing to intermediate size, | → | = resizing to the longest sequence, O = zero padding or no padding for the texture-based approach, MCC = Matthews correlation coefficient).

cross validation strategy. From the three padding methods examined, resizing all volume stacks of the data collection to one intermediate size yields the best results for most network approaches except for the texture-based approach with the VGG-16 backbone, where resizing all lesions to the size of the largest volume performs best. Interestingly, the same algorithm workflow with the Resnet50 backbone performs differently in that regard. A hypothesis that can be drawn from the intermediate padding performing best is that this scale provides on the one hand roughly the same amount of information per sample while on the other hand also keeping the input size in a range where it can be processed better. For the 3D-RCNN, we only look at classification in this work, in contrast to the task in [4] which included the detection of lesions. For this target, the proposed adaptations to the workflow in terms of padding strategy and not resampling the data set during batch creation improves the performance of both predicting the stenosis degree and the revascularisation decision from an AUC of 0.89 to 0.92, and 0.80 to 0.90, respectively. Having a more powerful feature extractor network for the texture-based approach combined with slightly more data augmentation improves the AUC by 0.05 for classifying stenosis significance, and by 0.04 for classifying revascularisation decision. The method performs considerably better when using test augmentations than without. Our proposed approach performs similar to the other two approaches, outperforming them by a small margin with an AUC of 0.92/0.90 for predicting a significant stenosis/revascularisation decision. Interestingly, test augmentations only yield a small improvement. This suggests that the method already has all necessary information to predict the task at hand from two orthogonal slices.

4   Discussion

In this paper, we compared and improved three segmentation independent deep learning-based algorithms for predicting both significant stenosis degree and clinical revascularisation decision for lesions annotated with a start and end point. We obtained comparable results for each method. Our proposed method – a 2.5D approach – slightly outperforms the other approaches and requires fewer views compared to the method previously described in [5]. Therefore, a faster training

Model/Metric	AUC	Accuracy	F1-score	Sensitivity	Specificity	MCC
3D-RCNN[4, 9]	0.80	0.76	0.55	*0.72*	0.77	0.42
3D-RCNN[4][18]	0.90±0.05	0.84±0.10	0.63±0.10	0.65±0.13	0.90±0.12	0.53±0.11
2D[5][8*]→[VGG]	0.86±0.06	0.84±0.05	0.56±0.12	0.49±0.16	0.93±0.02	0.47±0.13
2D[5][18+][RES]	0.77±0.06	0.81±0.03	0.60±0.06	0.68±0.12	0.84±0.02	0.48±0.07
2D[5][18*][RES]	0.90±0.06	0.85±0.05	0.66±0.07	0.70±0.16	0.89±0.04	0.57±0.10
2.5D[18+]	*0.90±0.04*	0.87±0.05	0.65±0.05	0.60±0.11	0.94±0.04	0.58±0.06
2.5D[18*]	*0.90±0.04*	*0.88±0.05*	*0.67±0.06*	0.61±0.11	*0.95±0.04*	*0.60±0.07*

Table 2. Results for predicting the revascularisation decision on a lesion-level (Abbreviations as in Table 1).

procedure and inference is possible. In future work, we will examine whether this method is also capable of detecting lesions instead of just classifying them, and whether it is able to predict an abnormal FFR value.

Disclaimer The methods and information here are based on research and are not commercially available.

References

1. Mendis S, Davis S, Norrving B. Organizational update: the world health organization global status report on noncommunicable diseases 2014. Stroke. 2015;46(5):e121–e122.
2. Taylor CA, Fonte TA, Min JK. Computational fluid dynamics applied to cardiac computed tomography for noninvasive quantification of fractional flow reserve: scientific basis. JACC. 2013;61(22):2233–2241.
3. Wels M, Lades F, Hopfgartner C, et al. Intuitive and accurate patient-specific coronary tree modeling from cardiac computed-tomography angiography. In: The 3rd interactive MIC Workshop; 2016. p. 86–93.
4. Zreik M, et al. A recurrent CNN for automatic detection and classification of coronary artery plaque and stenosis in coronary CT angiography. IEEE Transactions on Medical Imaging. 2018;38(7):1588–1598.
5. Tejero-de Pablos A, et al. Texture-Based classification of significant stenosis in CCTA multi-view images of coronary arteries. In: MICCAI. Springer; 2019. p. 732–740.
6. Zheng Y, Tek H, Funka-Lea G. Robust and accurate coronary artery centerline extraction in CTA by combining model-driven and data-driven approaches. In: MICCAI. Springer; 2013. p. 74–81.
7. Cimpoi M, Maji S, Vedaldi A. Deep filter banks for texture recognition and segmentation. In: Proceedings of the IEEE conference on computer vision and pattern recognition; 2015. p. 3828–3836.
8. He K, Zhang X, Ren S, et al. Deep residual learning for image recognition. In: Proceedings of the IEEE conference on computer vision and pattern recognition; 2016. p. 770–778.
9. Denzinger F, et al. Coronary artery plaque characterization from CCTA scans using deep learning and radiomics. In: MICCAI. Springer; 2019. p. 593–601.

Abstract: Unsupervised Anomaly Localization Using Variational Auto-Encoders

David Zimmerer[1], Fabian Isensee[1], Jens Petersen[1], Simon Kohl[1], Klaus Maier-Hein[1]

German Cancer Research Center (DKFZ), Heidelberg, Germany
d.zimmerer@dkfz.de

An assumption-free automatic check of medical images for potentially over-seen anomalies would be a valuable assistance for a radiologist. Deep learning and especially Variational Auto-Encoders (VAEs) have shown great potential in the unsupervised learning of data distributions. In principle, this allows for such a check and even the localization of parts in the image that are most suspicious. Currently, however, the reconstruction-based localization by design requires adjusting the model architecture to the specific problem looked at during evaluation. This contradicts the principle of building assumption-free models. We propose complementing the localization part with a term derived from the Kullback-Leibler (KL)-divergence. For validation, we perform a series of experiments on FashionMNIST as well as on a medical task including >1000 healthy and >250 brain tumor patients. Results show that the proposed formalism outperforms the state of the art VAE-based localization of anomalies across many hyperparameter settings and also shows a competitive max performance. This work was previously presented at MICCAI 2019 [1].

References

1. Zimmerer D, Isensee F, Petersen J, et al.; Springer. Unsupervised anomaly localization using variational auto-encoders. Proc MICCAI. 2019;.

© Springer Fachmedien Wiesbaden GmbH, ein Teil von Springer Nature 2020
T. Tolxdorff et al. (Hrsg.), *Bildverarbeitung für die Medizin 2020*,
Informatik aktuell, https://doi.org/10.1007/978-3-658-29267-6_43

Abstract: Coronary Artery Plaque Characterization from CCTA Scans Using DL and Radiomics

Felix Denzinger[1,2], Michael Wels[2], Katharina Breininger[1], Anika Reidelshöfer[3], Joachim Eckert[4], Michael Sühling[2], Axel Schmermund[4], Andreas Maier[1]

[1]Pattern Recognition Lab, Friedrich-Alexander-University Erlangen-Nuremberg, Erlangen, Germany
[2]Computed Tomography, Siemens Healthcare GmbH, Forchheim, Germany
[3]University Clinic Frankfurt, Frankfurt am Main, Germany
[4]Cardioangiological Centrum Bethanien, Frankfurt am Main, Germany
felix.denzinger@fau.de

Assessing coronary artery plaque segments in coronary CT angiography scans is an important task to improve patient management and clinical outcomes, as it can help to decide whether invasive investigation and treatment are necessary. In this work, we present three machine learning approaches capable of performing this task. The first approach is based on radiomics, where a plaque segmentation is used to calculate various shape-, intensity- and texture-based features under different image transformations. A second approach is based on deep learning and relies on centerline extraction as sole prerequisite. In the third approach, we fuse the deep learning approach with radiomic features. On our data the methods reached similar scores as simulated fractional flow reserve (FFR) measurements, which - in contrast to our methods - requires an exact segmentation of the whole coronary tree and often time-consuming manual interaction. In literature, the performance of simulated FFR reaches an AUC between 0.79-0.93 predicting an abnormal invasive FFR that demands revascularization. The radiomics approach achieves an AUC of 0.86, the deep learning approach 0.84 and the combined method 0.88 for predicting the revascularization decision directly. While all three proposed methods can be determined within seconds, the FFR simulation typically takes several minutes. Provided representative training data in sufficient quantities, we believe that the presented methods can be used to create systems for fully automatic non-invasive risk assessment for a variety of adverse cardiac events [1].

Disclaimer The methods and information here are based on research and are not commercially available.

References

1. Denzinger F, et al. Coronary artery plaque characterization from CCTA scans using deep learning and radiomics. In: Proc MICCAI; 2019. p. 593–601.

© Springer Fachmedien Wiesbaden GmbH, ein Teil von Springer Nature 2020
T. Tolxdorff et al. (Hrsg.), *Bildverarbeitung für die Medizin 2020*,
Informatik aktuell, https://doi.org/10.1007/978-3-658-29267-6_44

Quantitative Comparison of Generative Shape Models for Medical Images

Hristina Uzunova[1], Paul Kaftan[1], Matthias Wilms[2], Nils D. Forkert[2],
Heinz Handels[1], Jan Ehrhardt[1]

[1]Institute of Medical Informatics, University of Lübeck, Germany
[2] Department of Radiology, University of Calgary, Canada
uzunova@imi.uni-luebeck.de

Abstract. Generative shape models play an important role in medical image analysis. Conventional methods like PCA-based statistical shape models (SSMs) and their various extensions have shown great success modeling natural shape variations in medical images, despite their limitations. Corresponding deep learning-based methods like (variational) autoencoders are well known to overcome many of those limitations. In this work, we compare two conventional and two deep learning-based generative shape modeling approaches to shed light on their limitations and advantages. Experiments on a publicly available 2D chest X-ray data set show that the deep learning methods achieve better specificity and generalization abilities for large training set sizes. However, for smaller training sets, the conventional SSMs are more robust and their latent space is more compact and easier to interpret.

1 Introduction

Generative models are widely used in medical image analysis to encode prior knowledge about plausible anatomical or physiological shape variations to either explicitly aid segmentation and registration tasks or for data augmentation purposes in deep learning approaches [1, 2]. A typical example of a widely used subclass of generative models are PCA-based statistical shape models (SSMs)[3]. SSMs learn a low-dimensional linear manifold of plausible shapes based on a training population. However, despite their success in many real-world applications, SSMs have a number of limitations: 1) They rely on point-based 1-to-1 correspondences between training shapes that usually need to be established in time-consuming and error-prone preprocessing steps. 2) Due to their linear nature, they frequently fail to adequately model the underlying complex shape manifold. 3) Many training samples are needed to model anatomical details, especially in multi-object scenarios. Over the years, several approaches have been proposed to alleviate the problems related to 2) and/or 3) via kernel PCA [4], wavelet-decomposition [5], or multi-resolution approaches [6].

H. Uzunova and P. Kaftan contributed equally to this work.

© Springer Fachmedien Wiesbaden GmbH, ein Teil von Springer Nature 2020
T. Tolxdorff et al. (Hrsg.), *Bildverarbeitung für die Medizin 2020*,
Informatik aktuell, https://doi.org/10.1007/978-3-658-29267-6_45

More recently, the research focus has shifted towards deep learning-based generative modeling using approaches like autoencoders (AEs). Like SSMs, AEs learn latent representations of the training data, to capture their natural variations in a low-dimensional space. As the AE's latent space distribution is unknown and possibly implausible, a variational extension of AEs (VAEs) [7] was introduced, in which the latent space is constrained in a more plausible way making them more suitable for shape modeling. Neural networks are generally able to learn complex non-linear functions that capture the large variability of medical data and thus can successfully cope with the challenges of flexibility and non-linearity. In addition, (V)AEs can operate directly on label images and correspondences do not have to be established explicitly. However, their training still requires huge amounts of data and they are not as easy to interpret as their more traditional counterparts, making it harder to assess their plausibility.

So far, traditional SSMs and deep learning-based methods have been rarely compared in a systematic and consistent manner. This works aims to close this gap by evaluating the performance and properties of two traditional approaches (SSMs and their locality-based extension [6] (LSSMs)) and two deep learning methods (AEs and VAEs) on a common, public data set.

2   Materials and methods

2.1   Statistical shape models

SSMs are built using a training set of n discrete, vectorized shape representations $\mathbf{X}_1 \ldots \mathbf{X}_n$. Here, each $\mathbf{X}_i \in \mathrm{R}^{dm}$ is composed of the d sub-coordinates of all m landmarks representing the object's shape in a d-dimensional space. The steps to create an SSM are: 1) Compute the mean shape $\mathbf{X}_\mu = 1/n \sum_{i=1}^n \mathbf{X}_i$. 2) Eigen-decomposition of the covariance matrix $\mathbf{C} = 1/n \sum_{i=1}^n (\mathbf{X}_i - \mathbf{X}_\mu)(\mathbf{X}_i - \mathbf{X}_\mu)^T$. By retaining only the eigenvectors $\mathbf{u}_1, \ldots, \mathbf{u}_p$ corresponding to the p largest eigenvalues $\lambda_1, \ldots, \lambda_p$ of $\mathbf{C}$, a p-dimensional affine subspace of maximum shape variation with translation vector $\mathbf{X}_\mu$ and orthonormal basis $\mathbf{U} = [\mathbf{u}_1, \ldots, \mathbf{u}_p] \in \mathrm{R}^{dm \times p}$ is created. Embedding space and affine subspace are connected via $\mathbf{X} = \mathbf{X}_\mu + \mathbf{U}\mathbf{z}$ and $\mathbf{z} = \mathbf{U}^T(\mathbf{X} - \mathbf{X}_\mu)$, where $\mathbf{z} \in \mathrm{R}^p$ is the low-dimensional latent space representation of $\mathbf{X} \in \mathrm{R}^{dm}$. Hence, by varying $\mathbf{z}$, new shapes can be sampled from the subspace.

2.2   Locality-based multi-resolution statistical shape modeling

In SSMs, the number of training samples n influences the flexibility of the model (= subspace size) because p is bounded by $min(n, dm)$. Usually, a small p means that the model mainly covers global shape variations. Therefore, additional flexibility can be introduced by breaking up global relations and assuming that local shape variations have limited effects in distant areas. This idea can be integrated into the traditional SSM framework by manipulating the covariances $C_{i,j}$ in $\mathbf{C}$ based on the distance between the points associated with them on the shape (here, covariances are reduced using a distance-related Gaussian function)[6]. By choosing a sequence of standard deviations for the Gaussian function $\tau_1 > \tau_2 > \ldots > \tau_r$ to differentiate distant and local shape parts, SSMs at different levels of locality are generated. Those models are then fused into a single affine subspace with global and local variability that exhibits a higher flexibility than a standard SSM [6].

2.3 Autoencoders

AEs are typically neural networks that learn a low-dimensional mapping of high--dimensional input data. They consist of two main parts: An encoder $Q(X)$, which maps the input X to a latent vector $\mathbf{z} \in \mathrm{R}^p$; and a decoder $P(\mathbf{z})$ that tries to reconstruct the input X given only $\mathbf{z}$. For simplicity, we assume that X is a shape describing image (e.g. label image). The latent space mapping makes AEs suitable for representation learning, since $\mathbf{z}$ assumably contains all of the important information for the representation of the input image. To ensure $X \approx P(Q(X))$, a so-called reconstruction loss based on the sum of differences or cross-entropy is usually used. Subsequently, unseen samples can be reconstructed by sending them through a trained encoder and decoder. New shapes can be generated by sampling random latent vectors $\mathbf{z}$ and applying a trained decoder $P(\mathbf{z})$. However, since the distribution of the latent space is unknown, a random sample can lie far away from the learned samples leading to unrealistic shapes.

2.4 Variational autoencoders

VAEs [7] are an extension of AEs addressing two main problems: 1) The AEs can simply learn the identity function; and 2) Drawing random samples from the latent space to generate new images might lead to implausible results, since the distribution of the latent space is unknown. VAEs overcome those issues by assuming a prior distribution $d(\mathbf{z})$ over the latent space, typically a normal distribution. To implement this in practice, the lower bound can be expressed as

$$\mathbb{E}\left[\log p(X|\mathbf{z})\right] - \mathcal{D}_{KL}\left[q(\mathbf{z}|X)||d(\mathbf{z})\right] \tag{1}$$

where $p(X|\mathbf{z})$ is the decoder's probability to reconstruct X from $\mathbf{z}$ and thus the first term is a reconstruction loss (as in AE); and $q(\mathbf{z}|X)$ is the encoders probability to map X to $\mathbf{z}$, constrained by the KL divergence $\mathcal{D}_{KL}$ between the latent space and the prior distribution $d(\mathbf{z})$. When $d(\mathbf{z}) \sim \mathcal{N}(0,1)$ and $\mathbf{z} \sim \mathcal{N}(\boldsymbol{\mu}(X), \boldsymbol{\sigma}(X))$, $\mathcal{D}_{KL}$ can be computed in closed form [7]. Unseen samples can still be reconstructed in a similar way to AEs. However, the main advantage is that new realistic shapes can be generated by sampling latent vectors from a normal distribution and decoding them.

3   Experiments and results

The goal of our experiments is to analyze and compare the properties of the four different modeling approaches discussed in Sec. 2 using a common data set. To this end, the publicly available 2D chest radiograph dataset from [8] is used. It contains 247 images with ground truth segmentations of five structures (left and right lung, left and right clavicle, and the heart). See [8] for details.

3.1   Specificity and generalization

In a first experiment, all four methods are compared in terms of generalization and specificity for different training set sizes [9]. the available 247 images are used in a 5-fold-cross-validation manner with varying training set sizes (min: 5, max: 113). the generalization ability is measured as the accuracy of reconstructed unseen test data sets as explained in sec. 2. for specificity, 100 normally distributed random samples are generated for each method. for all methods, we sample from $\backslash(\boldsymbol{\mu}_t, \boldsymbol{\sigma}_t)$, where $\boldsymbol{\mu}_t$ and $\boldsymbol{\sigma}_t$ are the estimated mean and standard deviation of the latent variables of the training data set. we use the average symmetric contour distance (ASCD) and the hausdorff distance (HD) as evaluation measures for both properties. the (V)AEs are modelled as neural networks, where the inputs/outputs are channel-wise one-hot-encoded label images. affine data augmentation is applied and a class-weighted dice loss is used as reconstruction loss, since the labels significantly vary in terms of size. the SSM are directly applied on the point coordinates of the corresponding contour landmarks given in [8].

The results for all four methods – AE, VAE, SSM, and LSSM – are shown in Fig. 1. Both deep learning methods show overall better results in terms of specificity. However, for small training set sizes (< 20), the LSSM model shows slightly improved generalization abilities and specificity, especially notable in terms of Hausdorff distances, since LSSM is constrained to roughly preserve the topological structures. When directly compared, the AE shows better results for generalization and the VAE for specificity. This corresponds to the intuition that the latent space of AEs does not have a known distribution. Thus, random sampling with a normal distribution leads to unrealistic images. Both models benefit from a larger latent space ($p =256$ vs. $p =512$). The two SSM models are far less specific than the AEs, but LSSM has similar generalization abilities. Overall, SSM has worse generalization abilities than LSSM, while the latter is less specific. A large drawback of the deep learning models is also apparent: For smaller training set sizes, the models are not able to reconstruct all labels, especially small labels like the clavicles. Thus, the percentage of labels not assigned is fairly high. When labels are missing, they are excluded from the evaluation. To sum up, for large training set sizes the (V)AE models offer the best trade-off between specificity and generalization abilities. For smaller training sets, SSMs are more robust, since they always generate all structures.

3.2   Latent space

In the second experiment, we analyze the latent space of the methods. to this end, all models are evaluated in terms of compactness (= size of the latent space p) [9]. for the traditional model, the latent space usually grows with the number of training images, resulting in mean values in the interval [3.4, 14.2] for the SSM and [45.6, 54.8] for the LSSM. these numbers indicate fairly compact latent spaces. for the (V)AE models, the latent space size needs to be chosen by the user. in our experiments, we tested $p = 512$ and $p = 256$ for all training set sizes, with differences more pronounced for smaller training sets (fig. 1). note, the SSM-based models operate on point coordinates whereas the autoencoders use label images, which might affect the size of the latent space needed to encode the variability. to further investigate the structure of the latent spaces of the methods, we linearly interpolate between the latent vectors of two randomly chosen images and project the interpolated vectors back to image space. the results for SSM and VAE are shown in fig. 2 and indicate that smooth interpolations are possible, leading to the conclusion that both latent spaces are well structured in accordance with their definition.

An important difference between the models is that, in contrast to SSMs, AEs do not guarantee that the latent vector of a reconstructed image matches the latent vector of the original image. For our next experiment, we, therefore, calculate the distance $dist(\mathbf{z}, \mathbf{z}')$, where $\mathbf{z}$ is the encoding of the input image: $\mathbf{z} = Q(X)$ and $\mathbf{z}'$ is the encoding of the reconstructed image: $\mathbf{z}' = Q(X'), X' = P(\mathbf{z})$, where Q and P are the trained encoder and decoder, respectively. The average

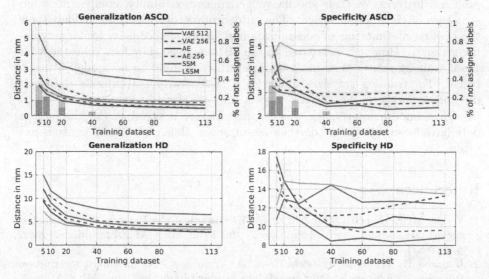

Fig. 1. Generalization ability and specificity of the four models – SSM, LSSM, VAE and AE – for varying training set sizes (lower values are better). Top: average symmetric contour distance; bottom: Hausdorff distance. The bars indicate the overall average percentage (right y axis) of labels not generated during calculation (purple: AE, blue; VAE). Dashed lines indicate smaller latent space size (256) for the VAE and AE models.

Fig. 2. Projected latent interpolation between two shapes. Top: SSM; bottom: VAE.

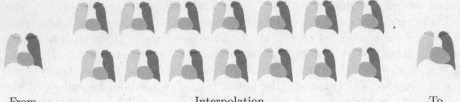

From   Interpolation   To

over all training data is computed for the best models (123 training images and 512 latent size) in a 5-fold-cross-validation manner. For the VAE we set $dist(\cdot, \cdot)$ to the Euclidean distance. Since the AE latent space is not normally distributed, the Mahalanobis distance is applied and distances are averaged over 100 training images. As baseline, we approximate the mean pairwise distance of the latent encodings of the training data. Values obtained are: VAE $dist(\mathbf{z}, \mathbf{z}')=1.16$ (baseline 1.89); AE $dist(\mathbf{z}, \mathbf{z}')=11.16$ (baseline 16.57). The reconstructed images get encoded close to their original latent vector, but the vectors substantially differ, indicating an ambiguity of the latent space.

4   Discussion and conclusion

In this work, we analyzed and compared four generative shape modeling approaches in terms of their specificity, generalization ability, compactness and structure of their latent space. The autoencoding deep learning models show the best results in terms of generalization ability, and specificity for large training set sizes. However, compared to the SSM models, they lack robustness for small training sets, where small or rare structures tend to be modelled incorrectly. For training set sizes under 20, LSSM clearly outperforms the other methods. Furthermore, the AE models are considerably less compact. Even though a smooth interpolation in the latent space is possible, (V)AEs lack or only have loose constraints on their latent space, thus their unambiguity is not given.

References

1. Wilms M, Ehrhardt J, Handels H. A 4D statistical shape model for automated segmentation of lungs with large tumors. In: Proc. MICCAI 2012. Springer; 2012. p. 347–354.
2. Uzunova H, Wilms M, Handels H, et al. Training CNNs for image registration from few samples with model-based data augmentation. In: Proc. MICCAI 2017. Springer; 2017. p. 223–231.
3. Cootes TF, Taylor CJ, Cooper DH, et al. Active shape models & their training and application. Comput Vis Image Underst. 1995 Jan;61(1):38–59.
4. Kirschner M, Becker M, Wesarg S. 3D active shape model segmentation with nonlinear shape priors. In: Proc. MICCAI 2011. Springer; 2011. p. 492–499.

5. Davatzikos C, Xiaodong Tao, Dinggang Shen. Hierarchical active shape models, using the wavelet transform. IEEE Trans Med Imaging. 2003 Mar;22(3):414–423.
6. Wilms M, Handels H, Ehrhardt J. Multi-resolution multi-object statistical shape models based on the locality assumption. Med Image Anal. 2017 May;38:17–29.
7. Kingma DP, Welling M. Auto-encoding variational bayes. In: Proc. ICLR; 2014. p. 1–14.
8. van Ginneken B, Stegmann MB, Loog M. Segmentation of anatomical structures in chest radiographs using supervised methods: a comparative study on a public database. Med Image Anal. 2006;10(1):19–40.
9. Davies RH, Twining CJ, Cootes TF, et al. A minimum description length approach to statistical shape modeling. IEEE Trans Med Imaging. 2002 May;21(5):525–537.

Abstract: FastSurfer
A Fast and Accurate Deep Learning Based Neuroimaging Pipeline

Leonie Henschel[1], Sailesh Conjeti[1], Santiago Estrada[1], Kersten Diers[1], Bruce Fischl[2,3,4], Martin Reuter[1,2,3]

[1]German Center for Neurodegenerative Diseases (DZNE), Bonn, Germany
[2]A.A. Martinos Center for Biomedical Imaging, MGH, Boston MA, USA
[3]Department of Radiology, Harvard Medical School, Boston MA,USA
[4]Computer Science and Artificial Intelligence Laboratory, MIT, Cambridge MA, USA
`martin.reuter@dzne.de`

Traditional neuroimage analysis pipelines involve computationally intensive, time-consuming optimization steps, and thus, do not scale well to large cohort studies. With FastSurfer [1] we propose a fast deep-learning based alternative for the automated processing of structural human MRI brain scans, including surface reconstruction and cortical parcellation. FastSurfer consists of an advanced deep learning architecture (FastSurferCNN) used to segment a whole brain MRI into 95 classes in under 1 min, and a surface pipeline building upon this high-quality brain segmentation. FastSurferCNN incorporates local and global competition via competitive dense blocks and competitive skip pathways, as well as multi-slice information aggregation that specifically tailor network performance towards accurate recognition of both cortical and sub-cortical structures. We demonstrate the superior performance of FastSurferCNN across five different datasets where it consistently outperforms existing deep learning approaches in terms of accuracy by a margin. Further, we perform fast cortical surface reconstruction and thickness analysis by introducing a spectral spherical embedding and by directly mapping the cortical labels from the image to the surface. Precisely, we use the eigenfunctions of the Laplace-Beltrami operator to parametrize the surface smoothly and quickly generate the final spherical map by scaling the 3D spectral embedding vector to unit length. For sustainability of the pipeline we perform extensive validation of FastSurfer: we measure generalizability to different scanners, disease states, as well as an unseen acquisition sequence, demonstrate increased test-retest reliability, and increased sensitivity to disease effects relative to traditional FreeSurfer. In total, we provide a reliable full FreeSurfer alternative for volumetric analysis (within 1 minute) and surface-based thickness analysis (within only around 1h + optionally 30 min for group registration).

References

1. Henschel L, Conjeti S, Estrada S, et al. FastSurfer – a fast and accurate deep learning based neuroimaging pipeline. CoRR. 2019;abs/1910.03866.

© Springer Fachmedien Wiesbaden GmbH, ein Teil von Springer Nature 2020
T. Tolxdorff et al. (Hrsg.), *Bildverarbeitung für die Medizin 2020*,
Informatik aktuell, https://doi.org/10.1007/978-3-658-29267-6_46

VICTORIA

An Interactive Online Tool for the VIrtual Neck Curve and True Ostium Reconstruction of Intracranial Aneurysms

Benjamin Behrendt[1], Samuel Voss[2,3], Oliver Beuing[4], Bernhard Preim[1], Philipp Berg[2,3], Sylvia Saalfeld[1,3]

[1]Department of Simulation and Graphics, University of Magdeburg, Germany
[2]Department of Fluid & Technical Flows, University of Magdeburg, Germany
[3]Forschungscampus STIMULATE, University of Magdeburg, Germany
[4]Institute of Neuroradiology, University Hospital of Magdeburg, Germany
sylvia.saalfeld@ovgu.de

Abstract. For the characterization of intracranial aneurysms, morphological and hemodynamic parameters provide valuable information. To evaluate these quantities, the separation of the aneurysm from its parent vessel is required by defining a neck curve and the corresponding ostium. A fundamental problem of this concept is the missing ground truth. Recent studies report strong variations for this procedure between medical experts yielding increased interobserver variability for subsequent evaluations. To make further steps towards consensus, we present a web application solution, combining a client based on HTML and JavaScript and a server part utilizing PHP and the Matlab Runtime environment. Within this study, participants are requested to identify the neck curve of five virtual aneurysm models. Furthermore, they can manipulate the ostium surface to model the original parent artery. Our application is now available online and easily accessible for medical experts just requiring an internet browser.

1 Introduction

The assessment of intracranial aneurysm (IA) rupture risk increasingly depends on morphological as well as hemodynamic parameters that are calculated based on the aneurysm sac [1, 2]. Furthermore, therapy planning requires a detailed knowledge of the individual IA neck size to select an appropriate treatment strategy and device, respectively [3]. In addition, a virtual separation of the IA from the parent vessel allows for the extraction of parameters from a 3D model rather than 2D projected images in the clinical routine that suffer from increased user- as well as image (i.e. the viewing angle of the 2D projections) dependency [4].

© Springer Fachmedien Wiesbaden GmbH, ein Teil von Springer Nature 2020
T. Tolxdorff et al. (Hrsg.), *Bildverarbeitung für die Medizin 2020*,
Informatik aktuell, https://doi.org/10.1007/978-3-658-29267-6_47

However, the separation between parent vessel and aneurysm sac (i.e. the ostium) strongly varies, which might lead to insufficient analyses and in consequence to unreliable conclusions. The separation of the IA from the healthy parent vessel is often realized using a (planar) cut-plane [5, 6], which might be error-prone for complex IA shapes. In previous work, we developed a semi-automatic extraction of an anatomical, bent neck curve [7], but the question about the correct neck curve remains unanswered.

Therefore, VICTORIA (VIrtual neck Curve and True Ostium Reconstruction of Intracranial Aneurysms) aims at a standardization of IA neck curve and ostium reconstruction. For the definition of these neck curves and ostia, highly experienced physicians are required. Since their availability for user studies is limited due to the clinical work load, we developed an easy accessable framework solely requiring a web browser. Thus, we can gather expert-knowledge from physicians as well as biomedical engineers. The study has been successfully launched at https://VICTORIA.cs.ovgu.de/.

2   Materials and methods

Within the VICTORIA study, participants are requested to identify the neck curve of patient-specific IA models extracted from 3D digital subtraction data. The extraction of surface models is described in our previous work [8].

2.1   VICTORIA web application

The study is conducted using a specialized web application, consisting of two parts: a client part (written in HTML and JavaScript), and a server part (written in PHP and using Matlab runtime environment). The VICTORIA study can be accessed via the internet using a web browser. Between client and server, the data is exchanged in the JSON format. The server stores user-submitted data in a relational database, thus allowing for easy sorting and filtering of the data, see Fig. 1.

In order to keep the motivation to participate high, the user is directly presented with five datasets and two tasks, respectively. For both tasks, a surface

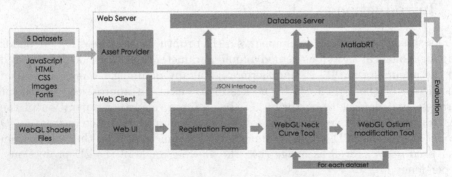

Fig. 1. Illustration of the different parts of the VICTORIA web application.

mesh of an IA and its parent vessel is shown. The rendering is performed using the WebGL2 API, thus allowing it to run in most current desktop browsers. The mesh is illuminated using the Phong lighting model to increase shape perception. The user has limited control over the camera (rotation, zoom and panning), ensuring that the neck region is always visible and centered in the image.

2.2   Neck curve definition

First, the user draws a neck curve onto the vessel mesh by selecting surface vertices, see Fig. 2. To connect the selected vertices into a circular path, the surface triangle mesh is interpreted as a bidirectional graph. The shortest paths between the selected points are then calculated using the A* algorithm by Hart et al. [9]. However, the A* algorithm is only designed to find the shortest path between two points, not the shortest path connecting a list of unordered points. To prevent having to force users to select the points in order and thus sacrificing usability, the list of points has to be sorted automatically. Here, a distance matrix stores the length of the shortest path between all points. Whenever a new point is added to the matrix, the distances to all other points are determined using A*. To sort the list of points, we begin with a list containing only one randomly chosen point. As long as there are points that have not been added to the list, we take the last entry, look up the closest point (based on the distance matrix) that has not been added yet, and add it to the back of the list. After all points have been processed, the resulting list contains the shortest path connecting all neck points selected by the user. The last and first point in the list will only be connected if their distance is shorter than the longest path between any of the other adjacent points in the list. This prevents the neck curve from closing before the user has finished adding all desired points. In case the resulting neck curve does not match the users' expectation additional points can be added.

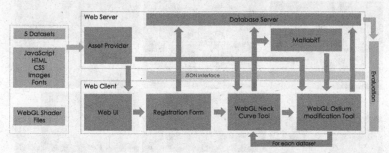

Fig. 2. The different steps of the ostium definition. (A) 3D visualization of the surface model with WebGL. (B) The user can interactively select points on the aneurysm surface. The points are automatically selected (see also inlay). (C) If the points are close to each other, the neck curve is automatically closed. (D) In the second step, an automatic ostium triangulation is provided. (E) The user can hover over the points and the active point is highlighted. (F) the point can be moved (including a reduced movement of its neighbors) until the user is satisfied with the ostium shape.

The sorting and path finding algorithm are implemented in JavaScript and are performed entirely on the client side. Even on less powerful devices, they run interactively without any noticeable delay.

2.3   Ostium creation and manipulation

After submitting the neck curve, the server calculates the associated ostium surface mesh. This step is implemented in Matlab, motivated by previous work [7] as well as to provide additional geometric functionalities and to spare the client's PC performance. To ensure the general applicability, we use the Matlab runtime environment and provide it at our linux server. The Matlab script receives the previously selected surface meshes and downsamples them to a predefined threshold. The process is illustrated in Fig. 3. For the illustration, the neck curve points are resampled to 32 points. The ostium triangulation is analytically defined and centered around the origin (z-coordinates equal 0). Next, the analytically defined border points are replaced by the neck curve points and simple Laplacian smoothing (50 iterations, $\sigma = 1.0$) is applied to all vertices except the border points, resulting in the smooth ostium surface (Fig. 3).

The second task consists of the adjustment of the previously calculated ostium surface. This is important to better approximate the inflow area for further postprocessing steps in order to better approximate the parent vessel's original geometry. During this task, only the backfaces of the vessel are rendered to reveal the ostium. The user can grab and drag any vertex of the ostium surface that is not part of its border. To keep the interaction as simple and straight-forward as possible, the vertices can only be moved in the direction of the average surface normal of the ostium. As moving one vertex at a time would be tedious, dragging one vertex by a distance of v also moves the surrounding vertices by a

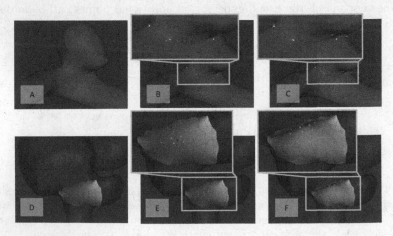

Fig. 3. Illustration of the ostium triangulation. The neck points are resampled to 32, p_1 - p_{32} (left). The pre-defined triangulation is centered around 0 with border points q_1 - q_{32} (center). Next, q_1 - q_{32} are replaced by p_1 - p_{32} and all points undergo Laplacian smoothing yielding the triangulated ostium surface.

distance of v_n based on their normalized Euclidean distance d_n to the original vertex. The parameter a controls the size of the affected area. We empirically determined a value of $\frac{1}{3}$ to result in an interaction that feels natural

$$v_n = v \cdot (max(0, d_n - (1 - a)) * a^{-1})^{0.75}$$

The second task can be considered optional, as it is possible for the user to directly accept and submit the ostium surface generated by the server without performing any modifications.

Finally, we implemented a registration form combined with a questionnaire. Users enter their name, e-mail address, occupation and employer, as well as answer questions about their experience with IAs. Thus, an examination of differences between user groups (e.g., physicians vs. engineers) can be conducted in the future.

3 Results

The VICTORIA study was implemented at the Otto-von-Guericke University, Magdeburg, Germany, and can be easily assessed at https://VICTORIA.cs.ovgu.de/. We tested this interactive survey sucessfully with three medical cooperation partners. They requested more hints and icons regarding the controlling of the application which we included. The neck curve definition requires approximately two minutes per case and less than ten minutes overall. The study requires the use of Mozilla Firefox or Google Chrome. Other, less commonly used browsers, such as Apple Safari or Microsoft Edge do not support the required WebGL technologies. The evaluation of the submitted ostia segmentations is not part of this work but ongoing research. In this work, the implementation of the web-based study is presented and the prototype does fulfill its purpose.

4 Discussion

Currently no ostium ground truth is available, yet it is required for many post-processing steps of IA models. We presented an approach that allows for an easy participation of international field experts and physicians by utilizing a combination of JavaScript, PHP and Matlab-programs, including 3D visualizations, editing and modification options.

Based on a ground truth ostium definition, a precise morphological evaluation of the 3D IA shape is further promoted, and it is highly beneficial for the quantification of hemodynamic flow simulations [10]. Furthermore, a 3D neck curve determination and subsequent parameter evaluation is superior to 2D analysis [4]. Particularly, since relevant blood flow parameters that are associated with rupture (e.g., normalized wall shear stress, shear concentration index, oscillatory shear index [11]) need to be calculated with high accuracy, wrong aneurysm-vessel-separation or high user-dependency can lead to clear variations regarding the analysis.

Furthermore, we expect our survey results to be utilized as ground truth data for deep learning-based ostium extraction approaches, e.g. similar to the MeshCNN network [12]. Finally, our architecture can be easily adapted to other medical image processing questions that require 3D models and user interaction.

Acknowledgement. This study was funded by the Federal Ministry of Education and Research in Germany within the Forschungscampus STIMULATE (grant number 13GW0095A) and the German Research Foundation (grant number SA 3461/2-1, BE 6230/2-1).

References

1. Detmer FJ, Chung BJ, Jimenez C, et al. Associations of hemodynamics, morphology, and patient characteristics with aneurysm rupture stratified by aneurysm location. Neuroradiology. 2019;61(3):275–284.
2. Niemann U, Berg P, Niemann A, et al. Rupture Status Classification of Intracranial Aneurysms Using Morphological Parameters. In: Proc. of IEEE Symposium on Computer-Based Medical Systems (CBMS); 2018. p. 48–53.
3. Paliwal N, Tutino V, Shallwani H, et al. Ostium ratio and neck ratio could predict the outcome of sidewall intracranial aneurysms treated with flow diverters. American Journal of Neuroradiology. 2019;40(2):288–294.
4. Wong SC, Nawawi O, Ramli N, et al. Benefits of 3D rotational DSA compared with 2D DSA in the evaluation of intracranial aneurysm. Acad Radiol. 2012;19(6):701–707.
5. Lauric A, Baharoglu MI, Malek AM. Ruptured status discrimination performance of aspect ratio, height/width, and bottleneck factor is highly dependent on aneurysm sizing methodology. Neurosurgery. 2012;71(1):38–46.
6. Xiang J, Natarajan SK, Tremmel M, et al. Hemodynamic–morphologic discriminants for intracranial aneurysm rupture. Stroke. 2011;42(1):144–152.
7. Saalfeld S, Berg P, Niemann A, et al. Semiautomatic neck curve reconstruction for intracranial aneurysm rupture risk assessment based on morphological parameters. Int J Comput Assist Radiol Surg. 2018;13(11):1781–1793.
8. Glaßer S, Berg P, Neugebauer M, et al. Reconstruction of 3D Surface Meshes for Bood Flow Simulations of Intracranial Aneurysms. In: Proc. of the Annual Meeting of the German Society of Computer- and Robot-Assisted Surgery (CURAC); 2015. p. 163–168.
9. Hart PE, Nilsson NJ, Raphael B. A formal basis for the heuristic determination of minimum cost paths. IEEE transactions on Systems Science and Cybernetics. 1968;4(2):100–107.
10. Berg P, Beuing O. Multiple intracranial aneurysms: a direct hemodynamic comparison between ruptured and unruptured vessel malformations. Int J Comput Assist Radiol Surg. 2018;13(1):83–93.
11. Cebral JR, Mut F, Weir J, et al. Quantitative characterization of the hemodynamic environment in ruptured and unruptured brain aneurysms. AJNR Am J Neuroradiol. 2011;32(1):145–151.
12. Hanocka R, Hertz A, Fish N, et al. MeshCNN: A Network with an Edge. ACM Trans Graph. 2019;38(4):90:1–90:12.

Abstract: Deep Probabilistic Modeling of Glioma Growth

Jens Petersen[1,2,3], Paul F. Jäger[1], Fabian Isensee[1], Simon A. A. Kohl[1*],
Ulf Neuberger[2], Wolfgang Wick[4], Jürgen Debus[5,6,7], Sabine Heiland[2],
Martin Bendszus[2], Philipp Kickingereder[2], Klaus H. Maier-Hein[1]

[1]Div. of Medical Image Computing, German Cancer Research Center
[2]Dept. of Neuroradiology, Heidelberg University Hospital
[3]Dept. of Physics & Astronomy, Heidelberg University
[4]Dept. of Neurooncology, Heidelberg University Hospital
[5]Div. of Molecular and Translational Radiation Oncology, Heidelberg Institute of
Radiation Oncology (HIRO)
[6]Heidelberg Ion-Beam Therapy Center (HIT), Heidelberg University Hospital
[7]Clinical Cooperation Unit Radiation Oncology, German Cancer Research Center
jens.petersen@dkfz.de

Existing approaches to modeling the dynamics of brain tumor growth, specifically glioma, employ biologically inspired models of cell diffusion, using image data to estimate the associated parameters. In this work, we propose to learn growth dynamics directly from annotated MR image data, without specifying an explicit model, leveraging recent developments in deep generative models. We further assume that imaging is ambiguous with respect to the underlying disease, which is reflected in our approach in that it doesn't predict a single growth estimate but instead estimates a distribution of plausible changes for a given tumor. In plain words, we're not interested in the question "How much will the tumor grow (or shrink)?" but instead "If the tumor were to grow (or shrink), what would it look like?". From a clinical perspective, this is relevant for example in radiation therapy, where a margin of possible infiltration around the tumor will also be irradiated. This is currently done in a rather crude fashion by isotropically expanding the tumor's outline, thus more informed estimates of growth patterns could help spare healthy tissue. In summary, our contributions are the following: 1. We frame tumor growth modeling as a model-free learning problem, so that all dynamics are inferred directly from data. 2. We present evidence that our approach learns a distribution of plausible growth trajectories, conditioned on previous observations of the same tumor. [1]

References

1. Petersen J, Jäger PF, Isensee F, et al. Deep probabilistic modeling of glioma growth. In: MICCAI 2019. vol. 11765 of LNCS. Springer; 2019. p. 806–814.

---

* now with DeepMind, the Karlsruhe Institute of Technology

© Springer Fachmedien Wiesbaden GmbH, ein Teil von Springer Nature 2020
T. Tolxdorff et al. (Hrsg.), *Bildverarbeitung für die Medizin 2020*,
Informatik aktuell, https://doi.org/10.1007/978-3-658-29267-6_48

Parameter Space CNN for Cortical Surface Segmentation

Leonie Henschel[1], Martin Reuter[1,2,3]

[1]German Center for Neurodegenerative Diseases (DZNE), Bonn, Germany
[2]A.A. Martinos Center for Biomedical Imaging, MGH, Boston MA, USA
[3]Department of Radiology, Harvard Medical School, Boston MA,USA
`martin.reuter@dzne.de`

Abstract. Spherical coordinate systems have become a standard for analyzing human cortical neuroimaging data. Surface-based signals, such as curvature, folding patterns, functional activations, or estimates of myelination define relevant cortical regions. Surface-based deep learning approaches, however, such as spherical CNNs primarily focus on classification and cannot yet achieve satisfactory accuracy in segmentation tasks. To perform surface-based segmentation of the human cortex, we introduce and evaluate a 2D parameter space approach with view aggregation (p^3CNN). We evaluate this network with respect to accuracy and show that it outperforms the spherical CNN by a margin, increasing the average Dice similarity score for cortical segmentation to above 0.9.

1 Introduction

Human cortical neuroimaging signals, such as cortical neuroanatomical regions or thickness are typically associated with the cortical surface. Thus, processing and analyzing these signals on geometric surface representations, rather than in a regular voxel grid, stays true to the underlying anatomy. As an example, smoothing kernels can be applied along the surface without the risk of blurring signal into neighboring structures such as cerebrospinal fluid (CSF), a neighboring gyrus, or the white matter (WM), which frequently occurs in a voxel grid. Here, these structures are in close proximity, while they are quite distant (e.g. neighboring gyrus) or non-existent (CSF, WM) on a cortical surface. Spherical coordinate systems have, therefore, become the standard for analyzing human cortical neuroimaging data [1]. Traditional algorithms are, however, computational expensive due to extensive numerical optimization and suffer from long run-times. This significantly limits their scalability to large-scale data analysis tasks. Therefore, supervised deep learning approaches are an attractive alternative due to their 2-3 orders of magnitude lower run-time. The new field of geometric deep learning offers great promise by providing ways to apply convolutional operations directly on a surface model. A subset of this field focuses on analyzing signals represented on spheres. However, these spherical convolutional neural networks (SCNNs) have mainly been proposed for classification

© Springer Fachmedien Wiesbaden GmbH, ein Teil von Springer Nature 2020
T. Tolxdorff et al. (Hrsg.), *Bildverarbeitung für die Medizin 2020*,
Informatik aktuell, https://doi.org/10.1007/978-3-658-29267-6_49

tasks with only one (the ugscnn [2]) being suitable for semantic segmentations. Traditional CNNs for voxel grid based segmentation tasks on the other hand are already well established and have thus been optimized to a great extent over the last few years. Potentially, a spherical signal can be mapped into the image space given an effective parameterization approach such as the mapping of the globe to a world map. A perfect (isometric) mapping between plane and sphere does, however, not exist leading to metric distortions and resulting in a non-uniform distribution of sample points which can affect regional segmentation quality. In this paper, we introduce a deep learning approach called parameter space CNN (p^3CNN; Fig. 1) for cortical segmentation. After reducing the problem from the sphere to a flat 2D grid via a latitude/colatitude parameterization a view aggregation scheme is used to alleviate errors introduced by distortion effects of a single parameterization. We finally train the network with multi--modal (thickness and curvature) maps and evaluate the results in comparison to a SCNN for segmentation (ugscnn) and the single view (parameterization) approach. We demonstrate that our p^3CNN achieves the highest accuracy on a variety of datasets.

2   Methodology

2.1   Network architecture

Within this paper we contrast a latitude/colatitude 2D parameterization (pCNN) and view aggregation scheme (p^3CNN) with an SCNN architecture [2] for semantic segmentation. For comparability, all networks are implemented with a consistent architecture, i.e. four encoding-decoding layers, same loss function, and equal number and dimension of convolutional kernels. All architectures are trained with a batch-size of 16 and an initial learning rate of 0.01 which is reduced every 20 epochs ($\gamma = 0.9$). After implementation in PyTorch all models are trained until convergence on one (p^3CNN) or eight (ugscnn) NVIDIA V100 GPUs to allow the aforementioned batch-size while maintaining comparability.

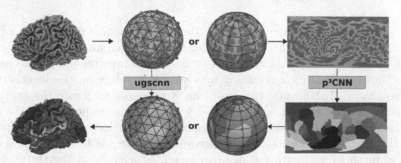

Fig. 1. Two segmentation networks are compared: a spherical CNN (ugscnn [2]) on the icosahedron (middle left) and our proposed view-aggregation on 2D spherical parameter spaces (p^3CNN, right). Both operate on curvature maps (top row) and thickness (not shown) for cortical segmentation of the cortex (bottom row).

2.1.1 Longitude/colatitude spherical parameterization Original signals, such as thickness, curvature and the cortical labels are defined on the left and right WM surfaces of each subject. First these surfaces are mapped to the sphere via a distortion minimizing inflation procedure [1]. We then map the cortical surface signals to a grid (i, j) in a 2D parameter space with 512×256 pixels (equal to 131072 vertices on the original sphere). To this end, we employ a longitude/colatitude coordinate system where each vertex position on the sphere (x, y, z) can be described by (i) the azimuthal angle $\varphi \in [0, 2\pi]$, (ii) the polar angle $\theta \in [0, \pi]$ and (iii) the radius r=100 via the spherical parameterization

$$x = r \, \sin \varphi \cos \theta, \quad y = r \, \sin \varphi \sin \theta, \quad z = r \, \cos \varphi \tag{1}$$

When sampling the (φ, θ) parameter space to the (i, j) grid, to avoid singularity issues at the poles, we shift the corresponding angles θ by half the grid width. After the transformation step, we sample the signal of interest (thickness, curvature or label map) at the given coordinates on the left and right hemisphere and project it onto the 2D parameter grid. The resulting parameter space "images" can then be fed into the multi-modal 2D deep learning segmentation architecture.

2.1.2 Parameter space CNN (pCNN) We use a DenseUNet [3] where each dense block consists of a sequence of three convolution layers with 64 kernels of size 3x3. Between the blocks, an index preserving max-pooling operation is used to half the feature map size. To enforce spherical topology while still permitting the use of standard convolution operations without loss of information at the image borders, we use a circular longitude padding. Prior to each convolution the left and right image borders are extended with values from the opposite side to provide a smooth transition. The horizontal borders are padded by splitting them in half and mirroring about the center (sideways) thereby modeling the transition across the poles. All networks are trained with two channels: thickness and curvature maps, which provide a representation of the underlying geometry of the cortex and are useful to e.g. locate region boundaries inside the sulcii.

2.1.3 View-aggregation (p³CNN) Due to the unequal distribution of grid points across the sphere in the longitude/colatitude parameterization, cortical regions mapping to the equator are less densely represented as those at the poles. Thus, segmentation accuracy may vary depending on the location of a given structure. To alleviate this problem, we propose to rotate the grid such that the poles are located along the x-, y- and z-axis, respectively. We then train one network per rotation and aggregate the resulting probability maps: (i) First, the label probabilities of each network are mapped to the original WM spherical mesh by computing a distance-weighted average of the three closest vertices on the sphere to each target vertex. (ii) Then, the three probability maps are averaged on a vertex-by-vertex basis to produce the final label map.

Due to the view aggregation across three parameter spaces, we term this approach p³CNN.

2.1.4 Spherical CNN The ugscnn [2] is selected for comparison with a geometric approach. Therein a linear combination of parameterized differential operators weighted by a learnable parameter represents the convolutional kernel. To allow well-defined coarsening of the grid in the downsampling step, the spherical domain is approximated by an icosahedral spherical mesh. Here, we use an icosahedron of level 7 as the starting point (163842 vertices) to approximate the original FreeSurfer sphere (average number of vertices: 132719) as close as possible.

2.1.5 Mapping The cortical thickness signal, the curvature maps and class labels defined in the subject's spherical space need to be mapped to the respective mesh architectures for both networks (i.e. icosahedron or polar grid). This is achieved via a distance weighted k-nearest neighbor regression and classification (i.e. majority voting). Equivalently, the final network predictions are mapped back to the subject's spherical space using the same technique. All evaluations are then performed in the original subject space, i.e., on the WM surface where the ground truth resides.

2.2 Evaluation

2.2.1 Surface-based dice similarity coefficient We evaluate the segmentation accuracy of the different models by comparing a surface-based Dice Similarity Coefficient (DSC) in the subject space on the original brain surface. With binary label maps of ground truth G and prediction P (1 at each labeled vertex, 0 outside), we modify the classic DSC as follows

$$DSC(G, P) = \frac{2\,area(G \cap P)}{area(G) + area(P)}, \; area(X) = \int_M X d_\sigma = a^T \cdot X \quad (2)$$

where $\cap$ is the element-wise product, and the *area* of a binary label X is its integral on the underlying Riemannian manifold M (here triangulated surface) which can be computed by the dot product of X and a where $a_i = \frac{1}{3}\sum T_i$, i.e. a third of the total area of all triangles T_i at vertex i. The DSC ranges from 0 to 1, with 1 indicating perfect overlap and 0 no similarity between the sets.

3 Results

We use five publicly available datasets (La5c [4], ADNI [5], MIRIAD [6], OASIS [7], ABIDE-II [8]) to train and evaluate our models. In total, 160 subjects balanced with regard to gender, age, diagnosis, and MR field-strength are used for training and 100 subjects for validation. Finally, we use 240 subjects from the Human Connectome Project (HCP) [9] as a completely independent testing set to measure segmentation accuracy. In our experiments, we utilize FreeSurfer [1] annotations of the cortical regions according to the "Desikan–Killiany–Tourville" (DKT) protocol atlas [10] as ground truth (Fig. 1). Fig. 2 represents the average

(left) and worst (right) DSC across all 32 cortical regions evaluated on the test
and validation set and pooled across hemispheres. The spherical CNN (green)
reaches the lowest DSC for all five datasets with an average DSC of 0.76. Introduction of our spherical parameterization approach (light blue, pCNN) already
outperforms the spherical CNN (green) with an up to 0.18 DSC point increase.
Note, that this improvement is already achieved in spite of the non-linear distortions induced by the latitude/colatitude parameterization. The view aggregation approach (dark blue, p³CNN) further increases the segmentation accuracy
and reaches the highest DSC for all six datatsets (all above 0.9). Further, our
proposed method improves the consistency of the segmentation accuracy. The
p³CNN has the lowest variation in segmentation accuracy across subjects with
a standard deviation of below 0.06 for each dataset (0.18 for ugscnn and 0.09
for pCNN). Notably, pCNN enhances the average lowest DSC score observed in
the test set by up to 0.4 DSC points (Fig. 2, right side). This indicates that
we do not only improve the average performance of the model but also raise
the prediction accuracy on error-prone regions and subjects. As for the average
DSC, aggregating the different views of the latitude/colatitude parameterization
(p³CNN) surpasses the pCNN approach raising the average worst DSC by another 0.1 DSC point. Interestingly, the variation across subjects is much lower
when using view aggregation compared to the single view network. Here, p³CNN
stays within the same range observed for the average DSC (0.03 to 0.08) whereas
the pCNN is less consistent (0.06 to 0.21). Possibly, errors introduced by unequal sampling at the pole and equator regions are compensated by inclusion
of information from the other two views in which the structures might be more
evenly sampled (different local attention).

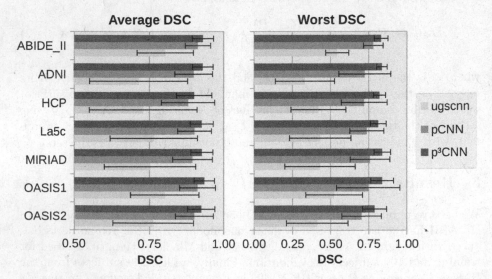

Fig. 2. Average (left) and Worst (right) DSC across the test sets. Highest accuracy is
achieved for latitude/colatitude parameterization with view aggregation (p³CNN).

4 Discussion

We introduce a novel method for cortical segmentation of spherical signals and compare it to a spherical-CNN for semantic segmentation. The presented approach is expected to generalize to other surface-based segmentation tasks. We showed that our view aggregation of spherical parameterizations (p³CNN) achieves a high average DSC of 0.92 for cortical segmentation and outperforms spherical CNNs. Geometric deep learning is still in its infancy and holds great potential for further optimizations. Yet, the promise of a non-distorted operating space is counter-balanced by high computational demands and challenging definitions of pooling and convolution operations. Furthermore, network architectures for 2D segmentations have improved significantly in the recent years, while spherical approaches are still lacking many of these innovations. Therefore, we recommend comparing all novel spherical or geometric CNN approaches not only to existing geometric methods but more importantly to view-aggregating 2D segmentation networks in the spherical parameter space as a baseline.

Acknowledgement. This work was supported by the NIH R01NS083534, R01-LM012719, and an NVIDIA Hardware Award. Further, we thank and acknowledge the providers of the datasets (cf. Section 3).

References

1. Fischl B. FreeSurfer. Neuroimage. 2012;62:774–781.
2. Jiang CM, Huang J, Kashinath K, et al. Spherical CNNs on unstructured grids. In: International Conference on Learning Representations; 2019. .
3. Huang G, Liu Z, van der Maaten L, et al. Densely connected convolutional networks. In: Proc IEEE CVPR. vol. 1; 2017. p. 3.
4. Poldrack RA, Congdon E, Triplett W, et al. A phenome-wide examination of neural and cognitive function. Scientific Data. 2016;3:160110.
5. Mueller SG, Weiner MW, Thal LJ, et al. Ways toward an early diagnosis in alzheimer's disease: the alzheimer's disease neuroimaging initiative (ADNI). Alzheimers Dement. 2005;1:55–66.
6. Malone IB, Cash D, Ridgway GR, et al. MIRIAD–Public release of a multiple time point alzheimer's MR imaging dataset. Neuroimage. 2013;70:33–36.
7. Marcus DS, Wang TH, Parker J, et al. Open access series of imaging studies (OASIS): cross-sectional MRI data in young, middle aged, nondemented, and demented older adults. J Cogn Neurosci. 2007;19:1498–1507.
8. Di Martino A, O'connor D, Chen B, et al. Enhancing studies of the connectome in autism using the autism brain imaging data exchange II. Scientific Data. 2017;4:170010.
9. Van Essen DC, Ugurbil K, Auerbach E, et al. The human connectome project: a data acquisition perspective. Neuroimage. 2012;62:2222–2231.
10. Klein A, Tourville J. 101 labeled brain images and a consistent human cortical labeling protocol. Front Neurosci. 2012;6:171.

Learning-Based Correspondence Estimation for 2-D/3-D Registration

Roman Schaffert[1], Markus Weiß[1], Jian Wang[2], Anja Borsdorf[2],
Andreas Maier[1,3]

[1]Pattern Recognition Lab, Friedrich-Alexander University, Erlangen, Germany
[2]Siemens Healthineers AG, Forchheim, Germany
[3]Erlangen Graduate School in Advanced Optical Technologies (SAOT)
roman.schrom.schaffert@fau.de

Abstract. In many minimally invasive procedures, image guidance using a C-arm system is utilized. To enhance the guidance, information from pre-operative 3-D images can be overlaid on top of the 2-D fluoroscopy and 2-D/3-D image registration techniques are used to ensure an accurate overlay. Despite decades of research, achieving a highly reliable registration remains challenging. In this paper, we propose a learning-based correspondence estimation, which focuses on contour points and can be used in combination with the point-to-plane correspondence model-based registration. When combined with classical correspondence estimation in a refinement step, the method highly increases the robustness, leading to a capture range of 36 mm and a success rate of 98.5 %, compared to 14 mm and 71.9 % for the purely classical approach, while maintaining a high accuracy of 0.43±0.08 mm of mean re-projection distance.

1 Introduction

Minimally invasive procedures rely on imaging techniques to enable the observation of and navigation to the operational site. Fluoroscopy, i. e. live X-ray imaging using a C-arm system, is commonly used for such applications. One drawback of the fluoroscopy is that important information may be missing. For instance, vessels are not visible without contrast agent, depth information is lost, and pre-operative planing markings are not available. To compensate for this, structures from pre-operative 3-D images are overlaid on top of the live images. For a meaningful overlay, the pose of the patient has to be known with a high accuracy. The pose can be estimated using 2-D/3-D registration. Although researchers have been focusing on automatic 2-D/3-D registration for decades, achieving reliable results remains challenging. A thorough review of existing 2-D/3-D registration methods is given by Markelj et al. [1].

With deep learning approaches gaining popularity in medical image processing [2], learning-based algorithms have been proposed. Miao et al. [3] train a

© Springer Fachmedien Wiesbaden GmbH, ein Teil von Springer Nature 2020
T. Tolxdorff et al. (Hrsg.), *Bildverarbeitung für die Medizin 2020*,
Informatik aktuell, https://doi.org/10.1007/978-3-658-29267-6_50

multi-agent deep convolutional neural network (DCNN) which performs image registration by repetitively selecting one from a set of possible small motion steps until the images are aligned. Liao *et al.* [4] train a correspondence matching for projections of randomly selected points of interest, rather than learning the whole registration task. Trilateration is then used to find the position in 3-D space. While this method achieves an improved performance, it demands a large training set and is only applicable to multi-view registration.

Recently, the point-to-plane correspondence (PPC) model-based registration was proposed, which achieves state-of-the-art accuracy and robustness [5]. The method establishes local correspondences using patch matching between the 2-D image and a projection of the 3-D image, and estimates a rigid motion using these. However, a large number of wrong correspondences may be present for challenging cases, e. g. large misalignments or repetitive structures, which prevent successful registration. A learning-based method was proposed to enhance registration performance by minimizing the impact of such correspondences [6]. However, the registration still relies on the established correspondences and a sufficient number of correct correspondences is needed.

In this paper, we follow an alternative direction and propose a learning-based correspondence estimation. We treat the task as a pixel-wise regression task and train a DCNN to predict the displacements of contour points, thereby defining correspondences between 2-D images. In contrast to natural images, multiple structures from different depths may be depicted in X-ray images at a single image point. As these structures may move differently, displacements cannot be unambiguously defined in 2-D images in the general case. Displacements are only unambiguous at contour points, where the viewing ray passes the object of interest once. Therefore, we focus on these points. We evaluate on spine data and show a highly increased registration robustness compared to patch matching. Although the accuracy is decreased for learning-based correspondence estimation, we show that a high accuracy can be retained by performing registration using learning-based and classical correspondence estimation consecutively.

2   Materials and methods

2.1   Point-to-plane correspondence model-based registration

The PPC model-based registration [5] is motivated by the intuition that (1) displacements in X-ray images can be best observed on contours of high-contrast objects and (2) displacements perpendicular to the contour can be easily detected, while displacements along the contour are difficult to measure locally due to the aperture problem. First, a set of apparent contour points $\{\mathbf{w}_i \in \mathbb{R}^3\}$ from the volume V, i. e. points corresponding to contours in the projected image, are extracted and projected onto the image plane as $\{\mathbf{p}_i \in \mathbb{R}^3\}$. Additionally, depth layer images (DLs) $\{\nabla I_d^{\text{proj}}\}$, i. e. gradient projection images of V from different depth intervals d, are rendered. In this work, the depth-layer-based contour point extraction is used [7], where apparent contour points are extracted based on the gradients $\{\nabla I_d^{\mathrm{proj}}\}$ and the depth of the contour points is retrieved by a depth-aware projection. For each $\mathbf{w}_i$, patch matching is performed between the $\{\nabla I_d^{\mathrm{proj}}\}$ which contains $\mathbf{w}_i$ and the gradients of the fluoroscopy image I^{FL}, namely ∇I^{FL}, leading to a match at position $\mathbf{p}_i'$. The patch matching is only performed along the projected gradient $\nabla I_d^{\mathrm{proj}}(\mathbf{p}_i)$, i.e. perpendicular to the contour. This is reflected in the PPC model, which is used to solve for the motion. For each $\mathbf{w}_i$, a constraint is defined which states that the point after the registration is located on a plane, which contains $\mathbf{p}'$ and is spanned by the two directions in which the motion is not known, namely along the contour and in depth. Under the small angle assumption, these constraints are expressed as a linear system of equations and a robust motion estimation is used [5]. The method is performed over multiple resolution levels to enable the search of correspondences over large distances. As wrong correspondences are present and the PPC model is approximative, the registration is performed iteratively on every resolution level. After each resolution level, the iteration leading to the highest quality based on image similarity and PPC distances after the motion estimation [5] is selected and results are rejected if a minimum similarity between the images is not achieved. In this work, three resolution levels are used, i.e. the lowest image scaling is 0.25. We denote the registration described here as registration using the PPC model and depth layer-based contour point extraction (DPPC).

2.2   Learning-based correspondence estimation

2.2.1   General setup In this work, we learn the correspondence estimation part of the registration framework. On the one hand, robust correspondence estimation is difficult to solve by hand. On the other hand, the learning task is kept comparably simple as e.g. no motion estimation or detection of distinctive structures needs to be learned. In contrast to natural images, for which many correspondence estimation techniques exist, the imaged structures appear as transparent in X-ray images. This poses a challenge for correspondence estimation, as a given image point may depict multiple structures from different depths. These structures may move differently, leading to ambiguous correspondences. Thus, we only estimate the motion at contour points, i.e. points for which the viewing ray intersects the structure of interest only once, leading to unambiguous displacements.

We train a DCNN which takes ∇I^{FL} and a gradient projection of V, ∇I^{proj}, as inputs and predicts a displacement for each contour point. More specifically, we train a FlowNet-S network [8] which predicts the displacement field F^{dsp} for contour points. FlowNet-S was originally proposed for optical flow estimation and has a encoder-decoder architecture with skip connections. Furthermore, the displacement field is estimated at multiple resolutions and is used in the subsequent higher resolutions as additional feature maps [8]. In contrast to optical flow, our displacements are only defined on contour points, and therefore only the values at contour points are considered.

2.2.2 Training procedure The training is performed for pairs of V and I^{FL} for which a ground truth (GT) registration T^{GT} is known. Multiple initial displacements T^{init} are generated and for each T^{init}, a set of contour points $\{\mathbf{w}_i\}$ and the respective projected points $\{\mathbf{p}_i\}$ are extracted. To generate the GT displacements, $\mathbf{w}_i$ are also projected under T^{GT}, and the displacement of the points in 2-D is computed. A binary mask image M is generated depicting the projected contour points and a vector field image $F_{\mathrm{GT}}^{\mathrm{dsp}}$ is used to store the displacements. We use the average endpoint error (EPE) over all contour points as a loss to train our network. As the loss is computed for multiple resolution levels in the network, we need to resample M and $F_{\mathrm{GT}}^{\mathrm{dsp}}$. In the former, a contour pixel for a lower resolution is set if the pixel contains at least one contour point at the full resolution, which corresponds to a max pooling operation. As $F_{\mathrm{GT}}^{\mathrm{dsp}}$ only contains meaningful values for contour pixels, it is downsampled by averaging only over these pixels. Data augmentation is performed by flipping the images horizontally, as well as performing planar translations and rotations to both ∇I^{FL} and ∇I^{proj} independently and adjusting M and $F_{\mathrm{GT}}^{\mathrm{dsp}}$ accordingly.

2.2.3 Integration into the registration framework The trained model is incorporated into the PPC-based registration as a replacement for patch matching. As the DCNN integrates information from multiple scales, the registration is performed only on full image resolution. In preliminary experiments, we find that a better performance is achieved by reducing the influence of slight contours, which are often caused by noise or by structures not well visible in I^{FL}. This is achieved by weighting the correspondences by the local gradient magnitude $\|\nabla I^{\mathrm{proj}}(\mathbf{p}_i)\|$. We denote the registration method using learning-based correspondence estimation as DPPC-CL. A similar weighting of contour points for training loss computation leads to a slight performance degeneration and is therefore not used. As DPPC achieves a high accuracy, we also combine the methods by performing DPPC-CL first, followed by DPPC using the two highest resolution levels. The resulting accurate method is denoted as DPPC-CL-A.

2.3 Evaluation setup

2.3.1 Methodology We utilize standardized evaluation metrics [9, 10]. The mean target registration error (mTRE) measures the displacement in 3-D space and is used to specify the initial error range to be tested. As we focus on single-view registration, the resulting accuracy is computed using the mean re-projection distance (mRPD), which measures the components of the displacements which can be observed from a given view. For robustness, we compute the success rate (SR), which is the overall ratio of successful registrations and the capture range (CR), which is the highest 1 mm subinterval of the initial error for which registration is successful in 95 % of cases. We use a success threshold of 2 mm, which corresponds to a highly accurate overview, as well as 5 mm in order to investigate robustness in case of lower registration accuracy.

2.3.2 Data We evaluate our approach for spine registration, which is challenging due to the repetitive structures, i.e. vertebrae and ribs. We use C-arm CT data and register the reconstructed volumes to the 2-D images used for reconstruction, so that T^{GT} is known from the system calibration with an accuracy of ≤ 0.16 mm projection error at the iso-center. The pixel spacing of the 2-D images is 0.61 mm, the volumes have isotropic voxel resolution of either 0.49 mm or 0.99 mm. The dataset contains 56 acquisitions from 55 patients of the thoracic and lumbar regions of the spine. As for some of the acquisitions, the registered structures are hardly visible, we manually select 6 acquisitions with a reasonable visibility as the test set on which registrations are performed (all with a voxel spacing of 0.49 mm). The remaining data is randomly split into 45 volumes for training and 5 volumes for validation. No patients are shared between the sets. For training, 10 initial transformations are generated per volume uniformly distributed in the range of $[0, 30]$ mm of mTRE, with translations up to 30 mm and rotations up to 15° for each motion component. Per transformation, 32 2-D images with different viewing directions are used to create training samples. Due to high achieved robustness, the evaluation is performed in the range of $[0, 45]$ mm of mTRE, and 450 initial displacements for each acquisition (translations up to 45 mm and rotations up to 22.5°). Single-view registration is performed on both the anterior-posterior and lateral views and the results are combined.

3   Results

The results are presented in Tab. 1 and Fig. 1. Compared to DPPC, DPPC-CL achieves a higher robustness, but a lower accuracy. DPPC-CL achieves SR_5 of 94.5 % and a CR_5 of 18 mm, compared to 72.0 % and 14 mm for DPPC. However, the $mRPD_5$ for DPPC is around 0.42 mm, while for DPPC-CL, it is around 1.51 mm. The low accuracy of DPPC-CL can also be observed if a success criterion of 2 mm is used, in which case the CR_2 is decreased to 4 mm, while the CR does not change for DPPC. Similarly, we observe (Fig. 1) that for DPPC-CL, an error below 10 mm mRPD is achieved for most cases, but a high accuracy cannot be achieved. For DPPC, either a very accurate result is achieved, or the error stays large. For the combined DPPC-CL-A, an mRPD of around 0.43 mm is achieved, as well as a high robustness, namely a SR of 98.5 % and a CR of 36 mm, regardless of the used success threshold.

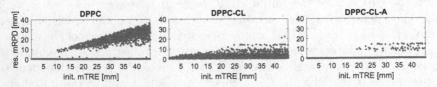

Fig. 1. Scatter plots depicting initial mTRE vs. resulting mRPD for each performed registration case for the compared methods.

Table 1. Evaluation results. Results for mRPD include mean and standard deviation. The success criterion in mm used to compute the respective measure is given as a subscript. Best results are highlighted in bold font.

Method	mRPD$_2$ [mm]	SR$_2$ [%]	CR$_2$ [mm]	mRPD$_5$ [mm]	SR$_5$ [%]	CR$_5$ [mm]
DPPC	**0.42±0.08**	71.9	14	**0.42±0.10**	72.0	14
DPPC-CL	1.03±0.42	72.6	4	1.51±1.02	94.4	18
DPPC-CL-A	0.43±0.08	**98.5**	**36**	0.43±0.08	**98.5**	**36**

4   Discussion

The results show that learning to establish correspondences between X-ray and rendered projection images is not only feasible, but leads to an increased robustness of the registration compared to classical patch matching. However, similar to other learning-based approaches [3, 4], DPPC-CL alone fails to produce competitive accuracy. This is compensated by a refinement step using DPPC. This way, DPPC-CL can increase the robustness of the method without sacrificing accuracy by bringing the misalignment into a range where DPPC works reliably.

To increase the accuracy of the method without relying on a refinement step, the use of multiple depth layers instead of the gradient projection image can be investigated. Also, the network can be trained directly with the objective to minimize the registration error, similar to the correspondence weighting scheme [6], encouraging the network to focus on the relevant displacement components. In this case, the method can also be combined with correspondence weighting or a learning-based contour point selection.

References

1. Markelj P, Tomaževič D, Likar B, et al. A review of 3D/2D registration methods for image-guided interventions. Med Image Anal. 2010;16(3):642–661.
2. Maier A, Syben C, Lasser T, et al. A gentle introduction to deep learning in medical image processing. Zeitschrift für Medizinische Physik. 2019;29(2):86–101.
3. Miao S, Piat S, Fischer P, et al. Dilated FCN for multi-agent 2D/3D medical image registration. In: AAAI; 2018. p. 4694–4701.
4. Liao H, Lin WA, Zhang J, et al. Multiview 2D/3D rigid registration via a point-of-interest network for tracking and triangulation (POINT^2). arXiv:190303896v3;.
5. Wang J, Schaffert R, Borsdorf A, et al. Dynamic 2-D/3-D rigid registration framework using point-to-plane correspondence model. IEEE Trans Med Imaging. 2017;36(9):1939–1954.
6. Schaffert R, Wang J, Fischer P, et al. Metric-Driven learning of correspondence weighting for 2-D/3-D image registration. In: GCPR; 2018. p. 140–152.
7. Wang J. Robust 2-D/3D registration for real-time patient motion compensation. FAU Erlangen-Nürnberg; to appear 2020.
8. Dosovitskiy A, Fischer P, Ilg E, et al. Flownet: learning optical flow with convolutional networks. In: IEEE ICCV; 2015. p. 2758–2766.
9. van de Kraats EB, Penney GP, Tomaževič D, et al. Standardized evaluation methodology for 2-D-3-D registration. IEEE Trans Med Imaging. 2005;24(9).

10. Mitrović U, Špiclin Ž, Likar B, et al.   3D-2D registration of cerebral angiograms: a method and evaluation on clinical images. IEEE Trans Med Imaging. 2013;32(8):1550–1563.

Abstract: Deep Learning Based CT-CBCT Image Registration for Adaptive Radio Therapy

Sven Kuckertz[1], Nils Papenberg[1], Jonas Honegger[2], Tomasz Morgas[2], Benjamin Haas[2], Stefan Heldmann[1]

[1]Fraunhofer Institute for Digital Medicine MEVIS, Lübeck, Germany
[2]Varian Medical Systems, Baden-Dättwil, Switzerland
sven.kuckertz@mevis.fraunhofer.de

Deformable image registration (DIR) is an important tool in radio therapy where it is used in order to align a baseline CT and daily low-dose cone beam CT (CBCT) scans. DIR allows the propagation of irradiation plans, Hounsfield units and contours of anatomical structures, respectively, which enables tracking of applied doses over time and generation of daily synthetic CT images. Furthermore, DIR allows to overcome segmentation of structures in CBCT images at each fraction. We present a novel weakly supervised deep learning based method for fast deformable registration of 3D images [1], targeting the challenges of multi-modal CT-CBCT registration that goes along with low contrast and artifacts in CBCT scans and extreme deformations of organs such as bladder.

The parameters of our convolutional neural network (CNN) are adapted for minimizing a loss function inspired from state-of-the-art iterative image registration. Therefore, our training is unsupervised and does not require any hard to obtain ground-truth deformation vector fields. Additionally, we include a weak supervision through ground-truth segmentations during training. We evaluate our proposed method on follow-up image pairs of the female pelvis including outlines of the bladder, rectum and uterus, showing that incorporating a measure for segmentation mask overlap during training enhances the alignment of organs with extreme deformations. Hence, our method outperforms state-of-the-art iterative DIR algorithms in terms of Dice overlap (in average 0.78 vs. 0.71) and average surface distance (3.10 mm vs. 4.17 mm), where both methods only use the image pair as input. Furthermore, it is nearly as good as iterative structure guided registration that depends on ground-truth segmentations, which first have to be generated after CBCT acquisition. Needing only one pass through the network, our method yields deformations over 100 times faster than conventional iterative algorithms (0.13 s vs. 15.39 s). Not requiring any segmentations of unseen image pairs, our framework additionally accelerates and facilitates the workflow of adaptive radio therapy.

References

1. Kuckertz S, Papenberg N, Honegger J, et al. Deep learning based CT-CBCT image registration for adaptive radio therapy. Proc SPIE. 2020;.

© Springer Fachmedien Wiesbaden GmbH, ein Teil von Springer Nature 2020
T. Tolxdorff et al. (Hrsg.), *Bildverarbeitung für die Medizin 2020*,
Informatik aktuell, https://doi.org/10.1007/978-3-658-29267-6_51

Learning-Based Misalignment Detection for 2-D/3-D Overlays

Roman Schaffert[1], Jian Wang[2], Peter Fischer[2], Anja Borsdorf[2], Andreas Maier[1,3]

[1]Pattern Recognition Lab, Friedrich-Alexander University, Erlangen, Germany
[2]Siemens Healthineers AG, Forchheim, Germany
[3]Erlangen Graduate School in Advanced Optical Technologies (SAOT)
`roman.schrom.schaffert@fau.de`

Abstract. In minimally invasive procedures, a standard routine of observing the operational site is using image guidance. X-ray fluoroscopy using C-arm systems is widely used. In complex cases, overlays of preoperative 3-D images are necessary to show structures that are not visible in the 2-D X-ray images. The alignment quality may degenerate during an intervention, e. g. due to patient motion, and a new registration needs to be performed. However, a decrease in alignment quality is not always obvious, as the clinician often focuses on structures which are not visible in the 2-D image, and only these structures are visualized in the overlay. In this paper, we propose a learning-based method for detecting different degrees of misalignment. The method is based on point-to-plane correspondences and a pre-trained neural network originally used for detecting good correspondences. The network is extended by a classification branch to detect different levels of misalignment. Compared to simply using the normalized gradient correlation similarity measure as a basis for the decision, we show a highly improved performance, e. g. improving the AUC score from 0.918 to 0.993 for detecting misalignment above 5 mm of mean re-projection distance.

1 Introduction

Imaging techniques are used in minimally invasive procedures to observe the operational site. One commonly used modality is fluoroscopy, i. e. live X-ray imaging with a C-arm system. Important structures, such as vessels, are not visible in X-ray images and overlays of pre-operatively acquired 3-D volumes can be used to visualize them. For the overlay, the patient pose needs to be estimated precisely and 2-D/3-D registration techniques are commonly used for this task. However, the accuracy of the overlay may degenerate during the procedure, e. g. due to patient motion, or motion of the C-arm in combination with an inaccurate calibration or out-of-plane registration errors, which become in-plane in the new view. In these cases, a new registration needs to be triggered. However,

© Springer Fachmedien Wiesbaden GmbH, ein Teil von Springer Nature 2020
T. Tolxdorff et al. (Hrsg.), *Bildverarbeitung für die Medizin 2020*,
Informatik aktuell, https://doi.org/10.1007/978-3-658-29267-6_52

manually detecting the misalignment is cumbersome, as the clinician is often focused on structures which are not visible in the X-ray images, such as vessels or pre-operative planning markings, and only these structures are visualized. While misalignment detection methods have been previously proposed (e. g. [1, 2]), the focus was mainly on detecting misregistrations, i. e. misalignment above a small threshold, without differentiating between small and large misalignment. However, during the intervention, it may be acceptable to tolerate some degree of misalignment before performing a re-registration in order to facilitate the workflow. Our goal is to aid the decision on performing a re-registration by providing information about the current degree of misalignment.

Recently, the point-to-plane correspondence (PPC) model-based registration was proposed [3]. Later, the robustness of the method was further enhanced by training a deep neural network (DNN) model to weight individual correspondences [4]. Based on this method, we propose to learn a misalignment detection method which can differentiate between different degrees of misalignment. The PPC correspondences are a natural starting point, as they represent local displacements, and therefore can be used to judge the overall misalignment. However, many wrong correspondences may be present, which do not represent the actual misalignment. Furthermore, all correspondences have to be assessed from a global perspective to estimate the overall misalignment. Therefore, we utilize the pre-trained correspondence weighting model. Starting from a global feature vector, a second network branch is added to predict the overlay quality. Compared to using the normalized gradient correlation (NGC) similarity measure, and demonstrate a highly improved classification performance.

2 Materials and methods

2.1 Registration using point-to-plane correspondences & learning correspondence weighting

The PPC model [3] follows the intuition that on the one hand, displacements in X-ray images are best observable for contour points of high-contrast structures which are visible in both images. On the other hand, the displacement component along the contour is difficult to determine using only local information.

In PPC model-based registration [3], correspondences are established between apparent contour points $\{\mathbf{w}_i \in \mathbb{R}^3\}$, i. e. points in the 3-D image V which represent contour points in the projection, and contours in the 2-D image I^{FL} using patch matching between ∇I^{FL} and gradient projection images from different depth intervals d of V, $\{\nabla I_d^{\mathrm{proj}}\}$. As displacement along the contour is difficult to determine, the search is only performed perpendicular to the contour, leading to correspondences $\{\mathbf{p}_i' \in \mathbb{R}^3\}$. The PPC model states that each $\mathbf{w}_i$ after registration is located on a plane Π_i, which contains $\mathbf{p}_i'$ and is spanned by the two directions in which the displacement is not known, i. e. along the contour and in depth. Registration is performed by iteratively estimating correspondences and the motion to align $\{\mathbf{w}_i\}$ to $\{\Pi_i\}$ over multiple resolution levels [3]. In this work, contour point extraction based on projected gradients is used [5].

While PPC-based registration achieves state-of-the-art performance, the robustness can be further improved by a learning-based correspondence weighting scheme, which reduces the influence of wrong correspondences [4]. To achieve this, a PointNet [6] is trained to weight the individual correspondences with the training objective to minimize the registration error. A set of per-correspondence feature vectors $\{\mathbf{f}_i \in \mathbb{R}^6\}$ serves as input and weights for each correspondence are the output. Each $\mathbf{f}_i$ contains $\mathbf{w}_i$, the normal of Π_i, the point-to-plane distance, and the NGC image similarity as computed by patch matching.

2.2 Automatic misalignment detection

Different measures can be used to describe the accuracy of 2-D/3-D registration. We learn to predict misalignment with respect to the mean re-projection distance (mRPD) [7], as it represents the misalignment visible in the overlay.

PPC correspondences lend themselves to misalignment detection as they measure the local displacements. However, misalignment detection is difficult due to the presence of wrong correspondences, which are not representative of the actual displacement. Furthermore, the correspondences are approximations so that the measured distances may not be accurate. Displacements along contours are also not measured. This means that the distance between the projection of $\mathbf{w}_i$ and $\mathbf{p}'_i$ may not represent the actual misalignment, even for correct correspondences. Thus, all correspondences have to be considered at once to obtain an overall estimate for the misalignment. Therefore, we propose to use a pre-trained PointNet model for correspondence weighting as a starting point. In the basic version, the PointNet processes point sets by applying a multi-layer perceptron (MLP) to each point independently and combining the resulting descriptors to a global descriptor by max pooling over all points. This descriptor can e. g. be used for classification tasks. For point-wise predictions, the descriptor is instead concatenated to local descriptors for each point, and the resulting descriptors are again processed independently [6]. We start with the global descriptor from the correspondence weighting model and add an additional network branch, which is used to classify the misalignment by deciding whether it is above a given set

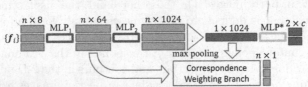

Fig. 1. Used PointNet architecture. Correspondence-wise feature vectors are depicted in orange (three correspondences shown), global vectors in red. The network is first trained for correspondence weighting (MLP$_1$, MLP$_2$, and the correspondence weighting branch). MLP$_1$ has the size of $8 \times 64 \times 64$ neurons and MLP$_2$ of $64 \times 64 \times 128 \times 1024$. Later, MLP* is added and is trained in a second step to classify whether the misalignment is above given thresholds $\{t_m\}$, where $c = \|\{t_m\}\|$. In our experiments, $c = 3$ and MLP* has a size of $1024 \times 128 \times 64 \times 6$.

of thresholds $\{t_m\}$. Multiple t_m are used to allow a more detailed feedback, allowing the clinician to decide on the acceptable misalignment depending on the current situation. See Fig. 1 for the used architecture.

During training, only the parameters of the newly added network branch are updated. We treat classifications for different t_m as independent tasks and train them using the focal loss [8]. The number of correspondences is fixed to 1024 for both training and testing, and a random subset of correspondences is selected if more correspondences are available. We focus on misalignments caused either by patient motion, or by C-arm motion in combination with inaccurate calibration or registration errors, which are out-of-plane in the original view, but in-plane in the new view. We assume that random initial misalignments are representative for such cases and perform training as well as evaluation based on randomly generated transformations. We compare the proposed method, denoted LRN, to detection based on image similarity thresholding (SMB). Similar to the image similarity used in the convergence criterion for the PPC-based registration framework [3], we compute the average NGC for patches around the projections of $\mathbf{w}_i$ between ∇I^{FL} and the $\nabla I_d^{\mathrm{proj}}$ of the depth interval d containing $\mathbf{w}_i$.

Training and validation is performed on the highest resolution level RL_0 (image scaling of 1.0) as well as RL_1 with a scaling of 0.5. The validation set is used to decide for one resolution level for both LRN and SMB. Furthermore, a receiver operator curve (ROC) for the validation set is used for both methods to find an operating point closest to the perfect classifier. The actual evaluation is performed for his operating point.

2.3 Data

We evaluate our method for a spine dataset. For each acquisition, a volume of interest (VOI) is defined which contains the spine while excluding as much of other structures as possible. Target points for registration error computation are defined uniformly distributed in the VOI.

For training, C-arm CT acquisitions are used, where combinations of the reconstructed volumes and the 2-D images used for reconstruction are considered. Overall, 59 volumes of the lumbar and thoracic regions of the spine are used. The volumes have different resolutions, with an isotropic voxel spacing of 0.49 mm or 0.99 mm. The 2-D images have a pixel spacing of 0.61 mm. The ground truth (GT) alignment is known with the calibration accuracy of below 0.16 mm projection error in the iso-center. The acquisitions are randomly split into a training set containing 47 volumes and a validation set containing 12 volumes. The same sets were used to train the original correspondence weighting model. The 2-D images are preprocessed to closer resemble fluoroscopic images. For each volume, 16 views are used. Correspondences are generated for each view for 60 different misalignments in the range of $[0, 20]$ mm of the mean target registration error (mTRE) [7]. Overall, 11520 cases are generated, with 9944 true positives (TP) for $t_m = 2$ mm, 7550 for $t_m = 5$ mm and 3847 for $t_m = 10$ mm.

For evaluation, a cadaver dataset with real fluoroscopic images is used. C-arm CT volumes are acquired and used as the 3-D images. Then, fluoroscopic images are acquired using C-arm poses for which an accurate calibration was performed first. In this work, the anterior-posterior and lateral views are evaluated. The dataset consists of 33 acquisitions from 13 cadavers. The volumes have a voxel spacing of 0.48 mm. The 2-D images have a pixel size of 0.62 mm. For each view, 80 misalignments in the range of $[0, 20]$ mm of mTRE are considered. Overall, 5280 cases are generated, with 4565 TP for $t_m = 2$ mm, 3449 for $t_m = 5$ mm and 1776 for $t_m = 10$ mm.

3   Results

For the validation set, we observe that RL_1 outperforms RL_0 for $t_m \geq 5$ mm for both LRN and NGC. For $t_m = 5$ mm, LRN achieves an AUC of 0.991 for RL_1 and 0.984 for RL_0, and NGC an AUC of 0.906 for RL_1 and 0.839 for RL_0. For $t_m = 10$ mm, LRN achieves an AUC of 0.977 for RL_1 and 0.933 for RL_0, and NGC an AUC of 0.780 for RL_1 and 0.671 for RL_0. For $t_m = 2$ mm, the results for RL_0 and RL_1 are comparable, with LRN achieving an AUC 0.990 and 0.991, respectively, and NGC an AUC of 0.967 on both resolution levels. As overall, RL_1 outperforms RL_0, we choose RL_1 for further evaluation.

For the test set, we compute the area under curve (AUC), recall, precision, and balanced accuracy metrics (Tab. 1). We observe that LRN outperforms SMB for all measures and values for t_m, but especially for larger t_m. For example, an AUC of 0.994 (LRN) vs. 0.987 (SMB) is achieved for $t_m = 2$ mm. While for $t_m = 5$ mm, the AUC is only slightly decreased to 0.993 for LRN, it is decreased to 0.918 for SMB. In general, larger t_m lead to decreased performance for both methods, but more drastically for SMB. The only exception being the recall for LRN, which is 0.947 for $t_m = 5$ and 0.954 for $t_m = 10$. However, recall cannot be considered without considering precision. We observe (Fig. 2) that the NGC is decreased for misalignment up to around 5 mm of mRPD and does not change considerably from there on. In contrast, the confidence scores estimated by LRN cover a wider range of values of the mRPD, enabling the differentiation between larger misalignments.

4   Discussion

We demonstrate that the learning-based LRN outperforms SMB by a large margin for the task of misalignment detection, especially for differentiating between

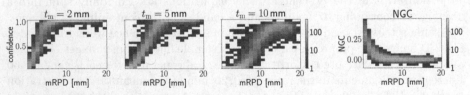

Fig. 2. Histograms showing the number of cases for different values of mRPD and the corresponding confidence of the network for detecting misalignment above the given t_m, as well as the NGC similarity measure. All cases in the test set are considered.

Table 1. Evaluation of classification performance for LRN and NGC for different t_m and the resolution level RL_1.

t_m [mm]	Method	AUC	Recall	Precision	Bal. Acc.
2	LRN	**0.994**	**0.958**	**0.996**	**0.966**
2	SMB	0.987	0.924	0.993	0.942
5	LRN	**0.993**	**0.947**	**0.981**	**0.957**
5	SMB	0.918	0.908	0.896	0.855
10	LRN	**0.981**	**0.954**	**0.851**	**0.935**
10	SMB	0.790	0.797	0.537	0.725

larger degrees of misalignment, where the similarity used by SMB does not reflect the changes in misalignment anymore. This shows that while the similarity measure can be used to distinguish between a very good registration and a small misalignment, it cannot be used to differentiate between larger degrees of misalignments. Here, using PPC correspondences in combination with a learning-based prediction is clearly advantageous. By allowing the detection of different levels of misalignment, a more detailed feedback can be given to the clinician, who then can decide at which point a new registration is needed.

In the future, the method should be validated on real interventional data for typical misalignment cases. To further increase the performance of the method, additional features can be used or the simultaneous use of features both from the initially successful registration and the current overlay can be investigated. Also, the proposed method can be combined with a multi-start registration strategy to enable an early selection of promising initial positions.

References

1. Mitrović U, Špiclin Ž, Likar B, et al. Automatic detection of misalignment in rigid 3D-2D registration. In: CLIP; 2013. p. 117–124.
2. Varnavas A, Carrell T, Penney G. Fully automated 2D–3D registration and verification. Med Image Anal. 2015;26(1):108–119.
3. Wang J, Schaffert R, Borsdorf A, et al. Dynamic 2-D/3-D rigid registration framework using Point-To-Plane correspondence model. IEEE Trans Med Imaging. 2017;36(9):1939–1954.
4. Schaffert R, Wang J, Fischer P, et al. Metric-Driven learning of correspondence weighting for 2-D/3-D image registration. In: GCPR; 2018. p. 140–152.
5. Wang J. Robust 2-D/3D registration for real-time patient motion compensation. FAU Erlangen-Nürnberg; to appear 2020.
6. Qi CR, Su H, Mo K, et al. PointNet: deep learning on point sets for 3d classification and segmentation. In: CVPR; 2017. p. 652–660.
7. van de Kraats EB, Penney GP, Tomaževič D, et al. Standardized evaluation methodology for 2-D-3-D registration. IEEE Trans Med Imaging. 2005;24(9):1177–1189.
8. Lin TY, Goyal P, Girshick R, et al. Focal loss for dense object detection. In: ICCV; 2017. p. 2980–2988.

Deep Groupwise Registration of MRI Using Deforming Autoencoders

Hanna Siebert[1,2], Mattias P. Heinrich[1]

[1]Institute of Medical Informatics, University of Lübeck
[2]Graduate School for Computing in Medicine and Life Sciences, University of Lübeck
siebert@imi.uni-luebeck.de

Abstract. Groupwise image registration and the estimation of anatomical shape variation play an important role for dealing with the analysis of large medical image datasets. In this work we adapt the concept of deforming autoencoders that decouples shape and appearance in an unsupervised learning setting, following a deformable template paradigm, and apply its capability for groupwise image alignment. We implement and evaluate this model for the application on medical image data and show its suitability for this domain by training it on middle slice MRI brain scans. Anatomical shape and appearance variation can be modeled by means of splitting a low-dimensional latent code into two parts that serve as inputs for separate appearance and shape decoder networks. We demonstrate the potential of deforming autoencoders to learn meaningful appearance and deformation representations of medical image data.

1 Introduction

The analysis of large image datasets can be facilitated by automatic methods for groupwise image registration. Thus, multiple images can be concurrently registered within a single optimization procedure taking into account all available image information. Groupwise image registration as well as analysing anatomical shape variation often require deformable templates representing the variability of a medical dataset. With the help of deformable templates, shape can be represented as a geometric deformation between a template and an input image. For this purpose it is essential that meaningful appearance and deformation models are used, which represent the underlying variability of the dataset appropriately (i.e. by jointly modeling shape and appearance).

Various image registration algorithms have been proposed to map large sets of images into a common coordinate system. A method to build an average anatomical model which provides an average intensity and an average shape within a single image has been presented in [1]. In [2], the problem of anatomical template construction has been addressed by introducing an iterative algorithm that simultaneously estimates the transformations and an unbiased template. Using deep-learning-based methods, speed and accuracy of groupwise image registration can be improved significantly. Deep groupwise registration networks have

© Springer Fachmedien Wiesbaden GmbH, ein Teil von Springer Nature 2020
T. Tolxdorff et al. (Hrsg.), *Bildverarbeitung für die Medizin 2020*,
Informatik aktuell, https://doi.org/10.1007/978-3-658-29267-6_53

the ability to take a group of moving images and a template image based on PCA as inputs and output warped moving images [3, 4].

An approach called 'deforming autoencoders' (DAE) has been introduced in [5] that proposed a new concept for disentangling the factors of variation within the dataset. More precisely, shape is separated from appearance in an unsupervised manner. An implicit decoupling of deformation and appearance information has already been used to learn low-dimensional probabilistic deformation models for image registration in [6], which aimed to analyse the deformations directly from training images.

Recently, a model has been proposed to jointly estimate a registration network and a deformable template in an unsupervised setting [7]. The approach of DAE as well follows the deformable template paradigm by considering that object instances are obtained by deforming a template through dense, diffeomorphic deformation fields, but is different in that it models shape and appearance variation in terms of a low-dimensional latent code that is learnable from images.

We apply and modify DAE in such a way that it is suitable for medical image analysis. Anatomical shape and appearance variation is modeled with the help of a low-dimensional latent code which is split into two separate parts that are fed into separate decoder networks with the aim of predicting shape and appearance estimates for new input images.

2   Materials and methods

For our model, we build on the architecture of deforming autoencoders [5] shown in Fig. 1 where appearance and deformation functions are synthesized by independent decoder networks. Image generation is interpreted as a synthesis of appearance on a template followed by a subsequent deformation. This warping step induces the observed shape variability. The reconstructed image is obtained by warping the template image generated by the appearance decoder with the warping field estimated by the shape decoder.

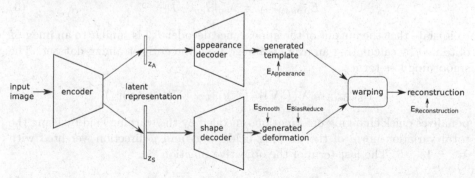

Fig. 1. DAE: A joint encoder network provides a latent code representation of appearance and shape that is divided into two parts, which serve as input for the appearance and shape decoder networks. Image generation is achieved by spatial warping of appearance with estimated deformation.

2.1   Architecture

A joint encoder network provides a low-dimensional latent code representing appearance and shape. This latent code is divided into two parts which serve as input for the appearance and shape decoder networks. In order to achieve a plausible deformation field, a 'differential decoder' is considered that generates the spatial gradient of the warping field instead of using a shape decoder that directly predicts the local warping field. A spatial transformer module [8], that employs differentiable bilinear interpolation, is used to warp the appearance part based on the shape code.

The architecture of the encoder and decoder networks closely follows that of DenseNet-121 [9], but without the 1×1 convolutional layers inside each dense block and with instance normalisation.

2.2   Training

Our objective function is a slight modification of the loss function used in [5]. It consists of four terms that restrict the model in such a way that reconstruction errors as well as implausible deformation fields are taken into account. Compared to the loss function of [5], the function used here has an additional term that includes a consideration of the generated templates and uses the more robust ℓ_1 norm as reconstruction loss. Thus, the objective function can be expressed as

$$E_{\text{DAE}} = E_{\text{Reconstruction}} + E_{\text{Appearance}} + E_{\text{Smooth}} + E_{\text{BiasReduce}} \qquad (1)$$

where the reconstruction loss

$$E_{\text{Reconstruction}} = \|I_{\text{recon}} - I_{\text{in}}\|_1 \qquad (2)$$

measures the ℓ_1 norm between the input image I_{in} and the reconstructed output image I_{recon}. Another ℓ_1 measure weighted with $\lambda_{\text{ap}} = 0.1$ is used for

$$E_{\text{Appearance}} = \lambda_{\text{ap}} \|I_{\text{ap}} - \bar{I}\|_1 \qquad (3)$$

to initiate that the output of the appearance decoder I_{ap} is similar to an image $\bar{I}$ obtained by calculating an average image from the entire training dataset. The smoothing loss term

$$E_{\text{Smooth}} = \lambda_{\text{tv}}(\|\nabla W_x(x,y)\|_1 + \|\nabla W_y(x,y)\|_1) \qquad (4)$$

penalizes quick changing deformations encoded by the warping field by using the total variation norm of the warping fields in x- and y-direction weighted with $\lambda_{\text{tv}} = 1e-6$. The last term of the objective function

$$E_{\text{BiasReduce}} = \lambda_{\text{br}} \|\bar{W} - W_0\|^2 \qquad (5)$$

with $\lambda_{\text{br}} = 1e-2$ measures the mean squared error between the average deformation grid and an identity mapping grid as a further regularisation of the warping field.

To show the benefits of the described model for medical applications, we use a MRI dataset available at https://www.kaggle.com/adalca/mri-2d. It consists of intensity-normalized and affinely aligned middle slice of brain scans which are resampled and zero-padded to a size of 128×128 for our experiments.

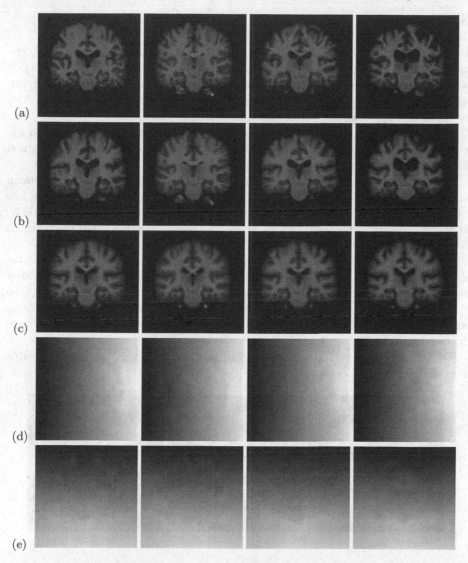

Fig. 2. Results for different images of testset with latent dimension $z_A = 1$ in our DAE approach: from top to bottom rows: input images (a), reconstructed output images (b), decoded appearance (c), decoded deformation in x-direction (d), and decoded deformation in y-direction (e). It can be seen that the reconstruction closely resembles the input (as desired) and most of the geometric differences are indeed encoded in the deformations, hence the estimated appearance is similar across patients.

Training is performed for 1000 epochs with a training dataset containing 208 images using the Adam optimizer and an initial learning rate of $2e-4$. For evaluation of our trained model we use 141 test images.

3 Results

In Fig. 2 we show the results for several test images when limiting the dimension of the latent representation for appearance to $z_A = 1$ in order to encode a canonical appearance for the dataset. Besides the reconstructed output images, we visualize the decoded appearance predicted by the appearance decoder network and the decoded deformation in x- and y-direction.

To point out the effects of an increased appearance latent code dimension z_A, we compare the the the reconstruction performance and the diversity of the obtained appearance representations for $z_A = 1$ and $z_A = 16$.

For evaluation of the DAE's reconstruction performance the overall mean squared error (MSE) between input image and reconstructed output image has been calculated. Maintaining the dimension $z_A = 1$ we achieve MSE = 0.0032. If the dimension is increased to $z_A = 16$, the reconstruction error improves to MSE = 0.0028.

As shown by the comparison of the average learned appearance images for $z_A = 1$ and $z_A = 16$ in Fig. 3 (a) and (b), the variability of the generated appearance representations increases with larger latent code dimensions z_A. To demonstrate that the generated appearance images are more meaningful than an average image, we compare the average learned appearance image to the average testset image in Fig 3 (c).

Inference of the trained autoencoder for a single images takes about 45 ms on GPU (Quadro P6000).

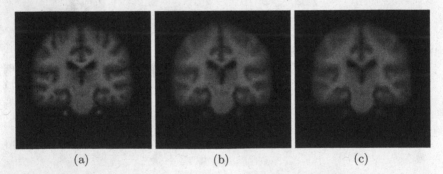

(a)   (b)   (c)

Fig. 3. Comparison of average appearance image generated with $z_A = 1$ (a), average appearance image generated with $z_A = 16$ (b), and average input image (c). Compared to the baseline (simple averaging) both settings of our DAE model yield visually sharper atlases. When using a smaller latent space for the appearance part a convincing disentanglement is reached and most variability is captured by the spatial transformations.

4   Discussion

We applied the model of DAE to MRI scans and showed its suitability for medical purposes. Our model learned to reconstruct an input image and to model a canonical appearance and deformation fields. Appearance and deformation have been successfully decoupled in an unsupervised learning framework leading to plausible representations of anatomical variability. Regularisation by means of warping associated terms in the objective function has achieved smooth and understandable deformation fields. We empirically found that using a much smaller part of the latent vector (as little as a one-dimensional scalar) is sufficient to represent appearance variations and at the same leads to better deformation estimates and thus sharper mean atlas images.

The method can be used for unsupervised groupwise image registration and could prospectively facilitate the analysis of anatomical shape variations. Further improvements could be reached when considering a more exhaustive study of the employed hyper-parameters.

Future work will include an extension of our experiments to 3D and a direct comparison to conventional groupwise registration algorithms as well as pairwise deep learning based registration.

References

1. Guimond A, Meunier J, Thirion JP. Average brain models: A convergence study. Computer Vision and Image Understanding. 2000;77(2):192 – 210.
2. Joshi S, Davis B, Jomier M, et al. Unbiased diffeomorphic atlas construction for computational anatomy. NeuroImage. 2004;23:S151 – S160.
3. Che T, Zheng Y, Sui X, et al. DGR-Net: Deep groupwise registration of multispectral images. In: Chung ACS, editor. Information Processing in Medical Imaging. Cham: Springer International Publishing; 2019. p. 706–717.
4. Che T, Zheng Y, Cong J, et al. Deep group-wise registration for multi-spectral images from fundus images. IEEE Access. 2019;7:27650–27661.
5. Shu Z, Sahasrabudhe M, Güler RA, et al. Deforming Autoencoders: Unsupervised disentangling of shape and appearance. In: European Conference on Computer Vision; 2018. p. 664–680.
6. Krebs J, Delingette H, Mailhe B, et al. Learning a probabilistic model for diffeomorphic registration. IEEE Transactions on Medical Imaging. 2019;38(9):2165–2176.
7. Dalca A, Rakic M, Guttag J, et al. Learning conditional deformable templates with convolutional networks. In: Advances in neural information processing systems; 2019. p. 804–816.
8. Jaderberg M, Simonyan K, Zisserman A, et al. Spatial transformer networks. In: Advances in neural information processing systems; 2015. p. 2017–2025.
9. Huang G, Liu Z, v d Maaten L, et al. Densely connected convolutional networks. In: 2017 IEEE Conference on Computer Vision and Pattern Recognition (CVPR); 2017. p. 2261–2269.

Robust Open Field Rodent Tracking Using a Fully Convolutional Network and a Softargmax Distance Loss

Marcin Kopaczka[1], Tobias Jacob[1], Lisa Ernst[2], Mareike Schulz[2], René Tolba[2], Dorit Merhof[1]

[1]Institute of Imaging and Computer Vision, RWTH Aachen University
[2]Institute of Laboratory Animal Science, RWTH Aachen University
marcin.kopaczka@lfb.rwth-aachen.de

Abstract. Analysis of animal locomotion is a commonly used method for analyzing rodent behavior in laboratory animal science. In this context, the open field test is one of the main experiments for assessing treatment effects by analyzing changes in exploratory behavior of laboratory mice and rats. While a number of algorithms for automated analysis of open field experiments has been presented, most of these do not utilize deep learning methods. Therefore, we compare the performance of different deep learning approaches to perform animal localization in open field studies. As our key methodological contribution, we present a novel softargmax-based loss function that can be applied to fully convolutional networks such as the U-Net to allow direct landmark regression from fully convolutional architectures.

1 Introduction and previous work

In translational medicine and neurological and psychatric research, experiments on animals are an important step during pre-clinical trials. During these experiments, a number of clinical and behavioral parameters are assessed to determine treatment effects. One of the most commonly used animal experiments is the open field test, in which the animal is placed into an open experimental environment and its exploration behavior is assessed. The animal's position, orientation and movement speed are recorded with a top-mounted camera and evaluated. Since the open field test is a widely used experimental setting, a number of methods and tools have been introduced to allow automated quantitative analysis. Notable examples include the MiceProfiler [1], The Noldus EthoVision software [2] and the Live Mouse Tracker [3]. While well-established and robust, the image analysis methods used in these tools are using established image processing and pattern analysis algorithms which do not reflect current advances in deep learning research. Therefore, we will assess how different current advances in fully convolutional networks can contribute to a robust and computationally effective localization of rodents in open field experiments which is the key requirement for all subsequent tasks.

© Springer Fachmedien Wiesbaden GmbH, ein Teil von Springer Nature 2020
T. Tolxdorff et al. (Hrsg.), *Bildverarbeitung für die Medizin 2020*,
Informatik aktuell, https://doi.org/10.1007/978-3-658-29267-6_54

2   Materials and methods

Here, we will describe all methods used for both ground truth generation and localization using deep learning methods. All research was performed on a set of open field recordings of single C57BL/6 mice which represent the most commonly used mouse strain in animal experiments.

2.1   Established methods for ground truth bootstrapping

Most current algorithms use well-established methods for animal localization such as background subtraction and morphological operations. While these methods are generally not as robust as modern approaches, their performance is usually sufficient for the task at hand due to the controlled environment in which the rodents are analyzed. We use these methods to create reference results that can also serve as automatically generated ground truth for our supervised deep learning algorithms which require annotated data for training. For our localization task, we require the centroid of the rodent which can be computed by segmenting the animal mask and computing the segmentation's centroid. To compute the segmentation, we perform background subtraction of the experimental box and thresholding followed by morphologically removing remaining noise. Subsequently, the largest remaining cluster is assumed to represent the mouse for which we compute the geometrical centroid.

2.2   Direct position regression using a VGG16 architecture

A common approach for image-based position regression is using a convolutional architecture to predict landmark positions. This is achieved by using a classification architecture and replacing the output layer with neurons for the x and y positions of the keypoint and subsequently training the net with a distance-based loss. In our case, we use the widely used VGG16 architecture [4] in which the last layer is adapted to predict x and y positions of the animal and train the network with an L1 loss. The network output can be directly interpreted as centroid coordinate prediction, thereby allowing end-to-end training with the centroid coordinates serving as target and eliminating the need for additional post-processing of the output.

2.3   Segmentation using a u-net architecture

Since our pipeline generates a segmentation mask for centroid computation, we can use the images and their masks to train a fully convolutional network to generate masks in which we subsequently compute the segmentation centroids. The most widely used fully convolutional architecture for semantic segmentation is the U-Net [5], which we modified to use a lower number of channels due to the nature of the problem and used residual blocks in the convolutional layers. The network was subsequently trained with a cross-entropy loss to obtain segmentation predictions for frames from the video recordings.

2.4   Direct landmark regression with a u-net and a softargmax loss

Fully convolutional networks such as the U-Net can be trained to directly predict landmark positions. This is achieved by a recently proposed specialized loss function that implements a differentiable approximation to the argmax function. [6]

$$soft\text{-}argmax(x, \beta) = \frac{\sum_{i,j} \exp(\beta x_{i,j}) \cdot \left(i \ j \right)}{\sum_{i',j'} \exp(\beta x_{i',j'})} \qquad (1)$$

in which β is a heat map intensity factor and i, j are the pixel coordinates. For large β, equation 1 converges towards the *argmax* function

$$argmax(x) = \lim_{\beta \to \infty} soft\text{-}argmax(x, \beta) = \left(i_{max}, j_{max} \right) \qquad (2)$$

where (i_{max}, j_{max}) is the coordinate of the pixel with the largest intensity in the heat map. By multiplying with the vector (i, j), we can establish a correspondence between pixel positions and actual coordinates.

However, training with just this loss function prooved numerically instable. Therefore, we present an extension of the above-described loss function to improve localization performance and to stabilize the training by inducing a hint to the actual mouse position. Our full loss for regressing the ground-truth position (y_0, y_1) is defined as:

$$p = \frac{\exp\left(x - x_{max}\right)}{\sum_{i,j} \exp(x_{i,j} - x_{max})}$$

$$L_{sharpness} = -\log p_{y_0, y_1}$$

$$\tilde{y}_0 = \sum_{i,j} p_{i,j} \cdot i$$

$$\tilde{y}_1 = \sum_{i,j} p_{i,j} \cdot j$$

$$L_{distance} = |\tilde{y}_0 - y_0| + |\tilde{y}_1 - y_1|$$

$$L = L_{sharpness} + L_{distance}$$

where x is the two dimensional net output. The value of $p_{i,j} \in [0,1]$ is interpreted as probability of the mouse being at a certain position (i,j). The estimated position including subpixel interpolation is $(\tilde{y}_0, \tilde{y}_1)$. The subtraction of x_{max} guarantess the result of the exponentiation to be finite. $L_{distance}$ is based on the softargmax loss [6]. This function is distance-aware and therefore well suitable for localization training. It penalizes probabilities based on their distance to the ground truth positions. The $L_{sharpness}$ term is based on the cross entropy loss, except normalizing over pixels not the channels. Additionally, it improves training speed and robustness by directly enlarging the probability of the correct position. We compute the loss at two positions in the network, once at the bottleneck stage and once at the end of the upsampling stage as our preliminary experiments have shown that this approach increases training time and prediction precision. The overall loss which is backpropagated through the network is the sum of both partial losses. The full architecture is shown in Fig. 1.

3   Experiments and results

To evaluate our loss function, we first generated a ground truth of segmentations and centroids from a set of 70 videos comprising 10000 individual frames departed in 10 subsets. Subsequently, all deep learning methods were validated using ten-fold cross validation.

Fig. 2 shows the results of the three implemented architectures. The basic VGG architecture delivers the least stable results, while both U-net-based approaches show a clearly higher precision. Results show that our proposed combined loss improves the detection accuracy beyond the default cross-entropy-based U-Net architecture while at the same time allowing direct training using landmark positions as ground truth, thereby eliminating the need for additional postprocessing steps to obtain the centroids from the segmentation masks. The median error of our proposed architecture is 1 pixel on a 512 x 384 pixel input and a mouse-size of 35 pixels. In contrast, the cross-entropy-based U-Net achieves a median precision of 1.5 pixels and the VGG regression architecture achieves 5 pixels.

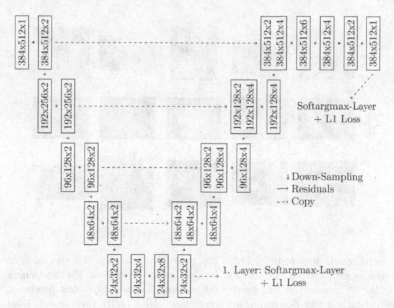

Fig. 1. Our proposed U-Net architecture with two instances of the distance and sharpness loss applied at the bottleneck and final stages.

Fig. 2. Quantitative results of the three implemented architectures. The error is measured as pixel distance to the automatically generated ground reference. Lower values are better.

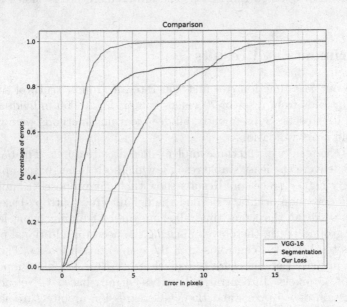

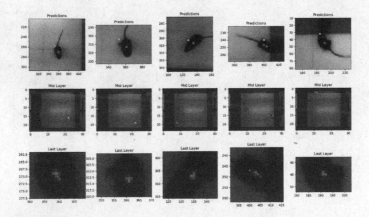

Fig. 3. Softargmax loss results. From top to bottom: final positions $(\tilde{y}_0, \tilde{y}_1)$ overlays on zoomed-in crops from the output images, map overlay of the bottleneck stage, map overlay on zoomed-in full resolution images. Yellow: positions predicted at the botleneck stage on the downsampled input size. Red: fully upsampled, final result. Green: ground truth (y_0, y_1). Best viewed electronically.

An analysis of the results of the two loss functions shows that already the loss that is applied to the bottleneck stage allows precise detection which is subsequently refined by the upsampling stages. Sample results are shown in Fig. 3.

4 Discussion and outlook

We evaluated a set of different deep learning methods for automated rodent localization in open field scenarios. Next to established architectures, we introduced a novel loss function that allows direct coordinate localization using fully convolutional architectures. Results show that our proposed approach outperforms other common approaches in terms of localization accuracy. Future work will include enhanced behavior analysis of rodent locomotion. Furthermore, we will investigate extending our architecture towards other tasks in medical imaging, for example multi-position and multi-class localization.

Acknowledgement. This research was fully funded by the German Research Foundation (DFG), project ID: ME 3737/18-1 and 651874.

References

1. De Chaumont F, Coura RDS, Serreau P, et al. Computerized video analysis of social interactions in mice. Nat Methods. 2012;9(4):410.
2. Noldus LP, Spink AJ, Tegelenbosch RA. EthoVision: a versatile video tracking system for automation of behavioral experiments. Behavior Research Methods, Instruments, & Computers. 2001;33(3):398–414.
3. De Chaumont F, Ey E, Torquet N, et al. Live mouse tracker: real-time behavioral analysis of groups of mice. BioRxiv. 2018; p. 345132.
4. Simonyan K, Zisserman A. Very deep convolutional networks for large-scale image recognition. arXiv preprint arXiv:14091556. 2014;.
5. Ronneberger O, Fischer P, Brox T. U-net: convolutional networks for biomedical image segmentation. In: International Conference on Medical image computing and computer-assisted intervention. Springer; 2015. p. 234–241.
6. Honari S, Molchanov P, Tyree S, et al. Improving landmark localization with semi-supervised learning. In: Proceedings of the IEEE Conference on Computer Vision and Pattern Recognition; 2018. p. 1546–1555.

Deep OCT Angiography Image Generation for Motion Artifact Suppression

Julian Hossbach[1,2], Lennart Husvogt[1,3], Martin F. Kraus[1,4],
James G. Fujimoto[3], Andreas K. Maier[1]

[1] Pattern Recognition Lab, Friedrich-Alexander-Universität Erlangen-Nürnberg
[2] SAOT, Friedrich-Alexander-Universität Erlangen, Germany
[3] Biomedical Optical Imaging and Biophotonics Group, MIT, Cambridge, USA
[4] Siemens Healthineers AG, Erlangen
julian.hossbach@fau.de

Abstract. Eye movements, blinking and other motion during the acquisition of optical coherence tomography (OCT) can lead to artifacts, when processed to OCT angiography (OCTA) images. Affected scans emerge as high intensity (white) or missing (black) regions, resulting in lost information. The aim of this research is to fill these gaps using a deep generative model for OCT to OCTA image translation relying on a single intact OCT scan. Therefore, a U-Net is trained to extract the angiographic information from OCT patches. At inference, a detection algorithm finds outlier OCTA scans based on their surroundings, which are then replaced by the trained network. We show that generative models can augment the missing scans. The augmented volumes could then be used for 3-D segmentation or increase the diagnostic value.

1 Introduction

Optical coherence tomography (OCT) enables a cross-sectional and non-invasive imaging of the eye's fundus in axial direction and thus, by depicting the retina's anatomical layers, results in a high diagnostic value in ophthalmology. A further significant increase for the examination is offered by the OCT angiography (OCTA), which exhibits the microvasculature of the retina and choroid. For example, microaneurysms, caused by diabetic retinopathy, can be identified in OCTA images [1].

One popular, solely image based, OCTA imaging technique relies on the varying reflectance of the flowing red blood cells over time, while the signal of surrounding tissue is almost stationary. By decorrelating 2 or more OCT scans, acquired over a short period of time at the very same location, vessels are enhanced and form an OCTA scan [2]. While the acquisition of a single OCT image, also called B-scan, is rapidly done by combining 1-D axial scans in lateral direction, a stack of B-scans is considerably slower.

As OCTA is derived from image changes over successively acquired B-scans, other origins of image differences than blood flow can result in artifacts. One

© Springer Fachmedien Wiesbaden GmbH, ein Teil von Springer Nature 2020
T. Tolxdorff et al. (Hrsg.), *Bildverarbeitung für die Medizin 2020*,
Informatik aktuell, https://doi.org/10.1007/978-3-658-29267-6_55

cause of such artifacts is motion, which leads to a misalignment of the B-scans of consecutive volumes. The origin of the motion can be rooted in pulsation, tremor and microsaccades, involuntary executed by the subject. Misalignment can lead to high decorrelation values and manifest as white stripes in en-face projections (along axial direction) of the OCTA volume [3]. Another source of artifacts, showing as black lines in the projection, is blinking, which results into lost OCT scans and therefore no OCTA image at that location.

More elaborated OCTA algorithms, like the Split-spectrum Amplitude Decorrelation Angiography, can compensate for motion in the axial direction but still relies on several aligned structural B-scans and quarters the axial resolution [4]. A recent algorithm consists of a Deep Learning (DL) pipeline for the extraction of angiographic information from a stack of OCT B-scans [5]. As both methods rely on matching B-scans, they are prone to the aforementioned artifacts. We propose a new generative DL based strategy to replace detected erroneous OCTA B-scans using an image-to-image translation architecture from a single OCT scan. Exhibiting these blind spots of conventional algorithms can increase the usability for physicians and improve further processing like vessel segmentation.

2   Materials and methods

2.1   Defect scan detection

The first step to replace defect OCTA scans is the detection algorithm, which triggers the OCT-OCTA translation network for identified angiographic scans.

Threshold based detection is commonly used, thus we adapt this approach to include the aforementioned artifacts. The summed flow signal of OCTA scans is calculated for each B-scan and compared to an upper and lower value. Instead of global thresholds, local limits $\theta_{l/u}$ are determined with $\theta_l = \mu_{16} - \eta\sigma_{16}$ and $\theta_u = \mu_5 + \tau_u\sigma_5$ for the lower and upper bound, respectively. The mean μ_x and the variance σ_x is calculated over $x - 1$ nearest B-scans and the scan itself. For the lower bound, a broader neighborhood is considered, as well as the parameter $\eta = 0.029$ was selected less strict as this threshold only filters blank scans. With $\tau_u = 0.0255$ and a higher sensitivity to local changes, θ_u detects motion corrupted scans and outliers.

2.2   Data set and processing

The next step we process our data such that it can be used for the OCT-OCTA translation network. The data for this project consists of 106 volumetric OCTA scans, which were each generated from 2 structural volumes. The volume size is $500 \times 500 \times 465/433$ (number of B-scans, lateral and axial) pixels over an area of 3×3 mm or 6×6 mm for 54 and 52 volumes, respectively. The data is split into a training, validation and test data sets of 91, 15 and 10 volumes and zero padded to a mutual axial size of 480 pixels to compensate for the varying dimensionality. Each B-scan is normalized to the range of 0 to 1 using the global maximum value.

The information on vessels in OCT scans is likely not depended on the global B-scan, but rather locally encoded. Therefore, we can crop the B-scans along the lateral axis into patches of size 480×128 pixels to reduce the input size for the neural network (NN). During training we randomly select 100 patches per OCT-OCTA B-scan pair, which passed the detection algorithm, to augment the data. At inference, the input B-scan is cropped into 5 overlapping patches, such that the first and last 8 columns can be removed at the composition of the outputs.

Patches where the depicted structures were cropped by the top or bottom image margins due to the curvature of the retina were removed.

2.3   OCT-OCTA translation

After the detection and outlier rejection, the remaining data is used to train a supervised NN for image-to-image translation.

To achieve such domain transform, U-Nets [6] has been shown to be suitable. The layout of the developed U-Net is illustrated in Fig. 1. In the encoding section, after an initial convolution, two blocks are used to each halve the spatial input resolution. Each block consists of 2 dense blocks, which concatenates the block's input with its output along the channel direction after a convolution as input for the next layer. The transition block learns a 1×1 convolution and reduces the width and height by average pooling (2×2). The latent space is decoded by 2 decoding layers with an upsampling operation and final 1×1 convolution with a sigmoid activation. Each decoding layer is built from a residual layer followed by a nearest neighbor interpolation (not in the last layer) and a convolution to avoid upsampling artifacts. If not stated otherwise, the kernel size is 3×3 pixels, and every convolution is followed by leaky ReLU (slope 0.1) as non-linearity and batch normalization.

The training process minimized the L2 norm between the generated patch and the ground truth. For a few training epochs, a further preprocessing step smooths the target OCTA images with a $3 \times 3 \times 3$ median filter to reduce the speckle noise in the target data and to enforce a higher focus on vessel information. In addition, from related work, it can be expected that speckle noise is also reduced in DL generated OCTA scans [5].

3   Results

The evaluation is 3 folded. First, we evaluate the generated OCTA B-scans from the test data by comparing them with the ground truth at intact locations. Secondly, we look at the en-face projection of the fake angiographic volume and its reference. Due to the anatomical structure of the choroid, the amount of blood vessels leads to noisy OCTA signals without hardly any recognizable individual vessels in the ground truth. In projections of our OCTA data, this leads to a reduced contrast of the vessels in upper layers. Therefore, we segment the vitreous as upper bound and the inner plexiform layer as lower bound using the OCTSEG-tool [7] of two volumes and only use the area in between for the evaluation of the projection. Finally, the detected defect scans are replaced and evaluated.

The first row of Tab. 1 shows the mean absolute error (MAE), mean square error (MSE) and the structural similarity (SSIM) between the generated scan and the ground truth, averaged over all intact test B-scans. Example B-scans are depicted in Fig. 2. The top left image shows the input OCT scan, to its right, the target angiographic image is shown. In the row below, the output image and the absolute difference to the ground truth are displayed. As expected from Liu et al. [5], the result has reduced noise structure.

	MAE	MSE	SSIM
B-scans:	0.019	0.002	0.761
Seg. proj. 1:	0.0096	0.0001	0.9978
Seg. proj. 2:	0.0138	0.0002	0.9896
Unseg. proj.:	0.0096	0.0001	0.93

Table 1. The table shows the mean absolute error (MAE), mean squared error (MSE) and the structural similarity (SSIM) for all test B-scans, the 2 segmented projections and the remaining unsegmented projections.

The image metrics of the segmented projections are written in Tab. 1 in the second and third row, the metric of the unsegmented volumes in the last row. In the 3rd and 4th row of Fig. 2, the segmented projection of the OCT, target and output volume are exhibited. Regarding also the less noisy structure, it can

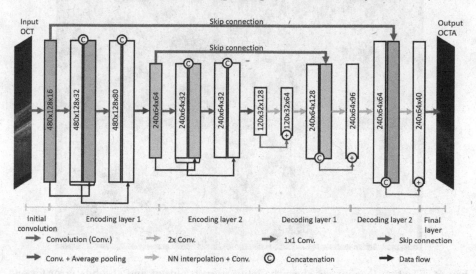

Fig. 1. Layout of the utilized U-Net for image translation with Dense Blocks and average pooling of 2×2 in the encoding part. The decoder combines nearest neighbor interpolation and residual blocks for upsampling.

be concluded that not only speckle noise is diminished, but also smaller vessels. Nonetheless, all major vessels are extracted accurately.

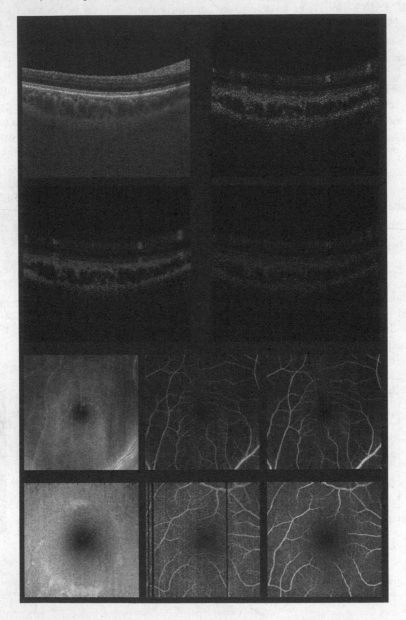

Fig. 2. The first four images show the input, target, output and absolute error for one example B-scan. The projections of the segmented volumes are shown below in order input, target and completely generated output. Note the artifacts are removed in the generated projection.

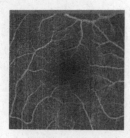

Fig. 3. The defect scans of the projection in Fig. 2 were replace with the generated ones. On top, the line marks the detected defect (red) and intact (green) scans.

The target projection of the second example in Fig. 2 clearly shows several artifacts as a result of blinking. In Fig. 3, we used the lower threshold to detect the defect scans and merge the network's result into the detected gaps, which are marked with the red stripe on top.

4   Discussion and conclusion

Based on a single intact OCT scan, the NN can approximate useful OCTA images. Major vessels have a sharper edge and seemingly a better contrast. Smaller vessels are not extracted accurately, but this might be rooted in the fact, that a single structural scan is insufficient for such details. As a result, inserted scans can be identified, when compared to the neighborhood. Furthermore, our approach still needs a correct input B-scan, otherwise the artifacts will remain.

As the requirements for our approach only comprise a single scan at locations with artifacts and the network with its preprocessing, an integration into the OCTA imaging workflow is easily possible and can improve the image quality easily.

Acknowledgement. We gratefully acknowledge the support of NVIDIA Corporation with the donation of the Titan Xp GPU used for this research.

References

1. de Carlo T, Romano A, Waheed N, et al. A review of optical coherence tomography angiography (OCTA). Int J Retina Vitreous. 2015;1(5).
2. Zhang A, Zhang Q, Chen C, et al. Methods and algorithms for optical coherence tomography-based angiography: a review and comparison. J Biomed Opt. 2015;20(10):100901.
3. Spaide R, Fujimoto J, Waheed N. Image artifacts in optical coherence angiography. Retina. 2015;35(11):2163–80.
4. Jia Y, Tan O, Tokayer J, et al. Split-spectrum amplitude-decorrelation angiography with optical coherence tomography. Opt Express. 2012;20(4):4710–25.
5. Liu X, Huang Z, Wang Z, et al. A deep learning based pipeline for optical coherence tomography angiography. J Biophotonics. 2019;12(10):e201900008.
6. Ronneberger O, Fischer P, Brox T. U-Net: convolutional networks for biomedical image segmentation. MICCAI. 2015;9351:234–241.
7. Mayer M, Sheets K. OCT segmentation and evaluation GUI. PRL FAU Erlangen. 2012;Available from: https://www5.cs.fau.de/de/forschung/software/octseg/.

Open Source Simulation of Fixational Eye Drift Motion in OCT Scans

Towards Better Comparability and Accuracy in Retrospective OCT Motion Correction

Merlin A. Nau[1,*], Stefan B. Ploner[1,*], Eric M. Moult[2], James G. Fujimoto[2], Andreas K. Maier[1]

[1]Pattern Recognition Lab, Friedrich-Alexander-Universität Erlangen-Nürnberg
[2]Department for Electrical Engineering and Computer Science and Research Laboratory for Electronics, Massachusetts Institute of Technology, Cambridge, USA
*both authors contributed equally
stefan.ploner@fau.de

Abstract. Point-wise scanning modalities like Optical Coherence Tomography (OCT) or Scanning Laser Ophthalmoscopy suffer from distortions due to the perpetual motion of the eye. While various motion correction approaches have been proposed, the absence of ground truth displacements or images entails a lack of accurate and comparable evaluations. The purpose of this paper is to close this gap by initiating an open source framework for the simulation of realistic eye motion and corresponding artificial distortion of scans, thereby for the first time enabling the community to a) create datasets with accessible ground truth and b) compare the correction of identical motion patterns in data acquired with different scanners or scan patterns. This paper extends previous work on simulation of fixational eye drift via a self-avoiding random walk in a potential to a continuous domain in time and space, allowing the derivation of smooth displacement fields. The model is demonstrated by presenting an examplary motion path, whose properties resemble reported properties of recordings in current literature on fixational eye motion. Furthermore, the artificial distortion of scans is demonstrated by showing a correspondingly distorted image of a virtual raster scan modeled according to the properties of an existing OCT scanner. All experiments can be reproduced and adapted to arbitrary scanner- and raster scan pattern-properties in the publicly available framework. Beyond that, the open source code provides a starting point for the community to integrate extensions like saccadic or axial eye motion.

1 Introduction

Raster scanned ophthalmic imaging modalities like optical coherence tomography (OCT) and Scanning Laser Ophthalmoscopy (SLO) suffer from distortion

© Springer Fachmedien Wiesbaden GmbH, ein Teil von Springer Nature 2020
T. Tolxdorff et al. (Hrsg.), *Bildverarbeitung für die Medizin 2020*,
Informatik aktuell, https://doi.org/10.1007/978-3-658-29267-6_56

due to the perpetual motion of the eye even during fixation. Martinez-Conde et al. categorize the motion in small-amplitude tremor, slow drift and occasional high-amplitude micro-saccadic motion [1]. One research direction to correct for this motion is to retrospectively register multiple scans and thereby reduce the contained motion. However, registration accuracy cannot be directly evaluated, because neither ground truth displacements nor motion-free reference data is available. This limits evaluation to reproducibility studies [2], which are limited by the accuracy of the underlying features and avoided in most publications due to the large amount of required repeated scans. Convenient yet accurate evaluations could be facilitated via simulation of eye motion and subsequent application to existing scans. A simulation could not only provide the underlying ground truth displacements, but also allow the comparison of identical motion in images of different scanners, scan patterns or scan quality. While distortion in the underlying scans is less of a problem in orthogonal raster scan motion correction appraoches [2], especially lag bias approaches [3] should be applied to the input scan before adding simulated distortion to avoid an adverse evaluation bias from correcting the initial distortion.

As a starting point for a full model for fixational eye motion, this paper proposes an extensible model for the simulation of drift eye motion. A promising approach based on a self-avoiding random walk in a potential has been previously investigated by Engbert et al. [4] and is described in more detail in the next paragraph. The approach has been reused by Azimipour et al. to simulate motion in AO-SLO and OCT images [3]. In this work, the authors published a simulated displacement field and a script to distort existing scans along with example images. However, the motion simulation itself is not publicly available, limiting the reuse to a single displacement field of a model that cannot be adapted.

The model describes the motion as a random walk in a grid, which is influenced by two potentials that alter the behavior of the random walk to better equate fixational drift eye motion. To model a point of fixation, the squared distance from a cell (i, j) to the center (i_0, j_0) is used as a potential according to

$$u_{i,j} = \lambda \cdot \left(\left(\frac{i - i_0}{i_0} \right)^2 + \left(\frac{j - j_0}{j_0} \right)^2 \right) \tag{1}$$

where λ is a user defined scaling factor. To achieve self-avoidance, an activation potential is tracked for each cell following Freund and Grassberger's model for a random walk in a swamp [5]. The activation is updated after each step by increasing the visited cell's activation by 1 and decaying the others according to

$$h_{i,j} \mapsto (1 - \epsilon) \cdot h_{i,j} \tag{2}$$

where $h_{i,j}$ is the activation of grid cell (i, j) and ϵ describes the decay.

While Engbert et al. validated their model on a macroscopic scale, the approach has limitations for the application to raster scanned images. Since the resulting displacement field is directly generated by the steps of the random walker, the frequency of the motion is directly connected to the sampling frequency. The movement in a grid leads to an unrealistic distribution of step directions limiting the use for evaluation of motion correction approaches. The use of grid cell coordinates and discrete step numbers instead of metric spatial and temporal units does not allow direct transfer to scans and properties of the path cannot directly be compared with measurements from literature. Lastly the lack of an open source implementation hinders the use of the model. To overcome these limitations, we propose a new, continuous, metric and open source drift eye motion model in Section 2, compare properties of example movements with literature in 3, and discuss advantages and limitations of the model in 4.

2   Materials and methods

While the herein proposed model conceptually follows the previously described model, it was adapted with the following key changes: The transferral of the discrete model from steps in a grid to a continuous domain allows random walking directions and step sizes which is further described in 2.1, the fitting of a continuous curve through the previously simulated steps to allow arbitrary sampling frequencies for the same underlying motion as described in 2.2, and, last but not least, the consistent use of metric units that allow direct use of simulated displacements for the distortion of images.

2.1   Random walk in a continuous domain

Starting at a location normally distributed around the center with standard deviation σ_{start}, the walker operates in a square continuous domain with an opening angle α specified in degree and performs steps with a frequency of f_{step} until the simulation period T is reached. Each step is sampled from a probability distribution defined by two components. The first component describes the velocity as a direction drawn from a uniform distribution and a step size d drawn normally distributed with mean μ_{step} and standard deviation $\sigma_{\text{step}}/\sqrt{w_{\text{step}}}$ according to the formula

$$\exp\left(0.5 \cdot \left(\frac{d - \mu_{\text{step}}}{\sigma_{\text{step}}}\right)^2 \cdot w_{\text{step}}\right) \tag{3}$$

The exponential weight w_{step} is described at the end of this section.

The second component is defined by the sum of the fixation potential and visited activation. The fixation potential is evaluated for the target location according to (1), except that i and j are treated as continuous variables. The visited-activation is still discretized in a grid whose side lengths are defined by a resolution k and the field size of the walker domain. To correctly retain the self-avoidance property for arbitrary step sizes and grid resolutions, it is not sufficient to determine the activation only at the target location. Instead, a line is drawn between the walkers start and target locations to determine the crossed cells, and the maximum activation is used. The starting cell is excluded unless the walker stays in the same cell, because it was just increased in the previous iteration and thus would usually dominate the activation of the other cells. The potentials are then transformed to a probability through inversion, resulting in the formula

$$\left(\max_{(k,l)\in L} \{h_{k,l}\} + u(x,y)\right)^{-w_{\text{pot}}} \tag{4}$$

where L are the cells on the connecting line between the start and target location of the current step, x, y are the coordinates of the target location, u is the continuous potential analogous to (1) and w_{pot} is another exponential weight.

The probability distribution is then defined by the product of both components and normalized appropriately. The weights w_{step} and w_{pot} can be used to pronounce the probabilities, i. e. large weights will make the selection of highest probabilities more likely up to a maximum selection, whereas the distribution becomes uniform as the weights approach zero.

Since it is impossible to directly draw samples from the previously described distribution, drawing is performed as a two step process: First, C candidate locations are sampled using (3) in a monte-carlo fashion. Secondly, a candidate is chosen by weighted random selection with probabilities computed according to (4). The probabilities defined by (3) are inherently taken into account in this decision through the density of the candidate locations. A map showing the sum of both potentials after the random walk described in Section 3 is shown in Fig. 1, as well as a visualization of the probability distribution sampling.

After the step, the activation of the crossed cells in L are incremented by 1 and the remaining cells are relaxed according to (2).

2.2   B-spline path representation for arbitrary sampling in time

To be able to freely choose the sampling frequency of a virtual scanner independantly from the motion simulation, a cubic B-spline is fitted through the

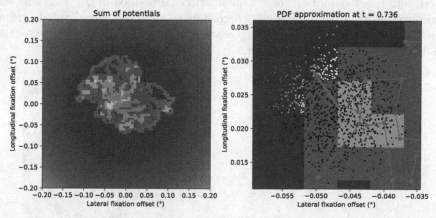

Fig. 1. Left: Summed potentials after the run described in Section 3. The activation of visited cells is apparent in the center, whereas the fixation potential causes the increased values in the periphery. Right: Visualization of the random selection. The background grid shows the potential sum, the circles represent step candidates with brightness corresponding to probability, the central arrow displays the selected step.

Table 1. Simulation setup for the reported run.

T	3.7 s	σ_{start}	0	f_{step}	250 Hz
μ_{step}	0.005 $^\circ$	σ_{step}	0.0025 $^\circ$	w_{step}	1
C	1000	k	202.5 $\cdot$ 1/$^\circ$	λ	20
ϵ	0.1	w_{pot}	4	f_{step}	400 kHz
α	0.4				

simulated walker locations. While this doesn't change the random walker's behavior on macro scale, this leads to continuous motion between the steps. This is reasonable, because eye movements are limited by inertia. The spline can then be sampled with a frequency $f_{sampling}$ until the scan duration T is reached.

3 Results

Tab. 1 lists the parameters for the simulation of the path displayed in both figures. The simulated curve exhibits an average speed of 1.46 $^\circ$/s with a standard deviation of 0.54 $^\circ$/s, which is in line with fixational eye motion measurements reported in [6]. Also the overall spread of the viewing direction is very similar.

The OCT angiography image shown in Fig. 2 was acquired with a swept source OCT scanner previously described in [7]. Key properties are a vertical cavity surface emitting laser (VCSEL) with a center wavelength of 1050 nm and an A-scan rate of 400 kHz. The image was acquired over a field size of 3×3 mm at a resolution of 500^2 pixels with 5 B-scan repeats. The number of A-scans discarded during flyback is 87. The whole acquisition thus takes almost 3.7 s. The image was first motion corrected using an orthogonal raster scan based, retrospective motion correction algorithm described in [2]. This scan was then distorted by virtually sampling according to all in this paragraph described scan parameters, with the sampling coordinates being shifted with respect to the described simulated eye motion.

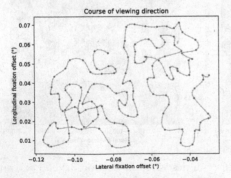
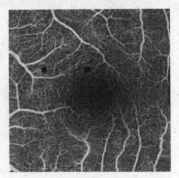

Fig. 2. Left: Path in the range 2.5 s to 3 s. Simulated steps displayed as blue dots, B-Spline with a subset of sampling points shown in orange. Right: Original and distorted image overlaid in red and cyan.

4   Discussion

In conclusion, the realism of the proposed fixational drift eye motion model is supported by both the visual impression of the artificially distorted scan in Fig. 2 and the aggreement of the properties derived from the motion curve with literature. Compared to the approach proposed by Engbert et al. [4], the motion is simulated in a both in time and space metric and continuous domain and the step frequency of the random walker, which is related to the frequency component of the simulated motion, is decoupled from the sampling frequency by sampling from a B-spline fitted through the simulated steps instead. The scripts for motion simulation and corresponding distortion of scans, available at https://github.com/sploner/eye-motion-simulation, provide a simpel yet effective approach to evaluate retrospective motion correction algorithms and establish a new level of both reproducibility and comparability, e. g. through the possibility to evaluate the correction of identical motion in different scan patterns, scanner speeds and scan qualities. Furthermore, the open source availability of the code allows custom extensions to the proposed model as needed. However, in its current state the approach lacks an integrated saccade model which would be a natural next step. Further possible extensions are the modeling of axial motion, head tilt, or a more exact model for warping the eye ball to the image plane. In addition, noise models could be integrated to allow additional evaluation of the stability of motion correction approaches towards noise.

Acknowledgement. The authors acknowledge funding from the German Research Foundation (DFG) through project MA 4898/12-1.

References

1. Martinez-Conde S, Macknik SL, Hubel DH, et al. The role of fixational eye movements in visual perception. Nat Rev Neurosci. 2004;5(3):229.
2. Ploner SB, Kraus MF, Husvogt L, et al. 3-D OCT motion correction efficiently enhanced with OCT angiography. Investig Ophthalmol Vis Sci. 2018;59(3-4):3922.
3. Azimipour M, Zawadzki RJ, Gorczynska I, et al. Intraframe motion correction for raster-scanned adaptive optics images using strip-based cross-correlation lag biases. PLoS One. 2018;13(10):e0206052.
4. Engbert R, Mergenthaler K, Sinn P, et al. An integrated model of fixational eye movements and microsaccades. Proc Natl Acad Sci U S A. 2011;108(39):E765–E770.
5. Freund H, Grassberger P. The red queen's walk. Physica A: Stat Mech Appl. 1992;190(3-4):218–237.
6. Ko Hk, Snodderly DM, Poletti M. Eye movements between saccades: measuring ocular drift and tremor. Vision Res. 2016;122(5):93–104.
7. Choi W, Potsaid B, Jayaraman V, et al. Phase-sensitive swept-source optical coherence tomography imaging of the human retina with a vertical cavity surface-emitting laser light source. Opt Lett. 2013;38(3):338–340.

Abstract: Multi-Task Framework for X-Ray Guided Planning in Knee Surgery

Florian Kordon[1,2,3], Peter Fischer[1,2], Maxim Privalov[4], Benedict Swartman[4], Marc Schnetzke[4], Jochen Franke[4], Ruxandra Lasowski[2], Andreas Maier[1], Holger Kunze[2]

[1]Pattern Recognition Lab, Department of Computer Science, Friedrich-Alexander-Universität Erlangen-Nürnberg, Erlangen, Germany
[2]Advanced Therapies, Siemens Healthcare GmbH, Forchheim, Germany
[3]Faculty of Digital Media, Hochschule Furtwangen, Furtwangen, Germany
[4]Department for Trauma and Orthopaedic Surgery, BG Trauma Center Ludwigshafen, Ludwigshafen, Germany
florian.kordon@fau.de

X-ray imaging is frequently used to facilitate planning and operative guidance for surgical interventions. By capturing patient-specific information prior to and during the procedure, such image-based tools benefit a more reliable and minimally invasive workflow at reduced risk for the patient. To this end, typical assessment involves geometric measurements of patient anatomy, verification of correct positioning of surgical tools and implants, as well as navigational guidance with help of anatomical landmarks and bone morphology. However, performing the involved steps manually is prone to intra-/inter-rater variability and increases the task complexity for the surgeon. To remedy these issues and using femoral drill site planning for medial patellofemoral ligament reconstruction as an example, we present a framework which allows fully-automatic localization of anatomical landmarks, segmentation of bone structures, and prediction of ROIs for geometric line features on X-ray images [1]. We exploit recent advances in sequential deep learning architectures in form of deep stacked hourglass networks to refine predictions based on the learned residual information between intermediate estimates. We propose an extension to a multi-task learning approach to incorporate cross-task information and introduce a novel adaption of gradient normalization for automatic task weighting in stacked network architectures. On 38 clinical test images the framework achieves a median localization error of 1.50 mm for the femoral drill site and mean IOU scores of 0.99, 0.97, 0.98, and 0.96 for the femur, patella, tibia, and fibula respectively. The demonstrated approach consistently performs surgical planning at expert-level precision without a need for manual correction.

References

1. Kordon F, Fischer P, Privalov M, et al. Multi-task localization and segmentation for x-ray guided planning in knee surgery. Proc Med Image Comput Comput Assist Interv. 2019; p. 622–630.

© Springer Fachmedien Wiesbaden GmbH, ein Teil von Springer Nature 2020
T. Tolxdorff et al. (Hrsg.), *Bildverarbeitung für die Medizin 2020*,
Informatik aktuell, https://doi.org/10.1007/978-3-658-29267-6_57

Abstract: 3D Catheter Guidance Including Shape Sensing for Endovascular Navigation

Sonja Jäckle[1], Verónica García-Vázquez[2], Felix von Haxthausen[2],
Tim Eixmann[3], Malte Maria Sieren[4], Hinnerk Schulz-Hildebrandt[3,5,6],
Gereon Hüttmann[3,5,6], Floris Ernst[2], Markus Kleemann[7], Torben Pätz[8]

[1]Fraunhofer MEVIS, Institute for Digital Medicine, Lübeck, Germany
[2]Institute for Robotics and Cognitive Systems, Universität zu Lübeck, Germany
[3]Medizinisches Laserzentrum Lübeck GmbH, Lübeck, Germany
[4]Department for Radiology and Nuclear Medicine, UKSH, Lübeck, Germany
[5]Institute of Biomedical Optics, Universität zu Lübeck, Germany
[6]German Center for Lung Research, DZL, Großhansdorf, Germany
[7]Department of Surgery, UKSH, Lübeck, Germany
[8]Fraunhofer MEVIS, Institute for Digital Medicine, Bremen, Germany
sonja.jaeckle@mevis.fraunhofer.de

In endovascular aortic repair (EVAR) procedures fluoroscopy and conventional digital subtraction angiography are currently used to guide the medical instruments inside the patient. Drawbacks of these methods are X-ray exposure and the usage of contrast agents. Moreover, the fluoroscopy provides only a 2D view, which makes the guidance more difficult. For this reason, a catheter prototype including an optical fiber for shape sensing and three electromagnetic (EM) sensors, which provide the position and orientation information, was built to enable a 3D catheter guidance. In addition, a model was introduced to process the input data from the tracking systems to obtain the located 3D shape of the first 38 cm of the catheter [1]. First, a spatial calibration between the optical fiber and each EM sensor was made. This relationship can be used to locate the reconstructed shape of the catheter with the EM sensor poses by determining a rigid transformation. The shape localization method was evaluated using the catheter prototype in different shape measurements and the located 3D shapes were compared with the segmented shapes of the computed tomography scans. The experiments resulted in average errors from 0.99 to 2.29 mm and maximum errors from 1.73 to 2.99 mm. The accuracies are promising for using the 3D guidance based on an optical fiber and three EM sensors for EVAR procedures. Future work will be to reduce the necessary EM sensors for locating the shape of the catheter. Moreover, this catheter guidance method will be evaluated in a more realistic setting on vessel phantoms.

References

1. Jäckle S, García-Vázquez V, von Haxthausen F, et al. 3D catheter guidance including shape sensing for endovascular navigation. Proc SPIE. 2020;.

© Springer Fachmedien Wiesbaden GmbH, ein Teil von Springer Nature 2020
T. Tolxdorff et al. (Hrsg.), *Bildverarbeitung für die Medizin 2020*,
Informatik aktuell, https://doi.org/10.1007/978-3-658-29267-6_58

Erlernbarkeitsstudie eines vibrotaktilen Armbands für assistive Navigation

Hakan Calim[1], Andreas Maier[2]

[1]Regionales Rechenzentrum Erlangen Nürnberg
[2]Fakultät für Pattern Recognition, FAU Erlangen-Nürnberg
hakan.calim@fau.de

Kurzfassung. Für die Entwicklung eines assistiven Navigationssystems für blinde bzw. sehbehinderte Personen wurde in einem Experiment die Einsetzbarkeit eines vibrotaktilen Armbands als Tool für die Übertragung von Umgebungsinformationen untersucht. Das Tool wurde zunächst für die Navigation der Probanden durch einen Parcours eingesetzt; im Anschluss wurden mit einem Fragenkatalog Angaben zu Tragbarkeit und Einsetzbarkeit erfasst. Die Steuerung der Probanden erfolgte manuell über eine Kontrollapplikation auf einem Smartphone; dies soll in einer späteren Arbeit durch ein System mit Umgebungserkennung für assistive Navigation ersetzt werden. Die Bewegungen und Kollisionen mit Hindernissen im Parcours wurden mit vier Raumkameras erfasst; Durchlaufzeiten und Anzahl Kollisionen wurden ausgewertet. Das Armband wurde auch im Vergleich mit Blindenhund und Blindenstock bewertet. Die Ergebnisse zeigen, dass das Armband schon nach drei Durchgängen deutliche Verkürzungen der Durchlaufzeiten ermöglichte - vergleichbar wie beim geübten Einsatz von einem Blindenstock. Die Tragbarkeit des Armbandes wurde mit Mean Opinions Scores von sehbehinderten Personen als „gut" bis „exzellent" eingestuft. Das Armband eignet sich daher insgesamt als Tool für die weitere Entwicklung eines assisitiven Navigationssystems.

1 Einleitung

Die Navigation von Blinden bzw. Sehbehinderten Personen (BSP) im öffentlichen Straßenverkehr stellt eine große Herausforderung für assistive Navigationssysteme dar. Eine erste Entwicklung solcher Systeme begann 1969 Bach-y Rita et al. [1] mit einer nicht mobilen Kamera, die Umgebungsinformationen erfasste und über Sensoren, die an einem Stuhl befestigt waren, taktil über den Rücken an einen blinden Probanden übertrug. Diese Grundidee der Sensor Substitution mit taktilen Reizen [2] kann heute mit Hilfe von Computer Vision, Kamerasystemen und tragbaren Sensoren verbessert werden. In dieser Arbeit wird ein vibrotaktiles „VibroTac" Armband (VTA) von SENSODRIVE [3] untersucht, ob es sich generell als Tool für die Erzeugung von taktilen Vibrationsmustern für ein assistives Navigationssystem eignet. Die Entwicklung dieses Navigationssystems ist

© Springer Fachmedien Wiesbaden GmbH, ein Teil von Springer Nature 2020
T. Tolxdorff et al. (Hrsg.), *Bildverarbeitung für die Medizin 2020*,
Informatik aktuell, https://doi.org/10.1007/978-3-658-29267-6_59

derzeit noch im Aufbau und nicht Teil dieser Studie. Um die Einsetzbarkeit, Akzeptanz und Erlernbarkeit des Armbandes beurteilen zu können wurde ein Parcours aufgebaut; durch diesen Parcours wurden insgesamt 8 Testpersonen (2 BSPs und 6 normal sehende Personen mit verbundenen Augen) mit Hilfe des Armbandes navigiert und Zeit und Kollisionen während des Durchgangs gemessen. Die Navigation über taktile Vibrationsmuster wurde manuell mit einer Steuerapplikation des VibroTac Armbandes durchgeführt, soll aber später durch das Navigationssystem ersetzt werden. Jede Testperson beantwortete am Schluss noch einen Fragenkatalog für Feedback zu Akzeptanz und Erlernbarkeit. In der Literatur wurden bereits diverse Körperstellen auf ihre Eignung zur Übermittlung von taktilen Informationen an den Menschen untersucht [4]. In [5] wird ein Tongue Display Unit (TDU) vorgestellt, wo Informationen über einen Sensor auf der Zunge übertragen werden. Auf der Zunge ist zwar eine Auflösung von 12x12 Pixeln möglich, was an keiner anderen Körperstelle erreicht werden kann, doch wird das Sprechen durch die Nutzung erschwert, was sich auf die Akzeptanz des TDUs auswirkt. In [6, 7, 8] werden andere Körperstellen wie Bauch, Rücken oder Fuß als Körperstellen für Sensoren genutzt und Vibrationsmotoren eingesetzt um Richtungen zu signalisieren. Allerdings ist es in diesen Arbeiten nicht möglich besondere Eindrücke wie z.B. Drehen um die eigene Achse zu erzeugen. Das VibroTac Armband besteht aus 6 Vibrationsmotoren, die elastisch miteinander verbunden sind. Die Frequenz, Amplitude und Signalverlauf der einzelnen Motoren können separat angesteuert werden und dadurch verschiedene Vibrationsmuster am Handgelenk erzeugt werden. Die Applikation zur Erzeugung der Vibrationsmuster läuft auf einem Smartphone und die Kommunikation zum Armband erfolgt über Bluetooth. Da sich der Akku und die Steuereinheit der Vibrationsmotoren auf dem VTA befinden, kann das VTA ohne Bewegungseinschränkung (wie z.B. durch Kabel) am Arm getragen werden. Für den Parcours wurden aus der Applikation folgende Vibrationsmuster ausgewählt: Für das Signal „Gehen vorwärts" vibrierte der Vibrationsmotor im oberen Teil des VTA in kurzen Zeitabständen. Durch ein Neigen des Smartphones war es möglich den linken bzw. rechten Vibrationsmotor am VTA zu aktivieren; somit konnte ein Signal für einen „Schritt seitwärts" nach links oder rechts vermittelt werden. Eine Drehung um die eigene Achse nach links wurde über ein Vibrationsmuster signalisiert, das Reize rund um das Handgelenk gegen den Uhrzeigersinn erzeugte. Für eine Drehung nach rechts wurde ein Vibrationsmuster ausgewählt, wo jeder Vibrationsmotor angesteuert wird und so eine Art Klopfen am Armgelenk spürbar ist.

2 Material und Methoden

Für die Validierung des VTA wurde ein Parcours (Abb. 1) in einem Raum aufgebaut, wo das Vorwärtsgehen auf einem Gehweg, das Umgehen eines Hindernisses und das Vorbeinavigieren an zwei gegenüberliegenden parkenden Autos (wie in einer S-Kurve) nachgestellt wurden. Die Abschnitte des Parcours wurden von Tischen so abgegrenzt, dass ein Gang von 1,5m Breite entstand. Das Hindernis war 0,6m breit, die S-Kurve wurde mit Hilfe von 2 Hindernissen (das zweite Hindernis in einem Abstand von 2m zum ersten Hindernis) umgesetzt. Alle Abschnitte des Parcours wurden über vier Raumkameras aufgezeichnet. Alle vier Kamerasignale wurden bei der Auswertung mit Hilfe eines Schnittsystems synchronisiert und mit Zeitstempel versehen. Jede Testperson trug zusätzlich eine Bodycam am Körper, um jede Kollision eindeutig erfassen zu können. Da nur zwei BSPs für die Untersuchung zur Verfügung standen, wurden auch sechs Personen ausgewählt, die normal sehen können, aber während des Experiments die Augen komplett mit Augenklappen verbunden hatten. Eine der sehbehinderten Personen war von Geburt an blind und bewegt sich normal mit Hilfe eines Blindenhundes; die zweite BSP ist durch Beeinträchtigung des Sehens nach und nach fast blind geworden und verfügt nur noch über 5 Prozent Sehfähigkeit und verwendet einen Blindenstock. Diese Testperson trug während des Tests auch Augenklappen. Fünf der normalerweise sehenden Testpersonen hatten keinen Einblick in den Raum mit dem Parcours vor dem Test; die sechste Person wurde als Person für einen oberen Referenzwert ausgewählt und hatte kurz die Möglichkeit den Raum zu sehen, konnte sich allerdings nicht im Raum bewegen. Der Parcours war auch den BSPs völlig unbekannt. Die Autoren beabsichtigen die Wiederholung der Studie mit einer grösseren Anzahl von Testpersonen für eine statistisch relevante Auswertung in Verbindung mit dem fertigen Navigationssystem; hier sollte nur in einem ersten Ansatz die generelle Eignung des VTAs untersucht werden. Vor dem ersten (von insgesamt drei) Durchläufen wurde jeder Testperson ein Text mit einer ausführlichen Einweisung in die Vibrationsmuster vorgelesen. Gleichzeitig zum Text wurden am VTA die Vibrationsmuster abgespielt, so dass die Probanden alle Vibrationsmuster fühlen konnten und jedem Bewegungsmuster zuordnen konnten.

3   Ergebnisse

Es zeigte sich, dass jede Testperson mit dem VTA im dritten Durchgang bereits eine Verbesserung in der Zeit hatte verglichen zum ersten Durchlauf. Bei den beiden sehbehinderten Probanden war die Durchlaufzeit mit dem VTA fast so gut wie ein Durchlauf mit einem Blindenstock. Die BSPs hatten die insgesamt kürzesten Durchgänge (Abb. 2); das liegt vermutlich daran, dass sie gewohnt sind, sich blind zu bewegen und sich auf Hilfsmittel zu verlassen. Es war zu beobachten, dass die sehenden Testpersonen sich viel vorsichtiger und daher langsamer bei einem Durchgang bewegten und das Vibrationssignal genau abgewartet haben. Die zeitlichen Verbesserungen mit jedem Durchgang zeigen, dass das Erlernen der Vibrationsmuster und die Navigation durch das VTA gut möglich war. Unklar ist, wieviel Anteil an der Beschleunigung auf einen etwaigen „Lerneffekt" und das Merken der Strecke zurückzuführen sind und ob ein solcher „Lerneffekt" überhaupt eingetreten ist.

4   Diskussion

Abbildung 3 zeigt einen Vergleich der Durchlaufzeiten mit Blindenhund, Blindenstock oder VTA als Hilfsmittel. Als Probanden dienten die beiden BSPs und die Testperson mit kurzer Rauminformation als obere Referenzgrösse. Mit dem Blindenhund wurde nur ein Durchgang durchgeführt von der BSP, der der Blindenhund zugeteilt ist; beide BSPs machten jeweils einen Durchgang mit Blindenstock. Zwar ist die Durchlaufzeit für P2 mit Blindenhund die schnellste Zeit, aber die Durchgangszeiten von Blindenstock (im Bereich von 00:47.00 Sekunden bis 00:55.88 Sekunden) von P2 und P3 (beide BSPs) unterscheiden sich kaum von den kürzesten Durchlaufzeiten mit Armband (00:49.37 bis 00:53.67 Sekunden); P3 war mit Armband in einem Durchgang sogar schneller als mit Blindenstock, obwohl diese Testperson sich normalerweise mit dem Blindenstock als Hilfsmittel bewegt. Bei der Untersuchung der Anzahl von Kollisionen mit Hindernissen oder Abgrenzungen im Parcours zeigte sich, dass sich die wenigsten Kollisionen (nur eine Kollision im Durchlauf) beim Hilfsmittel Hund und auch beim Armband ergaben (Abb. 4). Erstaunlicherweise hatten die BSPs mehr Kollisionen im Parcours mit Blindenstock (4) als mit Armband (2-5) und auch im Vergleich mit

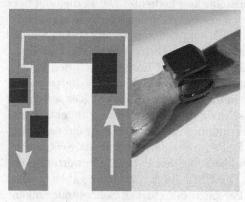

Abb. 1. Parcours und VTA.

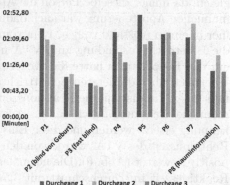

Abb. 2. Durchlaufszeit mit Armband.

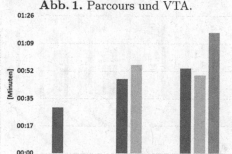

Abb. 3. Tools im Vergleich.

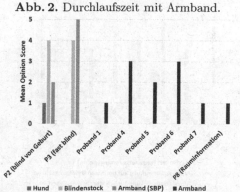

Abb. 4. Tools und Kollisionen.

den normalerweise sehenden Probanden; auch hier konnte man beobachten, dass ein BSP die Umgebung mit mehr Risikobereitschaft erkundete als Personen, die durch die ungewohnte Abdeckung der Augen sich in einer unbekannten Umgebung unsicher fühlten und sich vorsichtiger und genau nach Vibrationsmuster bewegten. Abbildung 5 zeigt die Auswertung der Fragen am Ende des Experiments zur Tragbarkeit (angenehm/unangenehm) des Armbandes, und zur Auswirkung auf den normalen Bewegungsablauf und Schrittgeschwindigkeit. Als Bewertungsskala dienten Mean Opinion Scores (MOS) [9] im Bereich von 1=mangelhaft, 2=mässig, 3=ordentlich, 4=gut und 5=exzellent. Insgesamt wurde dreimal „exzellent" vergeben (zweifach bzgl. Tragbarkeit und einmal für Bewegungsablauf); die Bewertung „gut" wurde insgesamt sechs mal angegeben. Was die Schrittgeschwindikeit mit Armband betrifft, so wurde die schlechteste Bewertung mit „mangelhaft" nur einmal vergeben; dies lag daran, dass die BSP gewöhnlich mit Blindenhund arbeitet und sehr schnell auf die Signale des Hundes reagieren kann. Die mögliche Schrittgeschwindigkeit in diesem ersten Experiment war abhängig von der manuellen Steuerung der Vibrationsmuster über die Smartphone App und hatte natürlich einen Einfluss auf die Reaktionszeit und damit Schrittgeschwindigkeit der Personen, allerdings war dieser Einfluss bei allen Probanden gleich, da immer dieselbe Person die Appsteuerung bediente. Die Bedienung der manuellen Appsteuerung war auch dadurch erschwert, dass diese Person sich immer in einem Abstand von ca. 1,5m vom VTA befinden musste, ansonsten wurde die Bluetooth Verbindung zum VTA unterbrochen. Durch das Hinterherfolgen auf die Testpersonen hatte die Steuerungsperson nicht immer gleich den vollen Überblick über die letzten Schrittrichtungen der Probanden. Dies hatte ebenfalls einen Einfluss auf die Reaktionszeit in diesem Experiment. Später soll diese manuelle Steuerung durch ein assistives Navigationssystem mit Umgebungserkennung ersetzt werden und diese Einschränkung aufheben. Die Frage nach der Reaktionszeit des VTAs wurde von den BSPs im Fragebogen mit MOS=4,5 sehr positiv bewertet (Abb. 6). Die normalerweise sehenden Personen bewerteten die Reaktionszeit im Durchschnitt mit 3,5. Die BSPs im Experiment gaben weiter an, dass sie das VTA mit MOS=4,5 an Personen mit starken Sehbehinderungen

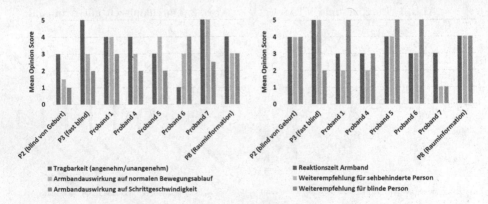

Abb. 5. Bewertung Tragbarkeit.   **Abb. 6.** Bewertung Einsetzbarkeit.

weiterempfehlen würden und mit MOS=3,5 für komplett blinde Personen empfehlen würden. Die nicht-BSP Probanden bewerteten eine Weiterempfehlung an BSPs mit einem durchschnittlichen MOS von 3,0.

5   Zusammenfassung und Ausblick

Diese Untersuchung hat gezeigt, dass durch den Einsatz des Armbandes schon nach wenigen Parcoursdurchgängen deutliche Verkürzungen der Durchlaufzeiten erreicht werden konnten und diese Zeiten vergleichbar waren zum geübten Einsatz vom Blindenstock. Die Tragbarkeit des Armbandes wurde mit Mean Opinions Scores von sehbehinderten Personen als „gut" bis „exzellent" eingestuft. Das Armband eignet sich daher insgesamt als Tool für die weitere Entwicklung eines assisitiven Navigationssystems und soll in weiteren Untersuchungen als Basis für die taktile Informationsübertragung dienen.

Danksagung. Die Firma SENSODRIVE GmbH hat die Arbeit mit einem vibrotaktilen Armband unterstützt; die Multimediagruppe des RRZE hat die videotechnische Erfassung des Experiments ermöglicht. Wir danken auch dem RRZE/FG-Netz für die Unterstützung mit (assistiver) Software.

Literaturverzeichnis

1. Bach-y Rita P, Collins CC, Saunders FA, et al. Vision substitution by tactile image projection. Nature. 1969;221(5184):963–964.
2. Visell Y. Tactile sensory substitution: models for enaction in HCI. Interacting with Computers. 2009;21(1-2):38–53.
3. SENSODRIVE GmbH. Vibrotactiles feedback - VibroTac;. Available from: https://www.sensodrive.de/produkte-leistungen/vibrotactiles-feedback.php.
4. Pawluk DTV, Adams RJ, Kitada R. Designing haptic assistive technology for individuals who are blind or visually impaired. IEEE Trans. 2015;8(3):258–278.
5. Kaczmarek KA. The tongue display unit (TDU) for electrotactile spatiotemporal pattern presentation. Scientia Iranica Trans D. 2011;18(6):1476–1485.
6. Kammoun S, Jouffrais C, Guerreiro T, et al. Guiding blind people with haptic feedback; 2012.
7. Katzschmann RK, Araki B, Rus D. Safe local navigation for visually impaired users with a time-of-flight and haptic feedback device. IEEE Trans Neural Sys and Rehab Eng : a publication of the IEEE Engineering in Medicine and Biology Society. 2018;26(3):583–593.
8. Velázquez R, Pissaloux E, Rodrigo P, et al. An outdoor navigation system for blind pedestrians using GPS and tactile-foot feedback. Applied Sciences. 2018;8(4):578.
9. Wikipedia. Mean opinion score;. Available from: https://de.wikipedia.org.

Visualizing the Placental Energy State in Vivo

Shyamalakshmi Haridasan[1], Bernhard Preim[1], Christian Nasel[2,3],
Gabriel Mistelbauer[1]

[1]Dept. Simulation and Graphics, Otto-von-Guericke University Magdeburg, Germany
[2]Dept. of Radiology, University Hospital Tulln, Karl Landsteiner University of
Health Sciences, Austria
[3]Dept. of Radiology and Nuclear Medicine, Medical University of Vienna, Austria
gmistelbauer@isg.cs.uni-magdeburg.de

Abstract. The human placenta is vital for the intrauterine growth and
development of fetus. It serves several vital functions, including the
transmission of nutrients and hormones from the maternal to the fetal
circulatory system. During pregnancy, partial infarcts, thrombosis or
hemorrhage within the placenta may affect or even reduce the functional
regions maintaining the exchange of hormones, oxygen and nutrients with
the fetus. This poses a risk to fetal development and should be monitored, since, at a certain point, the nutritious support might not be sufficient anymore. To assess the functional placental tissue, diffusion tensor
magnetic resonance imaging (DT-MRI) is used to discriminate different
levels of the placental functional state. Highly active regions contain
the so-called cotyledons, units that support the fetus with nutrients. In
case of their failure, the fetus gets deprived of sufficient nutritious support, which potentially leads to placental intrauterine growth restriction
(IUGR). The direct measurement of the functional state of the cotyledons could provide meaningful insight into the current placental energy
state. In this paper, we propose a workflow for extracting and visualizing
the functional state of a single cotyledon and a combined visualization
depicting the energy state of the entire placenta. We provide informal
feedback from a radiologist with experience in placental functional data
along 17 data sets.

1   Introduction

The human placenta plays a vital role during gestation by supporting the fetus
with the required nutrients, hormones and oxygen. This metabolic exchange between mother and fetus is done by many small units within the human placenta,
referred to as cotyledons [1]. As these units exhibit a high activity, they are well
perfused and found well visible in DT-MRI data sets, recognizable by a high
signal intensity and a toroidal shape. In case of failure, their activity decreases,
leading to a reduced signal intensity and an altered shape, but more important,
less energy is transferred to the developing fetus. Under this condition, the fetus could potentially start to suffer placental IUGR, thereby usually sparing the

© Springer Fachmedien Wiesbaden GmbH, ein Teil von Springer Nature 2020
T. Tolxdorff et al. (Hrsg.), *Bildverarbeitung für die Medizin 2020*,
Informatik aktuell, https://doi.org/10.1007/978-3-658-29267-6_60

most precious organ, the brain, while limiting further growth of other organs and body structures. Accordingly, placental DT-MRI demonstrated preservation of brain volume in growth-restricted fetuses who also suffered substantial reduction of the so-called putative functional placental tissue (PFPT), a term originally introduced by Nasel C. and Javor D. for regular appearing placental tissue [2, 3]. Further approaches to measure the amount of functional placental tissue were described, where placental perfusion was locally analyzed by partitioning the placenta with a Cartesian grid [4]. Additionally, the variation pattern of the regional placental oxygenation was found to coincide with the placental cotyledons when using BOLD MRI [5]. We present an in vivo visualization of functional placental compartments based on the assessment of PFPT-partitions measured using DT-MRI.

Though several factors may induce IUGR, placental insufficiency is the main reason for placental IUGR, which is a noteworthy challenge in maternal health care. Placental IUGR is related to an increased danger of perinatal mortality and dreariness. Generally, IUGR can be diagnosed by either estimating the fetal weight, amniotic fluid volume and abdominal volume [6]. High suspicion of IUGR is attained by the determination of a very low birth weight. A birth weight less than the tenth percentile, in a set of diagnostic observations and gestational age, is called small for gestational age (SGA). However, an estimated fetal weight judged below the tenth percentile does not always represent a placental pathology and, therefore, has to be carefully analyzed for other reasons of SGA. Falsely predicted SGA could yield negative aspects including unnecessary and frequent fetal examinations that might lead to iatrogenic premature birth. Evidence published so far indicates that idenfication of PFPT in single cotyledons is possible and potentially allows calculation of the global PFPT-volume, which, in turn, enables estimation of the energy state of the entire placenta. Therefore, a concise visualization of functional parts of the human placenta in vivo according to the PFPT-concept in order to differentiate placental IUGR from other pathologies is well motivated [2, 3, 7].

2   Materials and methods

Analyzing the so-called putative functional placental volume (PFPV)—the active placenta volume—might provide insight into the nutrition support of the fetus at a specific week of gestation [2]. We provide a visual representation that enables physicians to determine the current placental functional state. Our approach (Fig. 1) starts with the DT-MRI data set and a segmentation mask of the placenta that has been provided by an experienced radiologist. In the second step we manually segmented the cotyledons of the input data set. Thirdly, we compute the segmentation uncertainty and visualize all cotyledons together with the placenta. In the final step, we visually analyze each cotyledon individually and the placenta as aggregate to conclude on the overall energy support.

2.1   Input data

We retrospectively assessed 17 DT-MRI data sets from nine healthy and eight cases with placental IUGR. All other medical history, especially, the gestational week and age of the mothers, was not significantly different between the two groups. All DT-MRI data was acquired on a 1.5T clinical whole body MR-s-canner (Achieva Philips Medical Systems, Best, The Netherlands) at normal operating mode using a dual-b ($b0 = 0$ and $b1 = 750\,\mathrm{s/mm^2}$) SE-EPI sequence (TE/TR: 116/1066 ms; scan time: app. 1:30 min). A b1-value of $750\,\mathrm{s/mm^2}$ for diffusion sensitizing was chosen as trade-off between an optimal signal from the placenta in the abdomen while minimizing the scan duration in order to adjust for fetal motion [2, 3]. Up to 20 slices covering the whole placenta with a voxel size of $2.6 \times 2.6 \times 4\,\mathrm{mm}$ were measured and voxels containing placental tissue were labeled in extra image data sets, which were kept in spatial alignment with the original measurements during all processing steps. Due to the rather high spatial anisotropy of the voxels, isotropic resampling of images was performed to gain a resolution of 1 mm along all axes, which allowed use of additional morphological operations in order to improve the segmentation results [8]. Acquisition and assessment of the MRI data used for this retrospective analysis was approved by the local ethics committee (Ethics Committee of the Medical University of Vienna). Written, informed consent was obtained in all cases and the terms of clinical good practice according to the declaration of Helsinki and later amendments were obeyed [9, 10].

2.2   Segmentation

The placental cotyledons are assumed to have high signal intensity in DT-MRI possibly due to to their rather high perfusion in a healthy condition. We segmented all cotyledons by manually defining their contours in several axial slices using Livewire [11] in the medical imaging interaction toolkit (MITK) and subsequently interpolating these contours in intermediate slices.

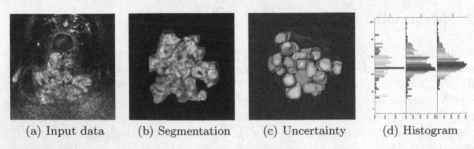

(a) Input data   (b) Segmentation   (c) Uncertainty   (d) Histogram

Fig. 1. Our proposed workflow. (a) shows the input data set with the placental mask and (b) displays the segmented placental cotyledons. Our proposed segmentation uncertainty visualization is displayed in (c) and the intensity histogram of the cotyledons in (d) using a diverging color map (RdYlBu).

Fig. 2. Color-coded segmentation uncertainty of the placental cotyledons, from green (uncertain) to tan (certain), with increasing certainty from left to right.

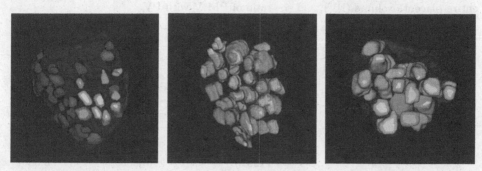

2.3   Visualization

Since a ground truth segmentation was not available, we provide an estimate of segmentation uncertainty by computing the ratio of the boundary voxels to the total number of voxels of a single cotyledon. A value closer to zero is considered to be certain and expresses the reliability of the computed PFPV. We visually

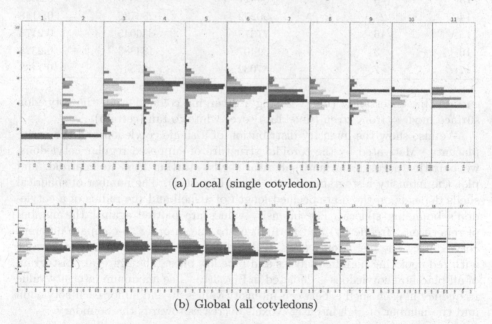

(a) Local (single cotyledon)

(b) Global (all cotyledons)

Fig. 3. (a) shows the intensity (y-axis) histograms of several spherical shells (top number) of a cotyledon, with increasing distance from the cotyledon's centroid. Since the intensity distribution changes from the first to the fourth shell, this cotyledon exhibits a toroidal shape and could be interpreted as regular. (b) displays the aggregate spherical histograms of all cotyledons of a placenta, using 17 shells. As the mean of the intensity distributions does not change with distance from the cotyledon centroids, the placenta is considered active but does not contain toroidal cotyledons.

Table 1. Comparison of nine healthy and eight pathological placentas. The columns represent: the number of cotyledons (# C), the volume of cotyledons (PFPV), the entire placenta volume (PV), and the ratio of PFPV with PV.

No.	# C	PFPV [mm^3]	PV [mm^3]	Ratio
1	18	114545	231962	0.4938
2	26	215852	355844	0.4938
3	18	15281	406465	0.2590
4	25	208384	319237	0.6527
5	19	147856	226229	0.6535
6	4	43789	470021	0.0931
7	14	112370	165069	0.6807
8	11	94805	164756	0.5754
9	11	38887	298910	0.1300
10	29	156664	488614	0.3206
11	5	22943	284193	0.0807
12	17	90850	364684	0.2491
13	9	84421	790935	0.1067
14	21	90279	286736	0.3148
15	16	77375	356045	0.2173
16	3	31407	134883	0.2328
17	7	67032	467547	0.1433

encode this uncertainty (Fig. 2) using a diverging color map for the cotyledon surface models, from green (uncertain) over white to tan (certain).

We also show the intensity distribution of a single cotyledon and the entire placenta. Motivated by the toroidal structure of supposed regular cotyledons, we partition a cotyledon into spherical shells, starting from its centroid, and plot the intensity histograms of each shell (Fig. 3(a)). The number of spherical shells depends on the user-specified length of a shell and the radius of a cotyledon's bounding sphere. The intensity values are plotted against the number of repetitions (frequency) and normalized to one in order to compare different cotyledons. The histogram colors denote the frequency of each intensity value with red depicting high frequencies and blue low ones. The aggregate histogram of all placental cotyledons is depicted in Fig. 3(b). The maximum intensity value frequency in each shell is between intensity values 40 and 60 for each cotyledon and the number of high intensity voxels decreases towards the boundary.

3   Results

We investigated 17 data sets (Tab. 1), which included nine healthy cases and eight suspected IUGR ones. For each case, we computed the number of cotyledons, the volume of cotyledons (PFPV), and the volume of the entire placenta.

In order to compare the PFPV across cases, we additionally computed the ratio of the PFPV with the volume of the entire placenta.

4 Discussion

As expected, the PFPV was found lower in patients with IUGR, which becomes especially clear when comparing case two (healthy placenta) with case ten (IUGR), having a PFPV of $215852 \, mm^3$ versus $156664 \, mm^3$, respectively. In case two 26 cotyledons were successfully differentiated while 29 cotyledons were identified in case ten. Even though the number of cotyledons may be comparably high in pathological placentas, they have less PFPV. This type of assessment could, therefore, help in early diagnosis of IUGR and could support taking adequate measures and treatments in order to reduce perinatal mortality.

References

1. Otake Y, Kanazawa H, Takahashi H, et al. Magnetic resonance imaging of the human placental cotyledon: proposal of a novel cotyledon appearance score. European Journal of Obstetrics and Gynecology and Reproductive Biology. 2019;232:82–86.
2. Javor D, Nasel C, Schweim T, et al. In vivo assessment of putative functional placental tissue volume in placental intrauterine growth restriction (IUGR) in human fetuses using diffusion tensor magnetic resonance imaging. Placenta. 2013;34:676–680.
3. Javor D, Nasel C, Dekan S, et al. Placental MRI shows preservation of brain volume in growth-restricted fetuses who suffer substantial reduction of putative functional placenta tissue (PFPT). Eur J Radiol. 2018;108:189–193.
4. Zun Z, Zaharchuk G, Andescavage N, et al. Non-Invasive placental perfusion imaging in pregnancies complicated by fetal heart disease using Velocity-Selective arterial spin labeled MRI. Sci Rep. 2017;7(16126):1–10.
5. Luo J, Turk E, Bibbo C, et al. In vivo quantification of placental insufficiency by BOLD MRI: a human study. Sci Rep. 2017;7(3713):1–10.
6. Do QN, Lewis MA, Madhuranthakam AJ, et al. Texture analysis of magnetic resonance images of the human placenta throughout gestation: a feasibility study. PLoS One. 2019;14:e0211060.
7. Miao H, Mistelbauer G, Karimov A, et al. Placenta maps: in utero placental health assessment of the human fetus. IEEE Trans Vis Comput Graph. 2017;23:1612–1623.
8. Basser PJ, Pajevic S, Pierpaoli C, et al. In vivo fiber tractography using DT-MRI data. Magn Reson Med. 2000;44:625–632.
9. World Medical Association. Declaration of helsinki: ethical principles for medical research involving human subjects; Accessed 2020/01/05. https://www.wma.net/policies-post/wma-declaration-of-helsinki-ethical-principles-for-medical-research-involving-human-subjects/.
10. European Medicines Agency. ICH topic e6 (r2): guideline for good clinical practice; Accessed 2020/01/05. https://www.ema.europa.eu/en/ich-e6-r2-good-clinical-practice.
11. Kang HW. G-wire: a livewire segmentation algorithm based on a generalized graph formulation. Pattern Recognit Lett. 2005;26:2042–2051.

Modularization of Deep Networks Allows Cross-Modality Reuse

Lesson Learnt

Weilin Fu[1,2], Lennart Husvogt[1,4], Stefan Ploner[1], James G. Fujimoto[4], Andreas Maier[1,3]

Pattern Recognition Lab, Friedrich-Alexander University
International Max Planck Research School Physics of Light (IMPRS-PL)
Erlangen Graduate School in Advanced Optical Technologies(SAOT)
Biomedical Optical Imaging and Biophotonics Group, MIT, Cambridge, USA
weilin.fu@fau.de

Abstract. Fundus photography and Optical Coherence Tomography Angiography (OCT-A) are two commonly used modalities in ophthalmic imaging. With the development of deep learning algorithms, fundus image processing, especially retinal vessel segmentation, has been extensively studied. Built upon the known operator theory, interpretable deep network pipelines with well-defined modules have been constructed on fundus images. In this work, we firstly train a modularized network pipeline for the task of retinal vessel segmentation on the fundus database DRIVE. The pretrained preprocessing module from the pipeline is then directly transferred onto OCT-A data for image quality enhancement without further fine-tuning. Output images show that the preprocessing net can balance the contrast, suppress noise and thereby produce vessel trees with improved connectivity in both image modalities. The visual impression is confirmed by an observer study with five OCT-A experts. Statistics of the grades by the experts indicate that the transferred module improves both the image quality and the diagnostic quality. Our work provides an example that modules within network pipelines that are built upon the known operator theory facilitate cross-modality reuse without additional training or transfer learning.

1 Introduction

In ophthalmology, fundus photography and optical coherence tomography angiography (OCT-A) are two widely used non-invasive imaging modalities. Fundus photography utilizes fundus cameras to provide 2D RGB images of the retinal surface of the eye, with 30° to 50° views of the retinal area at a magnification of ×2.5 to ×5 times [1]. OCT-A is a 3D imaging technique based on low coherence interferometry, and uses motion contrast to detect blood flow in the retina with micron-scale resolution [2, 3]. OCT-A data is often viewed as en face projections which present the 2D view of the retinal vasculature. In both imaging

© Springer Fachmedien Wiesbaden GmbH, ein Teil von Springer Nature 2020
T. Tolxdorff et al. (Hrsg.), *Bildverarbeitung für die Medizin 2020*,
Informatik aktuell, https://doi.org/10.1007/978-3-658-29267-6_61

modalities, characterization of the vasculature can strongly support diagnostical procedures. Processing and segmentation of retinal vessels from fundus images is a well-studied field, and several databases with manually labeled pixel-wise vessel annotations have been established [1]. With the recent advances in Deep Learning (DL) technologies, Convolutional Neural Networks (CNNs) are applied on the task and have achieved great success. However, OCT-A is a modality that has been developed fairly recently, and to the best of our knowledge, there is no vessel segmentation database with manual labels publicly available at the time of writing. This poses difficulties in DL-based algorithms for processing and segmentation of OCT-A data.

Despite that, the resolution of the images and the data distribution of the image intensities are different for the two imaging modalities, there exist structural similarities as presented in Fig. 2 (b) and Fig. 3 (a). Hence it is an instinctive idea to transfer DL-based algorithms which are designed and trained on fundus images to OCT-A data. However, deep networks are in general sensitive to the distribution of the input data, and even intra-modality transfer learning to another database normally requires fine-tuning. In the research direction of Precision Learning [4], prior knowledge of known operators is incorporated into the CNN architectures to improve the interpretability of the networks. On this basis, a network pipeline composed of two well-defined modules: a preprocessing net and a segmentation net, is constructed for the task of retinal vessel segmentation from fundus images [5]. A small U-Net is employed as the preprocessing net, and Frangi-Net is used to segment the vessels from the processed images. Modularization of the pipeline not only defines specific functions of network blocks, but also allows for flexible reuse of these modules across various tasks as we will show in the following.

In this work, we firstly train the pipeline in [5] for retinal vessel segmentation on the fundus image database DRIVE. Then we use the pretrained preprocessing module directly onto an OCT-A database composed of 20 2-D en face projection images. Due to the absence of ground truth data with clear vessels and clean background, an observer study based on five datasets involving five OCT-A experts is conducted. Feedback from the experts suggests that the images prepared with the pretrained preprocessing module have less noise and improved vessel network connectivity, and can thus potentially better assist the diagnosis procedure. This result indicates that the preprocessing module retains its edge-preserving denoising ability and is reusable across different imaging modalities.

2   Materials and methods

2.1   Preprocessing network

The preprocessing module is adopted from the network pipeline in [5], as shown in Fig. 1. In this workflow, a three-level U-Net with 16 filters in the input convolutional layer is employed as the preprocessing net, and an eight-scale Frangi-Net is used for segmentation. In the preprocessing part, a mean square error (MSE) regularizer is utilized to constrain the similarity between the input image and the preprocessed output. The overall pipeline is trained end-to-end on the fundus image database DRIVE as a retinal vessel segmentation task.

Each training batch contains 50 patches of size 168×168 pixels. Data augmentation techniques such as additive noise, rotation and scaling are employed for better generalization. The objective function consists of three main parts: weighted focal loss [6], ℓ_2-norm to confine the weights in U-Net, and the MSE similarity regularizer. Optimization is performed with Adam optimizer [7]. The learning rate is initialized to 5×10^{-5} and decays after each 10k steps. Early stopping is applied according to the validation loss curve.

2.2 Reader study

Retrospective data assessment by five experts is used for this study. In each experiment, three images are presented in random order, namely the raw OCT-A en face projection image, the output from the preprocessing net, and a blend of these two (50 % each). The experts are requested to grade the images from 1 (very good) to 5 (very bad) with respect to three aspects: image quality regarding to the noise level, vessel connectivity and the diagnosis quality. The observers are allowed to adjust the brightness and contrast of the given images. The mean score of each image type on each quality aspect over all experiments, as well as the corresponding inter-expert standard deviation are reported.

2.3 Database description

2.3.1   Fundus training database The Digital Retinal Images for Vessel Extraction (DRIVE) database which contains 40 RGB fundus images is used for training the network pipeline as a vessel segmentation task. All images in DRIVE are of size 565×584 pixels, and are provided with manual labels and Field of View (FOV) masks. The raw images are prepared with the pipeline of green channel extraction, illumination balance with CLAHE [8], and intensity standardization to (-1, 1). Note that the intensity of regions where vessel diameters are below 8 pixels normally have intensities between (-0.6, 0.6). The database is equally divided into one training and testing set, and a validation set containing four

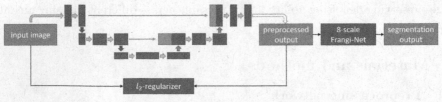

Fig. 1. The architecture of the retinal vessel segmentation network on fundus images. The preprocessing module is the U-Net on the left.

images is separated from the training set. During the training progress, a multiplicative pixel-wise weight map which is inversely proportional to the ground truth vessel diameter is generated for each image to emphasize on thin vessels. One representation from DRIVE is presented in Fig. 2 (a), the corresponding input and output of the preprocessing net are shown in Fig. 2 (b)-(c).

2.3.2 OCT-A testing database The testing OCT-A data in this study are acquired from a healthy 28-year-old male volunteer with an ultrahigh speed swept source OCT research prototype developed at the Massachusetts Institute of Technology and used by the New England Eye Center at Tufts Medical Center in Boston [3]. The database contains 20 en face OCT-A images of size 500×500 pixels, where 10 images have the field size of 3×3 mm and the other 10 images have the field size of 6×6 mm. Contrary to those in fundus images, vessels in OCT-A are represented as bright tubular structures in dark background. The pixel intensities of capillary regions range from 0 to around 1.5. To adjust the data range of the testing databases, the following linear intensity transform is applied on the OCT-A database: Firstly a threshold 4.0 is set, since the contrast in the big bright vessels are not of interest in this work. The images are inverted by multiplying -1 and then added with 0.5 such that the intensities in small vessel regions roughly match that in fundus images.

3 Results

Images in one representative experiment with enlarged Regions Of Interest (ROIs) are presented in Fig. 3. Direct visual impact indicates that in the preprocessed and the blend images, the noise level is reduced and the vascular structures are enhanced. These changes introduce cleaner boundaries and better-connected vessels. However, not all emerged vessels can be visually validated according to the given raw OCT-A image, i.e. some could be hallucinated by the preprocessing net. In addition, the high intensities within the thick vessels can be out of data range for the network and thus cause black responses in

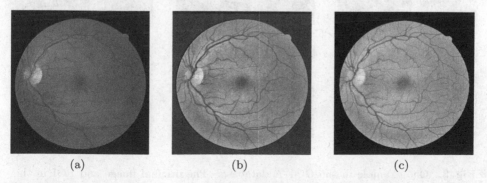

(a)   (b)   (c)

Fig. 2. The raw fundus image in (a). Input and output of the preprocessing network in (b) and (c), respectively. Example image is test01.TIFF from the DRIVE database.

Table 1. The mean and standard deviation of the observer study. IQ, VC, DQ refer to Image Quality regarding to noise level, Vessel Connectivity, and Diagnoistic Quality, respectively. The grades range from 1 (very good) to 5 (very bad).

	raw input	blend	output
IQ	3.0 ± 0.8	2.2 ± 0.6	2.2 ± 0.3
VC	3.1 ± 0.7	2.1 ± 0.5	2.2 ± 0.7
DQ	3.0 ± 0.8	2.0 ± 0.6	2.2 ± 0.5

the output. Blending of the raw image and the output of the preprocessing net could mitigate these issues. The visual impression of the three image types is confirmed with the statistical results of the observer study. Despite of the subjective influence which can be reflected by the inter-expert standard deviation, the output and the blend images achieve better scores than the raw input with respect to image quality, vessel connectivity as well as potential diagnosis quality, as shown in Tab. 1.

4　Discussion

In this work, we transfer a preprocessing net which is pretrained on the fundus database DRIVE directly onto OCT-A en face projection images without fur-

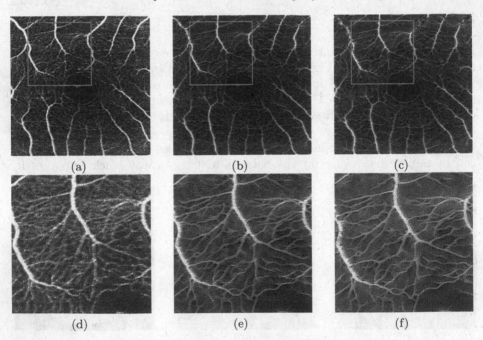

Fig. 3. One example in the OCT-A database. The original image and ROI in the yellow box shown in (a) and (d). The outputs from the preprocessing net in (c) and (f). The blend images in (b) and (c). Field size is 3×3 mm in the original image.

ther training. Direct visual inspection and an observer study indicate that the preprocessing network notably enhances the OCT-A images regarding to image quality, vessel connectivity and potential diagnosis quality. To the best of our knowledge, this is the first work of cross-modality CNN module transfer without further network fine-tuning or transfer learning. Despite the difference in input data distribution, the network performs a similar function on both modalities: balancing the contrast, reducing the noise level, and improving the vessel connectivity. This work provides one example of the successful reuse of modules within CNN pipelines which are constructed according to the known operator theory.

In the future, the image quality enhancement by the transferred net will be quantitatively validated with reconstructed high-resolution image of the OCT-A data. The preprocessing module could also be reused to improve the image quality in different data modalities. As an extension, pretrained modules from different network pipelines could be recombined for new tasks. Finally, the network could also be incorporated into an OCT-A reconstruction pipeline based on compressed sensing, where it could serve as a regularizer [9].

References

1. Srinidhi CL, Aparna P, Rajan J. Recent advancements in retinal vessel segmentation. J med Syst. 2017;41(4):70.
2. Husvogt L, Ploner S, Maier A. Optical coherence tomography. Springer, Cham; 2018. p. 251–261.
3. Choi W, Moult EM, Waheed NK, et al. Ultrahigh-Speed, swept-source optical coherence tomography angiography in nonexudative age-related macular degeneration with geographic atrophy. Ophthalmology. 2015;.
4. Maier AK, Syben C, Stimpel B, et al. Learning with known operators reduces maximum error bounds. Nature machine intelligence. 2019;1(8):373–380.
5. Fu W, Breininger K, Schaffert R, et al. A divide-and-conquer approach towards understanding deep networks. In: MICCAI. Springer; 2019. p. 183–191.
6. Lin TY, Goyal P, Girshick R, et al. Focal loss for dense object detection. In: Proceedings of the IEEE international conference on computer vision; 2017. p. 2980–2988.
7. Kingma DP, Ba J. Adam: a method for stochastic optimization. arXiv preprint arXiv:14126980. 2014;.
8. Zuiderveld K. Contrast limited adaptive histogram equalization. In: Graphics gems IV. Academic Press Professional, Inc.; 1994. p. 474–485.
9. Husvogt L, Ploner S, Moult EM, et al. Using medical image reconstruction methods for denoising of OCTA data. Invest Ophthal Vis Sci. 2019;60:3096.

U-Net in Constraint Few-Shot Settings

Enforcing Few-Sample-Fitting for Faster Convergence of U-Net for Femur Segmentation in X-Ray

Duc Duy Pham[1], Melanie Lausen[1], Gurbandurdy Dovletov[1],
Sebastian Serong[2], Stefan Landgraeber[2], Marcus Jäger[3,4], Josef Pauli[1]

[1]Intelligent Systems, Faculty of Engineering, University of Duisburg-Essen, Germany
[2]Department of Orthopedics and Orthopedic Surgery,
Saarland University Medical Center, Germany
[3] Department of Orthopedics, Trauma and Recontructive Surgery, St. Marien
Hospital Mülheim
[4] Chair of Orthopaedics and Trauma Surgery, University Hospital Essen, Germany
duc.duy.pham@uni-due.de

Abstract. In this paper, we investigate the feasibility of using a standard U-Net for Few-Shot segmentation tasks in very constraint settings. We demonstrate on the example of femur segmentation in X-ray images, that a U-Net architecture only needs few samples to generate accurate segmentations, if the images and the structure of interest only show little variance in appearance and perspective. This is often the case in medical imaging. We also present a novel training strategy for the U-Net, leveraging U-Net's Few-Shot capability for inter-patient consistent protocols. We propose repeatedly enforcing Few-Sample-Fitting the network for faster convergence. The results of our experiments indicate that incrementally fitting the network to an increasing sample set can lead to faster network convergence in constraint few-shot settings.

1 Introduction

In medical image analysis, segmentation is a crucial task for image based diagnostics and patient treatment planning. Since manual segmentation is tedious and expensive, computerized methods are an active topic of research. With the recent success of deep convolutional neural networks in computer vision tasks, Ronneberger et al.'s U-Net architecture [1] has also achieved state-of-the-art results for segmentation tasks in biomedical images and serves as base architecture for various extensions. Since training deep neural networks is a time consuming process, research towards a decrease in necessary number of iterations until convergence is of major interest. While Smith [2] proposes using cyclical learning rates for classification tasks, Schnieders and Tuvls [3] suggest combining specific loss functions to reduce the number of iterations until convergence. Both Shrivastava et al.'s work [4] and Loshchilov and Hutter's paper [5] suggest selecting hard examples online to increase optimization speed for object detection

© Springer Fachmedien Wiesbaden GmbH, ein Teil von Springer Nature 2020
T. Tolxdorff et al. (Hrsg.), *Bildverarbeitung für die Medizin 2020*,
Informatik aktuell, https://doi.org/10.1007/978-3-658-29267-6_62

and classification tasks, respectively. Our approach of training the U-Net in the medical domain is motivated as follows:

In contrast to natural images, in the medical domain, imaging for diagnosis is often applied according to a fixed protocol, in which there is only little variation in perspective, e.g. X-rays, CT and MRI. Consequently, fitting the U-Net to only few image samples may restrain the generalization capability of the U-Net in general, but since the application domain is heavily restricted by the protocols anyway, it should nevertheless produce adequate segmentation results for this application. In the following we refer to this procedure as Few-Sample-Fitting. Based on aforementioned considerations, we investigate the Few-Shot capability of U-Net in these constraint settings and propose a novel training strategy leveraging this property.

2 Materials and methods

2.1 U-Net

Ronneberger et al. [1] present a U-shaped fully convolutional network for segmentation tasks in medical images. It consists of a contracting path of subsequent convolutional and max-pooling layers, and an expanding path of transposed convolutional and ordinary convolutional layers. Skip connections, as proposed in Long et al's work [6], between layers of the same resolution level ensure a better localization capability in the decoding process and support a more stable gradient flow. Since this architecture is commonly used in medical image computing, where labeled data is scarce and expensive to acquire, we investigate, to what extend we can lower the amount of training data for a feasible segmentation in constraint few-shot settings. Furthermore, we apply our proposed training scheme on this particular architecture.

2.2 Training

On the one hand, we train the U-Net architecture in a conventional way, in which we divide the data set into training, validation and testing set. For training we use a Dice Similarity Coefficient based loss function, i.e.

$$\mathcal{L}_{\text{unet}} := 1 - \frac{2 \cdot \sum_p GT(p) \cdot y_{\text{unet}}(p) + \epsilon}{\sum_p GT(p) + \sum_p y_{\text{unet}}(p) + \epsilon} \tag{1}$$

where y_{unet} is the U-Net prediction, GT is the desired segmentation ground truth, $\epsilon > 0$ is a small positive number for numerical stability and p depicts a point in the prediction/ground truth image.

On the other hand, we propose an incremental Few-Sample-Fitting training scheme, as depicted in Alg. 3. We start with a small amount of training and validation samples, and incrementally increase the available number of samples, respectively. Starting with only two samples for training and validation, we train the U-net until convergence, thus basically overfitting on these few samples. By

---

Algorithmus 3 Incremental Few-Sample-Fitting Training Scheme.

---

initialize total Training Set $\mathcal{T}_{all}$ and Validation Set $\mathcal{V}_{all}$
initialize empty current Training $\mathcal{T}_{cur} \leftarrow \emptyset$ and Validation Set $\mathcal{V}_{cur} \leftarrow \emptyset$
while $\mathcal{T}_{all}$ not empty **do**
    move certain amount of samples from $\mathcal{T}_{all}$ to $\mathcal{T}_{cur}$
    move certain amount of samples from $\mathcal{V}_{all}$ to $\mathcal{V}_{cur}$
    while validation loss not converged **do**
        train network with samples from $\mathcal{T}_{cur}$
        monitor network with samples from $\mathcal{V}_{cur}$
    end while
end while

---

injecting new samples into training and validation set, the training and validation loss will presumably increase. Thus, the supposed minimum in the error
landscape at the current weight configuration vanishes, as the currently learned
weights have been specifically adapted for a training set, that did not consider the
newly inserted samples. We argue that by greedily overfitting to these supposed
minima and removing them from the estimated error landscape by additional
sample injection we can traverse the real error landscape faster in constraint
few-shot settings. We basically use the local minima found for each sample set
as improved initial starting point for searching the global minimum. A similar
practice can be observed in informed search algorithms, in which heuristics are
used to estimate the distance a goal. In this case we could interpret the difference of the loss after the injection of new samples as a heuristic. In case of a
great absolute difference, the current weight configuration is far away from the
global minimum, whereas a small loss change indicates a good configuration.

2.3   Experiments

In our experiments we use two inhouse data sets consisting of 38 x-ray images of
the hip joint each in anterior-posterior (AP) projection and 37 x-ray images in
frog-leg lateral (Lauenstein) view. Fig. 1 shows exemplary x-ray images of the
AP data set and the Lauenstein data set. As can be seen in the first two images
the AP data set shows more variance in field of view, whereas the Lauenstein
dataset is more standardized and therefore more restraint.

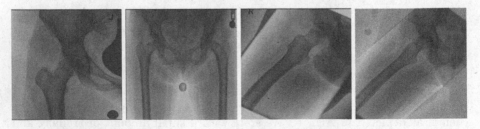

Fig. 1. Exemplary X-ray images of the AP data set (left images) and the Lauenstein
data set (right images).

Fig. 2. Achieved DSCs depending on number of training samples and training scheme for (a) AP data set and (b) Lauenstein data set.

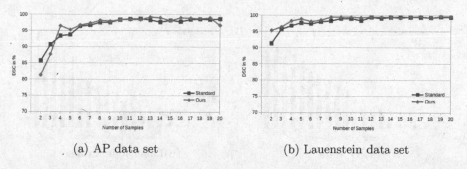

(a) AP data set   (b) Lauenstein data set

In a 5-fold cross-validation manner, we divided both data sets into training, validation and testing. Both training sets yielded 20 samples, and both testing sets had 6 images in each fold. For our experiments regarding minimal amount of required images, we incrementally increased the number of training samples for the conventional way of training and trained the U-Net from scratch to segment the right femur with the reduced available number of samples. We flipped images with prosthetics on the right side to guarantee a physiologically feasible right femur during training and inference. For each training set size, we measured the total number of iterations until validation convergence and the achieved DSC on the test set. In case of our proposed training method, we divided the data sets the same way and measured the same metrics, with the only difference that we applied our suggested training strategy. We resized the images to an input size of 256 × 256 and applied data augmentation by means of rotation and translation. Our U-Net implementation comprises 5 resolution levels and it's convolutional layers utilize kernels of size 3 × 3, starting with 64 kernels in the first resolution level and doubling in each deeper resolution level. We used Keras with Tensorflow backend as deep learning framework and used the provided early-stopping functionality to estimate convergence. Our experiments were run on a NVIDIA GTX 1080ti GPU.

3   Results

Fig. 2(a) shows the achieved DSCs with both training schemes for the AP data set and Fig. 2(b) the resulting DSCs for the Lauenstein data set. For both data sets, it is observable that with increasing number of training samples our proposed training scheme and the conventional training scheme lead to segmentations of similar quality. In the more diverse AP data set a stable DSC is achieved after about 10 training samples, whereas for the more contraint Lauenstein data set a consistent DSC is achieved after about 8 samples already. Fig. 2 shows exemplary segmentation results of both data sets depending on the training strategy for 10 training samples in total. Fig. 3 depicts the number of iterations needed for convergence depending on the number of samples, data set and training strategy. For our proposed training strategy we calculated the

Fig. 3. Needed number of iterations until convergence depending on number of training samples and training scheme for (a) AP data set and (b) Lauenstein data set.

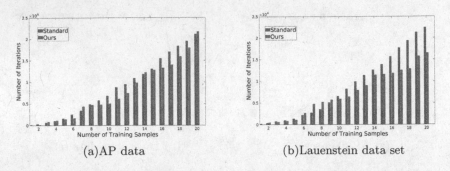

(a)AP data   (b)Lauenstein data set

total (accumulated) number of iterations until convergence, starting from one sample until the number of samples to be examined, to ensure comparability to the standard training scheme. In case of the AP data set (Fig. 3(a)), for most number of training samples, the needed number of iterations until validation loss convergence is lower for our proposed training scheme than the standard training scheme. A lower number of needed iterations can however not be guaranteed, even for larger amounts of training samples, as can be seen for 20 training samples. This seems to correlate with the lower achieved DSC, shown in Fig. 2(a). Regarding the Lauenstein data set (Fig. 3(b)), the gap of needed number of iterations between the standard and our proposed training scheme becomes even more apparent. In contrast to the AP data set, the lower number of needed iterations becomes more apparent the more training samples are available.

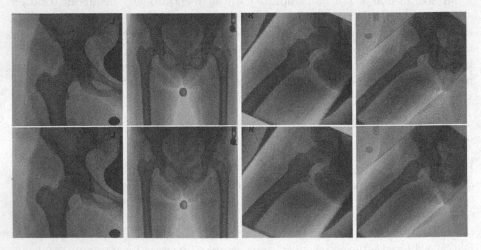

Fig. 4. Exemplary segmentation results with standard training (top) and proposed training (bottom) from the AP data set (left columns) and the Lauenstein data set (right columns) with 10 training samples.

4 Discussion

From the results we can draw two main conclusions. First, it is surprising, how well U-Net does regarding DSC, using either of both training schemes. Only 10 training samples are needed to already achieve DSC scores that are comparable to DSCs achieved by a model that has been trained with 20 samples. For these kind of very constraint settings, which often occur in medical imaging, overfitting U-Net does seem to work well. This leads to the second conclusion. The results show that leveraging this overfitting property during training can drastically reduce the number of needed iterations until convergence, especially when a larger number of training samples is used, particularly for more constraint settings, where drastic changes, e.g. in field of view (Fig. 1(a) and (b)) are not to be expected. However, it needs to be kept in mind, that although we can achieve good segmentation results by overfitting U-Net in both training strategies, the generalization capability is also drastically reduced. Therefore employing the proposed strategy and using only a small number of training samples in general should only be applied in constraint few-shot settings, in which only small variations within the data set are to be expected.

5 Conclusion

In this work we demonstrate that a U-Net architecture only needs few samples to generate accurate segmentations in constraint few-shot setting on the example of femur segmentation in x-ray. We additionally present a novel training strategy for the U-Net, which drastically reduces the number of iterations until convergence and therefore speeds up the training process.

References

1. Ronneberger O, Fischer P, Brox T. U-Net: convolutional networks for biomedical image segmentation. In: International Conference on Medical Image Computing and Computer-Assisted Intervention. Springer; 2015. p. 234–241.
2. Smith LN. Cyclical learning rates for training neural networks. In: 2017 IEEE Winter Conference on Applications of Computer Vision (WACV). IEEE; 2017. p. 464–472.
3. Schnieders B, Tuyls K. Fast convergence for object detection by learning how to combine error functions. In: 2018 IEEE/RSJ International Conference on Intelligent Robots and Systems (IROS). IEEE; 2018. p. 7329–7335.
4. Shrivastava A, Gupta A, Girshick R. Training region-based object detectors with online hard example mining. In: Proceedings of the IEEE conference on computer vision and pattern recognition; 2016. p. 761–769.
5. Loshchilov I, Hutter F. Online batch selection for faster training of neural networks. arXiv preprint arXiv:151106343. 2015;.
6. Long J, Shelhamer E, Darrell T. Fully convolutional networks for semantic segmentation. In: Proceedings of the IEEE conference on computer vision and pattern recognition; 2015. p. 3431–3440.

Abstract: Multi-Scale GANs for Memory-Efficient Generation of High Resolution Medical Images

Hristina Uzunova[1], Jan Ehrhardt[1], Fabian Jacob[2], Alex Frydrychowicz[2], Heinz Handels[1]

[1]Institute of Medical Informatics, University of Lübeck
[2] Department for Radiology and Nuclear Medicine, University Hospital of Schleswig-Holstein
uzunova@imi.uni-luebeck.de

Generative adversarial networks (GANs) have shown impressive results for photo-realistic image synthesis in the last couple of years. They also offer numerous applications in medical image analysis, such as generating images for data augmentation, image reconstruction and image synthesis for domain adaptation. Despite the undeniable success and the large variety of applications, GANs still struggle to generate images of high resolution. A reason for that is the fact that generated images are easier to distinguish from real ones at higher resolutions, which hinders the training process. Further reasons are computational demands and memory requirements of current network architectures.

We propose a memory-efficient multi-scale GAN [1] approach for the generation of high-resolution medical images in high quality. Our approach combines a progressive multi-scale learning strategy with a patch-wise approach, where low-resolution image content is learned first, and image patches at higher resolutions are conditioned on the previous scales to preserve global intensity information.

We demonstrate the ability to generate realistic images of unprecedented sizes on thoracic X-rays of size 2048^2 and 3D lung CTs of size 512^3. We also show that in contrast to common patch-based approaches, our method does not cause patch artifacts. Also, an experiment is designed to show that w.r.t. the growing side length of an isotropic 3D image, the memory requirements for popular GANs grow cubical, while they stay constant for any image size using our approach, making its application on arbitrarily large images computationally feasible.

References

1. Uzunova H, Ehrhardt J, Jacob F, et al. Multi-Scale GANs for memory-efficient generation of high resolution medical images. In: Proc MICCAI. vol. 6. Shenzhen, China; 2019. p. 112–120.

© Springer Fachmedien Wiesbaden GmbH, ein Teil von Springer Nature 2020
T. Tolxdorff et al. (Hrsg.), *Bildverarbeitung für die Medizin 2020*,
Informatik aktuell, https://doi.org/10.1007/978-3-658-29267-6_63

Epoch-Wise Label Attacks for Robustness Against Label Noise

Chest X-Ray Tuberculosis Classification with Corrupted Labels

Sebastian Gündel[1], Andreas Maier[1]

[1]Pattern Recognition Lab, FAU Erlangen-Nürnberg
sebastian.guendel@fau.de

Abstract. The current accessibility to large medical datasets for training convolutional neural networks is tremendously high. The associated dataset labels are always considered to be the real "ground truth". However, the labeling procedures often seem to be inaccurate and many wrong labels are integrated. This may have fatal consequences on the performance of both training and evaluation. In this paper, we show the impact of label noise in the training set on a specific medical problem based on chest X-ray images. With a simple one-class problem, the classification of tuberculosis, we measure the performance on a clean evaluation set when training with label-corrupted data. We develop a method to compete with incorrectly labeled data during training by randomly attacking labels on individual epochs. The network tends to be robust when flipping correct labels for a single epoch and initiates a good step to the optimal minimum on the error surface when flipping noisy labels. On a baseline with an AUC (Area under Curve) score of 0.924, the performance drops to 0.809 when 30% of our training data is misclassified. With our approach the baseline performance could almost be maintained, the performance raised to 0.918.

1 Introduction

Current research highlights the vast number of datasets where corresponding labels are partly incorrect. In the medical field this can be caused by many different reasons, e.g., errors in the labeling procedure when retrieving from the clinical reports. In addition, radiologists may misinterpret clinical images which lead to incorrect ground truth [1].

Different strategies can be applied to handle datasets with noisy labels: Additional radiologists re-annotate the dataset labels to check the variability between the original labels and the radiologists [2]. However, most datasets contain an extensive number of images and a small fraction can only be processed. Dealing with label noise in the training set, robust loss functions are

© Springer Fachmedien Wiesbaden GmbH, ein Teil von Springer Nature 2020
T. Tolxdorff et al. (Hrsg.), *Bildverarbeitung für die Medizin 2020*,
Informatik aktuell, https://doi.org/10.1007/978-3-658-29267-6_64

generated [3].

In this paper we implement a robust method to deal with this label noise in the training set on a binary class problem. By randomly attacking labels in each epoch, a fraction of noisy labels may be switched such that the network is trained with correct labels. We use tuberculosis classification based on CXR images and artificially insert label noise to analyse the effects of different noise ratios.

2   Materials and methods

2.1   Datasets

For pulmonary tuberculosis classification based on chest X-ray images, there are two public datasets available. The first, the Montgomery dataset contains 138 frontal images, 58 with and 80 without tuberculosis. The second dataset is derived from the Shenzhen hospital including 662 X-rays. Half of the images include tuberculosis, the other half has no evidence. The entire collection contains 800 CXR images [4].

For training purposes, we downsample all images to 256×256. We split the data collection into 70% for training, 10% for validation, and 20% for testing. For the experiments, we treat the corresponding dataset labels as clean without any ratio of noise.

2.2   Network and training setup

As convolutional neural network, we use a densly-connected model (DenseNet) with 121 layers [5]. We load the ImageNet pretrained weights before starting the training. The input image is accordingly normalized and provided in the

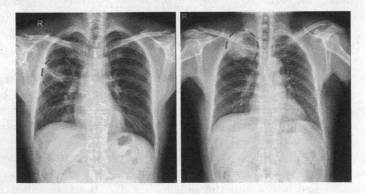

Fig. 1. Two example chest X-ray images with tuberculosis; Tuberculosis in the right middle lung (left) and tuberculosis in the right upper lung (right). More difficult cases may result in a wrong classification.

Table 1. AUC score when the labels were flipped with probability p_1 before training.

$p_1(e = 1)$	0.0	0.1	0.2	0.3	0.4	0.5
AUC	0.924	0.894	0.835	0.809	0.791	0.775

three input channels. The output layer of the network is reduced such that one sigmoidal unit is returned. During training we use the Adam optimizer [6] ($\beta_1 = 0.9$, $\beta_2 = 0.999$) and a learning rate of 10^{-4}. We stop the training and jump back to the best epoch if the validation accuracy does not improve after a patience of 8 epochs. We apply the binary cross-entropy function to predict the loss. Each batch is filled with 16 examples. The performance on the test set is evaluated with the area under ROC curve (AUC).

2.3 Label noise

Many medical datasets include incorrectly labeled data. As we assume to have a clean dataset, we artificially inject a portion of label noise to the data and measure the performance to see the effects on the performance. For all experiments, label noise is only applied to the training set. The labels of the validation set are kept such that we can retrieve our best model. An important factor to evaluate a model is to measure the performance on clean labels. Often, this clean test set can not be guaranteed as the whole dataset is corrupted. Since we artificially integrate label noise on the training data only, our model can be correctly evaluated and the returned performance scores can be considered as valid.

Assuming we have the clean labels l_i for all examples i, we define two flip probabilities $p_p = p(\hat{l}_i = 0|l_i = 1)$ and $p_n = p(\hat{l}_i = 1|l_i = 0)$. The two parameters describe how many labels are incorrect before we start the training process. In our experiments we simplify the problem such that the same ratio of positive and negative cases are flipped: $p_1(e = 1) = p_p = p_n$. First, we train our baseline model on the clean, original labels. We reach an AUC of 0.924. Inducing higher ratios of label noise the performance drops as can be seen in Tab. 1. Even if a high amount of labels are incorrect (e.g. $p_1(e = 1) = 0.5$), the model can classify many examples correctly.

2.4 Individual label attacks

The model is widely robust to a certain amount of label noise. We hypothesize that individual, epoch-wise label attacks make the model even more stable in terms of the classification performance. Therefore, we define a new probability $p_2(e = 1)$, which changes the label for a single epoch only. In this case the probability is tremendously smaller that a label is incorrect for the entire training process. We measure the performance based on different epoch-wise noise ratios $p_2(e = 1)$ when we have no prior label noise ($p_1(e = 1) = 0$).

In Tab. 2, we see that training with individual, epoch-wise attacks is significantly more robust than constant noise over the examples. Even if we flip in

Table 2. AUC score when the labels were flipped in each epoch with probability p_2.

$p_2(e = 1)$	0.1	0.2	0.3	0.4	0.5	0.6
AUC	0.901	0.917	0.888	0.905	0.639	0.475

each epoch with a probability $p_2(e = 1) = 0.4$, the performance can nearly reach the baseline performance. However, for experiments with $p_2(e = 1) \geq 0.5$, the performance significantly drops.

- Individual Label Attacks on Prior Label Noise: The main goal of this paper is to show that the individual and epoch-wise label attacks help to improve the classification performance when prior label noise is integrated in the training set. Fig. 2 visualizes the four scenarios which are possible for each label based on prior noise with p_1 and the epoch-wise label flips with p_2.
- Probability p_2 derivation: In most datasets, the label noise ratio is unknown. For the determination of the label flip probability p_2, we can derive the value without knowledge of the label noise ratio. For the p_2 determination we define a sample flip minimum and maximum. This can be derived from the binomial distribution

$$B(k|p, n) = \frac{n!}{k! \cdot (n - k)!} \cdot p^k (1 - p)^{n-k} \tag{1}$$

where k is the number of flips, $p = p_2$ the flip probability, and n the number of epochs. We use our previous experiments to see how many epochs are trained. An average training duration of 18 epochs is predicted ($n = 18$). For the prediction of the optimal p_2, we define 2 constraints:

- An example should be flipped at least once in the training ($B(k = 0) \approx 0$)

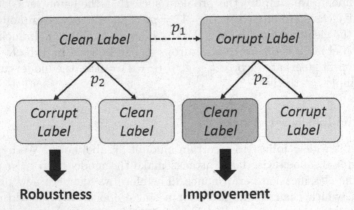

Fig. 2. Label Attack Strategy: The dataset includes prior noise with a certain noise rate (blue blocks). Flipping a label in one epoch ends up in one of the four scenarios: A corrupted/clean label derived from a clean label or a corrupted/clean label derived from a corrupted label (red blocks).

Table 3. AUC scores when the dataset labels were flipped with a certain probability p_1 before training and attacked with an epoch wise flip probability $p_2 = 0.25$.

$p_1(e=1)$	0.1	0.2	0.3	0.4	0.5
AUC	0.891	0.883	0.918	0.846	0.846
AUC gain	-0.003	+0.048	+0.109	+0.055	+0.071

– An example should be flipped less than a half in the training ($B(k \geq \frac{n}{2}) \approx 0$)

For simplification for the prediction p, we say that

$$B(k_1 = 0) = B(k_2 = \frac{n}{2})$$ (2)

This condition is fulfilled if the mean $\mu = p*n = \frac{k_1+k_2}{2}$. Thus, we can predict the epoch-wise flip probability

$$p_2 = \frac{k_1 + k_2}{2n} = \frac{9}{36} = 0.25$$ (3)

According to Equation 1, we get a probability $B(k_1 = 0) = 6 * 10^{-3}$ that an example is never flipped in the training and a probability $B(k_3 \geq \frac{n}{2}) = \sum_{k=\frac{n}{2}}^{n} \binom{n}{k} p^k (1-p)^{n-k} = 0.0193$ that an example is flipped in a half or more epochs. We hypothesize that this fraction of examples may not contribute to the training improvement under the condition that we have a noisy label for $B(k_1 = 0)$ and a clean label for $B(k_3 \geq \frac{n}{2})$. Thus, the real probability that an example may not contribute is a multiplication with p_1 or $(1 - p_1)$, respectively, which results in a significantly smaller value.

3 Results

We evaluated our method with a constant p_2 defined in Equation 3 under varying noise probabilities p_1. Tab. 3 shows the performance on the evaluation. We apply the noise on the same labels as is the experiments in Tab. 1. The best performance gain could be achieved with $p_1 = 0.3$, from an AUC score of 0.809 to 0.918. We can see that the performance for all noise ratios significantly improved compared to Tab. 1. Only for $p_1 = 0.1$, there is no improvement.

We analyse the epoch-wise labels based on the probability $p_1 = 0.2$. According to Fig. 2, the labels can be categorized in four groups. The probability of clean and corrupted labels for one epoch can be predicted with

$$p_{clean} = p_{cl|cl} + p_{cl|co} = (1 - p_1) * (1 - p_2) + p_1 * p_2 = 0.6 + 0.05 = 0.65$$ (4)

$$p_{corrupt} = p_{co|cl} + p_{co|co} = (1 - p_1) * p_2 + p_1 * (1 - p_2) = 0.2 + 0.15 = 0.35$$ (5)

The labels with probability $p_{cl|co}$, meaning that a noisy label is flipped to correct in an epoch, are responsible for the performance gain. We hypothesize that the additional epoch-wise noise with probability $p_{co|cl}$ is widely robust during training.

4   Discussion

We observed that individual label attacks help to improve the performance. Flip probability p_2 was calculated according to the binomial distribution. The number of epochs for the prediction varied during training depending, e.g., on the label noise. As we could not find out the exact number of epochs, we used the average duration over the past training runs. However, according to Tab. 2, the performance is robust for a wide range of p_2.

Moreover, we artificially inserted label noise prior to training. However, label noise may be biased, e.g., the probability of label noise on difficult examples is higher. This bias was not considered in our experiments. Effects on the performance may vary when label noise is directly derived from the dataset.

5   Conclusion

We showed that more label noise in the training decreases the performance on tuberculosis classification. We implemented a robust method to increase the performance when training with noisy labels. By flipping certain labels in each epoch, a fraction of noisy labels were converted to correct labels. These examples contributed to the training such that the performance significantly increased. Furthermore, the epoch-wise flips were widely robust during training, no significant performance drops existed when the epoch-wise label conversion strategy was integrated. This method can be extended and applied on multi-label problems.

References

1. Bruno MA, Walker EA, Abujudeh HH. Understanding and confronting our mistakes: the epidemiology of error in radiology and strategies for error reduction. RadioGraphics. 2015;35(6):1668–1676.
2. Rajpurkar P, Irvin J, Ball RL, et al. Deep learning for chest radiograph diagnosis: a retrospective comparison of the CheXNeXt algorithm to practicing radiologists. PLOS Medicine. 2018 11;15(11):1–17.
3. Zhang Z, Sabuncu M. Generalized cross entropy loss for training deep neural networks with noisy labels. In: Bengio S, Wallach H, Larochelle H, et al., editors. Advances in Neural Information Processing Systems 31; 2018. p. 8778–8788.
4. Jaeger S, Candemir S, Antani S, et al. Two public chest x-ray datasets for computer-aided screening of pulmonary diseases. Quantitative imaging in medicine and surgery. 2014 12;4:475–7.
5. Huang G, Liu Z, Weinberger KQ, et al. Densely connected convolutional networks. 2017 IEEE Conference on Computer Vision and Pattern Recognition (CVPR). 2016; p. 2261–2269.
6. Kingma D, Ba J. Adam: a method for stochastic optimization; 2014. Available from: http://arxiv.org/abs/1412.6980.

Abstract: How Big is Big Enough?
A Large-Scale Histological Dataset of Mitotic Figures

Christof A. Bertram[1], Marc Aubreville[2], Christian Marzahl[2], Andreas Maier[2], Robert Klopfleisch[1]

[1]Institute of Veterinary Pathology, Freie Universität Berlin, Germany
[2]Pattern Recognition Lab, F.-Alexander-Universität Erlangen-Nürnberg, Germany
christof.bertram@fu-berlin.de

Quantification of mitotic figures (MF) within the tumor areas of highest mitotic density is the most important prognostic parameter for outcome assessment of many tumor types. However, high intra- and inter-rater variability results from difficulties in individual MF identification and region of interest (ROI) selection due to uneven MF distribution. Deep learning-based algorithms for MF detection and ROI selection are very promising methods to overcome these limitations. As of today, few datasets of human mammary carcinoma are available. They provide labels only in small image sections of the whole slide image (WSI) and include up to 1,552 MF annotations [1].

Our research group has developed a large-scale, open access dataset with annotations for MF in 32 cases of canine cutaneous mast cell tumors [1]. Entire WSI were completely labeled by two pathologists resulting in 44,800 MF annotations. Of those, 5.5% were initially missed by expert WSI screening and added through a deep learning-based pipeline for identification of potential candidates.

For algorithmic validation, we used a two-stage approach (RetinaNet followed by cell classificator), which yielded a F1 score of 0.820. Through the algorithm-aided completion of the dataset we were able to increase the F1 score by 3.4 percentage points. Influence of the size of the dataset was assessed by stepwise reduction of the number of WSI and size (in high power fields, HPF) of the image sections used for training. With the number of included images, the F1 score moderately increased (3 WSI: 0.772; 6 WSI: 0.804; 12 WSI: 0.817; 21 WSI: 0.820). The size of the tumor area in training (ROI selected by an expert) had significant effects on the F1 score (5 HPF: 0.583; 10 HPF: 0.676; 50 HPF: 0.770; complete WSI: 0.820), which was determined in entire WSI of the test set. We emphasize the benefit of appropriate dataset size and complete WSI labeling.

Acknowledgement. CAB gratefully acknowledges financial support received from the Dres. Jutta & Georg Bruns-Stiftung für innovative Veterinärmedizin.

References

1. Bertram CA, Aubreville M, Marzahl C, et al. A large-scale dataset for mitotic figure assessment on whole slide images of canine cutaneous mast cell tumor. Sci Data. 2019;6(274):1–9.

© Springer Fachmedien Wiesbaden GmbH, ein Teil von Springer Nature 2020
T. Tolxdorff et al. (Hrsg.), *Bildverarbeitung für die Medizin 2020*,
Informatik aktuell, https://doi.org/10.1007/978-3-658-29267-6_65

Der Einfluss von Segmentierung auf die Genauigkeit eines CNN-Klassifikators zur Mimik-Steuerung

Ron Keuth, Lasse Hansen, Mattias P. Heinrich

Institut für Medizinische Informatik, Universität zu Lübeck, DE
ron.keuth@student.uni-luebeck.de

Kurzfassung. Die Erfolge von Faltungsnetzwerken (Convolutional Neural Networks, CNNs) in der Bildverarbeitung haben in den letzten Jahren große Aufmerksamkeit erregt. Die Erforschung von Verfahren zur Klassifikation von Mimik auf Bildern menschlicher Gesichter stellt in der Medizin eine große Chance für Menschen mit körperlicher Behinderung dar. So können beispielsweise einfach Befehle an einen elektronischen Rollstuhl oder ein Computerprogramm übermittelt werden. Diese Arbeit untersucht, ob und wie weit die Verwendung von Zusatzinformation (hier in Form von Segmentierungen von Gesichtspartien) beim Training eines CNN-Klassifikators die Genauigkeit bezüglich der Entscheidung für verschiedene Kiefer- und Lippenstellungen verbessern kann. Unsere Ergebnisse zeigen, dass die Genauigkeit des CNN-Klassifikators mit dem Detailgrad der verwendeten Segmentierungen zunimmt und außerdem bei Zuhilfenahme von Segmentierungen ein deutlich kleinerer Datensatz (60% der ursprünglichen Datenmenge) ausreicht, um ein ähnlich genaues CNN (im Vgl. zu einem ohne Zusantzinformation) zu trainieren.

1 Einleitung

Das Gesicht ist die Grundlage der menschlich-sozialen Interaktion – es ermöglicht den Ausdruck und die Interpretation von Gefühlen sowie die Identifikation von Personen. Gelingt es, das Gesicht für den Computer interpretierbar zu machen, eröffnet dies viele neue Anwendungen: z.B. in der Mensch-Computer-Interaktion, der Sicherheitstechnik und auch der Medizin. In den letzten Jahren ist es mit Ansätzen des maschinellen Lernens gelungen, in diesem Bereich neue Maßstäbe zu setzen. Eines der medizinisch relevantesten Anwendungsbeispiele stellt dabei die mögliche Steuerung von Systemen durch körperlich behinderte Menschen dar. Beispielsweise wurden elektronische Rollstühle entwickelt, die über die Form des Mundes einfache Befehle empfangen können [1]. Dazu ist die robuste Erkennung verschiedener Kiefer- und Lippenstellungen erforderlich. Ein CNN kann diese in Bildern klassifizieren. Eine interessante Fragestellung ist dabei, ob zusätzlich extrahierte Information, wie Segmentierungen von verschiedenen Gesichtspartien, einen CNN-Klassifikator weiter verbessern können.

© Springer Fachmedien Wiesbaden GmbH, ein Teil von Springer Nature 2020
T. Tolxdorff et al. (Hrsg.), *Bildverarbeitung für die Medizin 2020*,
Informatik aktuell, https://doi.org/10.1007/978-3-658-29267-6_66

1.1   Verwandte Arbeiten

Das Unterstützen von Klassifikationen durch eine bereits vorgenommene Abstraktion der Daten stellt keine neue Idee dar. Im Kontext von autonomen Systemen konnte bei der korrekten Planung der nächsten Aktion gezeigt werden, dass die Verwendung von verschiedenen Repräsentationen der Daten eine positive Auswirkung hat. Von allen untersuchten Repräsentationen hatte die Segmentierung dabei den größten Einfluss [2]. Eine Klassifikation von Gefühlen konnte durch die Verwendung von Landmarken verbessert werden. Die Klassifikation erfolgt hier über jeweils zehn Frames eines Videos. Durch die zeitliche Komponente wird die Klassifikation von Übergängen beim An- und Abflauen der Emotion stabilisiert. Dies wird zusätzlich durch die Verwendung einer LSTM-Einheit unterstützt [3]. Für unser konkretes Anwendungsbeispiel einer Mimiksteuerung für einen elektronischen Rollstuhl existiert bereits ein Ansatz, bei dem mit Kantendeteketion und K-means clustering zwei gesprochene Befehle anhand ihrer Lippenposition klassifiziert werden [1].

1.2   Eigener Beitrag

Wir zeigen, wie die Verwendung von Segmentierungen verschiedener Gesichtspartien während des Klassifikationsprozesses zu einer verbesserten Genauigkeit führt. Um den Einfluss der Segmentierung dabei exakt bestimmen zu können, werden drei Segmentierungen mit unterschiedlichen Anzahlen von Klassen verwendet. Weiterhin wird untersucht, ob die Segmentierung auch als alleinige Entscheidungsgrundlage ausreichend ist. In der Arbeit konnten wir feststellen, dass diese semantischen Zusatzinformationen ein erfolgreiches Training mit einem stark verringerten Umfang des Datensatzes ermöglichen. Dieser Aspekt ist vor allem für medizinische Problemstellungen interessant, da hier aufgrund strenger Datenschutzvorgaben oft nur wenige Daten vorliegen [4].

2   Material und Methoden

Die Klassifikation erfolgt mit einem ResNet18 [5] und umfasst zehn Mimiken, die verschiedene Kombinationen aus Kieferstellung und Lippenposition darstellen (vgl. Tab. 1). Dabei wurden die zehn untersuchten Mimiken durch den privaten

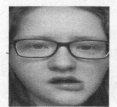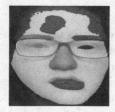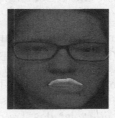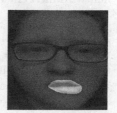

Abb. 1. Beispielbild für die Mimik „Kiefer halb geöffnet, Lippen rechts" mit den drei automatisch generierten Segmentierungen unterschiedlichen Detailgraden.

JAWGA-Datensatz vorgegeben. Dieser umfasst 690 Porträts von 66 verschiedenen Personen. Die Porträts wurden mit verschiedenen Kameras, meist mit einer Frontkamera eines Smartphones, aufgenommen. Aufgrund des eher geringen Umfangs des Datensatzes erfolgt das Training mit einer sechsfachen Kreuzvalidierung. Die in den folgenden Experimenten genutzten Segmentierungen von Gesichtspartien werden automatisch mit dem UNet [6] extrahiert. Dieses wurde auf dem Helen Facial Feature Datensatz [7] trainiert, der mit einer Grundwahrheit für Segmentierung erweitert wurde [8]. Der Datensatz umfasst 2000 Bilder von Porträts und weist eine große Diversität in Bezug auf Nationalität, Alter, Lichtverhältnisse, Posen und Mimik auf. Diese Diversität erlaubt eine ausreichende Generalisierungsleistung zu erreichen, um auch für den JAWGA-Datensatz erfolgreich Segmentierungen zu erstellen (vgl. auf JAWGA generierte Segmentierungen in Abb. 1).

Um den genauen Einfluss der Segmentierung bestimmen zu können, werden drei Segmentierungen mit unterschiedlichem Detailgrad und Klassenanzahl untersucht. Die einklassige Segmentierung umfasst nur den Mund und dient somit lediglich als Markierung der groben *region of interest*. Bei der Dreiklassigen wird dieser Bereich in Ober-, Unterlippe und Mundinneres unterteilt und bietet bereits eine detaillierte Entscheidungsgrundlage. Die Segmentierung mit neun Klassen umfasst zusätzlich zu den o.g. drei Klassen die Haut (des Gesichtes), die Nase, Augen und Augenbrauen (je links und rechts, vgl. Abb. 1) und bietet so beispielsweise mit der Nase einen Referenzpunkt zur Bestimmung der Lippenposition (mittig/links/rechts). Es wird untersucht, ob die Segmentierung als alleinige Eingabe für das CNN ausreichend ist oder ob das Bild selbst zusätzlich vorteilhaft ist. Letzteres wird mit der Konkatenation der Segmentierung an die Farbkanäle des Bildes realisiert.

2.1   Experimente

2.1.1   Vergleich der Klassifikatoren

Die Klassifikation auf dem Bild, die als Referenz dient, und die sechs verschiedenen Kombinationen von Segmentierungen und deren Verwendung während der Klassifikation (Seg1/Seg3/Seg9 + Bild) werden alle über 80 Epochen mit einer Batchgröße von 16 und dem Adam Optimierer (initiale Lernrate: 0.001) auf dem JAWGA-Datensatz trainiert. Anschließend werden die erreichten Genauigkeiten miteinander verglichen. Zusätzlich wird die Fehlerart- und verteilung berechnet und ebenfalls verglichen.

2.1.2   Einfluss der Trainingsdatenmenge

In dem zweiten Experiment wird untersucht, ob die Verwendung der verschiedenen Segmentierungen einen Vorteil bei dem Training des Klassifikators mit kleinen Datenmengen bringt. Dafür werden die 66 Personen des JAWGA-Datensatzes in sechs disjunkte Mengen aufgeteilt. Anschließend werden die verschiedenen Klassifikatoren in fünf Durchläufen trainiert. Dabei erfolgt das Training in jedem Durchlauf von Grund auf neu und umfasst eine weitere Menge für das Training. Die Generalisierungsleistung der Klassifikatoren wird dann – anders als mit der Kreuzvalidierung im

Tabelle 1. Erreichte Genauigkeit der verschiedenen Klassifikatoren auf den zehn Klassen (Mittelwert μ und Varianz σ^2). Die Varianz bezieht sich auf die Genauigkeit der sechs Durchläufe der Kreuzvalidierung.

Lippen	Kiefer	Bild	Seg1	B+Seg1	Seg3	B+Seg3	Seg9	B+Seg9
mittig	geschlossen	0.78	0.70	0.83	0.83	0.87	0.86	0.91
	halb geöffnet	0.76	0.68	0.79	0.82	0.84	0.87	0.89
	geöffnet	0.93	0.94	0.94	0.90	0.88	0.96	0.94
rechts	geschlossen	0.79	0.66	0.81	0.81	0.88	0.91	0.81
	halb geöffnet	0.91	0.72	0.82	0.88	0.89	0.93	0.91
	geöffnet	0.89	0.86	0.91	0.90	0.91	0.91	0.90
links	geschlossen	0.66	0.53	0.71	0.83	0.78	0.81	0.77
	halb geöffnet.	0.81	0.65	0.82	0.76	0.78	0.82	0.84
	geöffnet	0.96	0.82	0.90	0.94	0.85	0.90	0.90
Kuss	geschlossen	0.97	0.77	0.96	0.94	0.97	0.88	0.94
μ		0.846	0.733	0.849	0.861	0.867	0.886	0.890
$\sigma^2(\cdot 10^{-4})$		27.42	11.63	24.18	1.95	3.50	8.4	1.23

ersten Experiment – mit derselben letzten Menge, die nie im Training verwendet wurde, validiert. Die fünf Durchläufe sind für alle Klassifikatoren dabei immer identisch. Die Hyperparameter für das Training werden vom vorherigen Experiment unverändert übernommen.

3 Ergebnisse und Diskussion

3.1 Vergleich der Klassifikatoren

Aus dem Experiment geht hervor, dass die Verwendung einer Segmentierung einen positiven Einfluss auf die Genauigkeit des CNN-Klassifikators hat. Dabei lässt sich mit Genauigkeiten von $0.849, 0.867$ und 0.890 für die ein-, drei- und neunklassige Segmentierung eine Abhängigkeit zum Detailgrad der Segmentierung erkennen (vgl. Tab. 1). Bei dem Vergleich der CNN-Klassifikatoren, die dieselbe Segmentierung mit gleichem Detailgrad verwenden, kann bei der zusätzlichen Verwendung des Bildes eine höhere Genauigkeit von durchschnittlich 0.5% erreicht werden. Werden die klassenspezifischen Genauigkeiten in der Tab. 1 betrachtet, lässt sich eine leichte Tendenz erkennen, dass bei der Referenz und der Klassifikation unter Zuhilfenahme der einklassigen Mundsegmentierung eine höhere Differenz bei der Genauigkeit ähnlicher Mimiken auftritt. Extreme Mimiken (wie „Kiefer weit geöffnet", „Kussmund") erreichen stets die höchste Genauigkeit. Mit einer höherklassigen Segmentierung nimmt diese Differenz ab. Der Grund dafür ist die hohe Variabilität innerhalb einer Klasse im JAWGA-Datensatz. Diese Variabilität zwischen Personen erschwert die generelle Differenzierung von beispielsweise benachbarten Lippenpositionen und gestaltet sich – in Einzelfällen – selbst für den Menschen ohne Vergleich mit den Bildern der restlichen Klasse dieser Person als sehr schwierig. Solche schwer zu identifizierenden Bilder können z.B. durch die individuelle Auffassungen der Kategorisierungsbegriffe wie „geöffnet" und „halb geöffnet" begründet werden.

Tabelle 2. Aufschlüsselung der Fehler bei den Klassifikatoren. Der Nachbarschafts-fehler beschreibt die Verwechselung mit einer benachbarten Klasse. Beispielsweise „geschlossen" mit „halb geöffnet" bei der Kiefer- und „links" mit „mittig" bei der Lippenstellung. Der Fehlertyp „Kussmund" umfasst das Vertauschen des Kussmunds mit den Klassen „Kiefer geschlossen, Lippen mittig/links/rechts". Grobe Fehler umfassen alle anderen Klassifikationsfehler.

	Bild	Bild+Seg1	Seg1	Bild+Seg3	Seg3	Bild+Seg9	Seg9
Fehleranzahl	106	104	184	92	96	76	79
Nachbarschaft	73 (.69)	83 (.8)	139 (.76)	82 (.89)	78 (.81)	64 (.84)	60 (.76)
Kussmund	24 (.23)	16 (.15)	10 (.05)	6 (.07)	12 (.13)	7 (.09)	14 (.18)
grober Fehler	9 (.08)	5 (.05)	35 (.19)	4 (.04)	6 (.06)	5 (.7)	5 (.06)

In Tab. 2 wird die Fehlerverteilung aufgeschlüsselt. Je niedriger der Anteil von groben Fehlern ist, desto besser ist das Ergebnis des Klassifikators zu bewerten, da in diesem Fall nur noch bei der schwierigen Differenzierung benachbarter Klassen Fehler auftreten. Generell ist zu beobachten, dass bei steigender Genauigkeit auch der Anteil der groben Fehler sinkt, wenn eine Segmentierung vorliegt. Die höhere Robustheit durch Zuhilfenahme selbst von der einklassigen Segmentierung („Bild+Seg1") wird beim Vergleich mit der Klassifikation nur auf dem Bild deutlich. Obwohl eine ähnliche Gesamtgenauigkeit erreicht wird, kann die Anzahl der groben Fehler halbiert werden. Bei der korrekten Identifikation des Kussmundes ist die Klassifikation auf dem Bild mit der Segmentierung der Klassifikation auf der Segmentierung alleine deutlich überlegen („Kussmund"). Ein Grund dafür ist, dass sowohl bei der Klasse „Kiefer geschlossen, Lippen mittig" als auch beim „Kussmund" ähnliche Formen von segmentierten Pixeln erkennbar sind. Zudem reicht die Segmentierung alleine nicht aus, um die exakte Platzierung der Lippen zu bestimmen. Hier profitiert der Klassifikator bei Unsicherheiten vom Bild.

3.2 Einfluss der Trainingsdatenmenge

Bei der Klassifikation nur auf dem Bild ist eine deutliche Abhängigkeit von der Anzahl der Trainingsdaten erkennbar (vgl. Abb. 2). Steht dagegen die drei- oder

Abb. 2. Die Genauigkeit der verschiedenen Klassifikatoren auf dem Testdatensatz abhängig von der Größe des Trainingsdatensatzes.

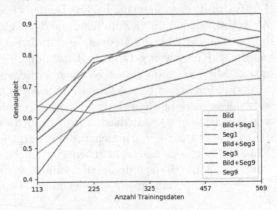

neunklassige Segmentierung zur Verfügung, so genügen zum Erreichen einer ähnlichen Genauigkeit deutlich weniger Daten, anstatt 569 reichen 325. Generell ist festzustellen, dass für das Erreichen einer besseren Genalisierungsleistung beim Training mit wenig Daten eine Segmentierung relevanter für die Klassifikation ist als das eigentliche Bild. Dies wird beim Vergleich von „Bild+Seg3" und „Seg3" deutlich. Die Genauigkeit eines Klassifikators, der auf dem Bild mit der Segmentierung arbeitet, ist stärker abhängig von der Anzahl der Trainingsdaten als eine Klassifikation auf der Segmentierung. Dem Klassifikator helfen also die bereits durch die Segmentierung abstrahierten Merkmale des Bildes. Dieser Umstand wird besonders bei der sehr geringen Anzahl von 113 Trainingsdaten deutlich. Hier erreicht die Klassifikation nur auf dem Bild lediglich eine Genauigkeit von $41,49\%$, während sich das Ergebnis, durch zusätzlich zu dem Bild generierte Segmentierung auf $55,04\%$ („Bild+Seg9") bzw. $63,22\%$ („Seg9") verbessert.

4 Zusammenfassung und Ausblick

Wir konnten zeigen, dass bei einer Mimikklassifikation durch ein CNN die Genauigkeit durch die Verwendung von automatischen Segmentierungen, in Abhängigkeit von deren Detailgraden, verbessert werden kann. Die besten Klassifikationsergebnisse durch das CNN erhalten wir, wenn wir Segmentierungen und reine Bildinformationen verbinden. Zudem konnten wir zeigen, dass eine detaillierte Segmentierung als Entscheidungsgrundlage für eine Klassifikation von unterschiedlichen Mimiken genügt. Diese indirekte Verwendung von Daten ist auf Grund der strengen Datenschutzvorgaben in der Medizin relevant. Wir konnten auch zeigen, dass die durch die Segmentierung abstrahierten Daten es erlauben, für das Training nur 60% des Datensatzes zu verwenden, um eine vergleichbare Genauigkeit zu erreichen. In Zukunft wäre ein Vergleich mit landmarkenbasierten Verfahren und anderen öffentlichen Mimikdatensätzen von Interesse.

Literaturverzeichnis

1. Ju JS, Shin Y, Kim EY. Vision based interface system for hands free control of an intelligent wheelchair. J Neuroeng Rehabil. 2009;.
2. Zhou B, Krähenbühl P, Koltun V. Does computer vision matter for action? arXiv preprint arXiv:190512887. 2019;.
3. Hasani B, Mahoor MH. Facial expression recognition using enhanced deep 3d convolutional neural networks. In: Proc IEEE comput soc conf comput vis pattern recognit workshops; 2017. p. 2278–2288.
4. Cho J, Lee K, Shin E, et al. Medical image deep learning with hospital PACS dataset. arXiv preprint arXiv:151106348. 2015;.
5. He K, Zhang X, Ren S, et al. Deep residual learning for image recognition. In: Proc IEEE comput soc conf comput vis pattern recognit; 2016. p. 770–778.
6. Ronneberger O, Fischer P, Brox T. U-Net: convolutional networks for biomedical image segmentation. In: Med Image Comput Comput Assist Interv; 2015. p. 234–241.

7. Le V, Brandt J, Lin Z, et al. Interactive facial feature localization. In: Proc IEEE Eur Conf Comput Vis; 2012. p. 679–692.
8. Smith BM, Zhang L, Brandt J, et al. Exemplar-Based face parsing. In: Proc IEEE comput soc conf comput vis pattern recognit; 2013. p. 3484–3491.

Imitation Learning Network for Fundus Image Registration Using a Divide-And-Conquer Approach

Siming Bayer[1], Xia Zhong[1], Weilin Fu[1], Nishant Ravikumar[2], Andreas Maier[1]

[1]Pattern Recognition Lab, FAU Erlangen-Nuremberg
[2]CISTIB, School of Computing and School of Medicin, University of Leeds
siming.bayer@fau.de

Abstract. Comparison of microvascular circulation on fundoscopic images is a non-invasive clinical indication for the diagnosis and monitoring of diseases, such as diabetes and hypertensions. The differences between intra-patient images can be assessed quantitatively by registering serial acquisitions. Due to the variability of the images (i.e. contrast, luminosity) and the anatomical changes of the retina, the registration of fundus images remains a challenging task. Recently, several deep learning approaches have been proposed to register fundus images in an end-to-end fashion, achieving remarkable results. However, the results are difficult to interpret and analyze. In this work, we propose an imitation learning framework for the registration of 2D color funduscopic images for a wide range of applications such as disease monitoring, image stitching and super-resolution. We follow a divide-and-conquer approach to improve the interpretability of the proposed network, and analyze both the influence of the input image and the hyperparameters on the registration result. The results show that the proposed registration network reduces the initial target registration error up to 95%.

1 Introduction

Retina blood vessels and their morphological features are important biomarkers for non-invasive monitoring of chronic and age-related diseases, such as diabetic retinopathy, glaucoma, or macular edema. In order to analyse the progression of diseases, image registration techniques are used to conduct longitudinal studies by comparing serially acquired intra-patient funducsopic images. Moreover, acquisitions from different viewpoints can be fused into one single image containing panoramic information of the retina. However, registration of retinal images remains a challenging task due to various factors, such as uneven illumination of textureless regions, large variety of the viewpoints on serially acquired fundus images and pathological changes to the anatomy of the retina.

A detailed review [1] of fundus image registration techniques shows that feature-based approaches are more frequently applied to resolve this task. In [2], a

© Springer Fachmedien Wiesbaden GmbH, ein Teil von Springer Nature 2020
T. Tolxdorff et al. (Hrsg.), *Bildverarbeitung für die Medizin 2020*,
Informatik aktuell, https://doi.org/10.1007/978-3-658-29267-6_67

graph matching method is combined with ICP to find correspondences between vascular bifurcations and register retinal vessels. A comparison of feature-based retina image registration algorithms using bifurcations, SIFT or SURF as features is presented in [3]. Those methods are accurate and are easy to interpret. A major limitation of conventional feature-based method is, that it consists of time consuming optimization methods. In order to address this limitation, [4] proposed a generative adverserial network (GAN) for the estimation the final dense deformation field. However, the network is only trained and tested on data, where the image pairs have large overlapping area. Moreover, the entire registration pipeline is mapped into one single network, and operates as a black-box. This makes it difficult to interpret and to analyze.

Recent advances towards better understanding of deep learning (DL) networks using precision learning [5] encourage the decomposition of an end-to-end DL framework into known operators. Previously, [6] proposed an imitation learning network for intra-operative brain shift compensation where the optimal displacement vectors of landmarks defined in the 'source' image domain are predicted directly from the underlying image pair to be registered (in order to map them to the 'target' image domain). In this work, we use a modified version of this network and propose a generalized method for feature-based fundus image registration. The image pairs used for training and evaluation of the proposed network vary in their appearance, and are used for different applications. In order to analyze the image registration network, we apply the concept of precision learning, following a divide-and-conquer strategy proposed in [7] for the identification of the critical components which affects the accuracy of the limitation learning network.

2   Materials and methods

2.1   Fundus image registration dataset (FIRE)

The FIRE dataset published in [8] is a public database for retina image registration containing 134 pairs of intra-patient fundus images[1]. Moreover, ten homologous landmark pairs on the vessel bifurcation points are manually annotated for each image pairs. All images are acquired in the same hospital with the same type of fundus camera. They have a resolution of 2912×2912 pixels and a field of view of $45° \times 45°$. In general, the image pairs can be divided into three categories with regard to the characteristics of the images:

2.1.1   Category A This category comprises 14 image pairs, which were collected during a longitudinal study with similar viewpoint. Due to pathological changes from disease progression image appearance between each pair of images varies greatly.

---

[1] Accessable via https://www.ics.forth.gr/cvrl/fire/

2.1.2   Category P In this part, 49 intra-patient image pairs from different view points were captured for the purpose of image stitching. The anatomical differences within one image pair is small.

2.1.3   Category S In this group, 71 image pairs were acquired for the application of super-resolution. Therefore, the images within each image pair are captured from a similar viewpoint. Anatomical differences or pathological changes within the retinal are invisible.

2.2   Imitation learning network for fundus image registration

We employ imitation learning for the task of pair-wise registration of fundus images. The core idea of imitation learning is to train a network to mimic the behavior of the demonstrator based on current observations. In the case of pair-wise registration, the demonstrator predicts the optimal displacement vectors for known correspondences.

- Observation Encoding: We use both the spatial position of the landmarks and the image features associated with each landmark as our observation encoding. The image features are defined as a concatenation of isotropic 2D patches around the landmarks on the input image. The 2D patches are extracted by resampling the original image with a isotropic spacial step size of S and a patch size of $C \times C$. For each point set, the normalized point spatial distribution is used as a part of observation encoding.
- Demonstrator and Augmentation: As the point correspondence of the landmarks is known in the training data, the displacement vectors between the homologous points in a source-target image pair are directly considered as the demonstrator. Each data set is augmented by varying the brightness and contrast relative to the original image. Additionally, we also transform the original image and point-pairs using random affine transformations.
- Network and loss: The network architecture of the proposed imitation network is illustrated in Fig. 1. The input to the network includes source and target images as well as their corresponding landmarks. To facilitate the training of a robust registration network, a multi-task network is applied to predict the translation of the source image, and the displacement vectors of each source landmark, simultaneously. The desired transformation of the source image can be estimated subsequently. The same loss function as proposed in [6] is employed as a weighted loss for both tasks.

2.3   Experimental analysis of imitation learning network

Our network is trained and tested with the fundus images pairs introduced in Section 2.1. A leave-one-out scheme was used to evaluate the registration performance of the imitation learning network on an independent held out test image-pair from the data set. While, within each fold of this leave-one-out scheme, the

133 image pairs were further split into training and validation sets using a ratio of 0.9 : 0.1. Both input images and the corresponding landmarks are augmented by creating 64 additional copies simultaneously. The Adam optimizer with a learning rate of 0.001 was used throughout all experiments for training.

In order to evaluate the generality and performance of the proposed method quantitatively, and understand the learning mechanism of the imitation learning architectures, e.g. to elucidate what the imitation network observes/learns, we conduct the following two experiments:

2.3.1   Experiment I In this experiment, we analyze the influence of the appearance of the input images on the registration result. Following a divide and conquer strategy proposed in [7], we divide the fundus image registration pipeline into two parts, namely, image preprocessing (including vessel segmentation) and image registration. Two different known operators are employed to resolve the task of image preprocessing prior to application of the imitation network. The preprocessing and vessel enhancement techniques used in this study are validated and well understood in the literature. First, histogram equalization and a Laplacian of Gaussian filter (LoG) are applied. It is a straightforward analytical method with high noise sensitivity. The second method for image preprocessing is adopted from [7], including a differentiable guided filter layer and an eight-scale Frangi-Net [9]. The CNN network pipeline for image preprocessing and segmentation is trained following the experiment setups in [7], and no further fine-tuning is conducted. Photographs in the FIRE database are standardized to (-1, 1) gray-scale images. To match the vessel diameters in the training data, images in FIRE are downsampled by a factor of four before fed into the network and upsampled after processing. Previous studies demonstrate, that the combination of a guided filter layer and Frangi-Net is a DL counterpart of the guided filter and the Frangi filter, on par with U-Net in terms of vessel segmentation accuracy. However, it has fewer parameters and higher interpretability due to the use of known operators within the learning framework. In both cases, the

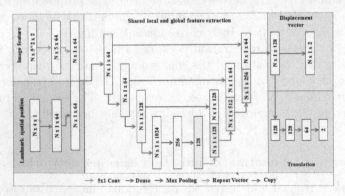

Fig. 1. Architectures of the imitation network for the direct estimation of the displacement vectors on landmarks.

output of the image preprocessing block is a gray-scale image with enhanced vessel structures, which can be used as the input of the imitation network. Hereby, C and S are fixed to 20 and 40.

2.3.2   Experiment II We use guided filter layer and Frangi-Net to preprocess the input image. The hyperparameters of the imitation network C and S are modified. C is fixed to 20 and 40, whilst S is changed. Here, the aim is to evaluate the influence of the hyperparameters on the registration result.

3   Results

Since annotated landmarks are provided as ground truth, we use target registration error (TRE) as the evaluation metric. The result of both experiments are presented in Fig.2. Initially, the TRE in pixels between the unregistered landmarks are 152.9 ± 66.34, 2518.9 ± 948.22, and 156.36 ± 155.21 for the image Category A, P, and S, respectively.

4   Discussion

The quantitative results in Fig. 2 shows our proposed network is able to recover 50%, 95%, and 75% of the initial displacement for image Category A, P, and S respectively. The results of *Experiment I* in Fig. 2a. indicates that input images preprocessed using Frangi-Net improve the registration performance of the network, for the image categories P and S, when $C = 20$ and $S = 40$. For the image Category A however, image preprocessing degrades the performance of the imitation network. Considering the characteristics of the input image of each Category, we can draw the following conclusions: for input image pairs with similar appearance (i.e. categories P and S), the imitation network focuses and learns primarily from the vascular structures of the retina. Thus, an accurate image preprocessing and segmentation method could benefit the overall performance of the registration step. In Category A where the input images

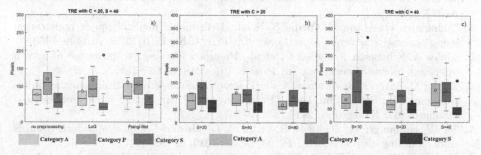

Fig. 2. TRE between landmark positions predicted from the source points and the corresponding target points. The results of the *Experiment I* are presented in Fig. a., whilst Fig. b. and Fig. c. show the results of *Experiment II*.

show a large variation in their appearance, the proposed network relies other image features besides the vasculature. Vessel enhancement and segmentation techniques such as LoG or Frangi-Net enhance vascular structures and suppress other information. Therefore, the application of those techniques on the input images affect the performance of the proposed registration network for Category A negatively.

In the result of *Experiment II* (Fig. 2b. and 2c.) the impact of the hyperparameters C and S are demonstrated. Small C values were found to be more suitable to predict the displacement vectors of the landmarks in all three categories, when the input images are preprocessed and segmented using the guided filter layer and Frangi-Net. This effect is more visible in categories A and P, where the overlapping area of the input images are large, i.e. the initial distance of the landmarks are small. In Category P, the results in both cases $C = 20, S = 40$ and $C = 40, S = 20$ are comparable. Furthermore, they outperform other hyperparameter combinations. To summarize, in *Experiments II C* can be considered as the resolution of the observation, whilst S represents the extent of the entire observation.

A comprehensive comparison between the proposed network and iterative fundus image registration methods will be performed in future studies. The registration accuracy of the proposed network could potentially be improved by automatically identifying the optimal values for the associated hyperparameters, namely, C and S, based on the characteristics of the input image paris to be registration. This will also be investigated in future studies.

References

1. Saha SK, Xiao D, Bhuiyan A, et al. Color fundus image registration techniques and applications for automated analysis of diabetic retinopathy progression: a review. Biomed Signal Process Control. 2019;47:288 – 302.
2. Deng K, Tian J, Zheng J, et al. Retinal fundus image registration via vascular structure graph matching. In: Int J Biomed Imaging; 2010. p. 13.
3. Hernandez-Matas C, Zabulis X, Argyros AA. An experimental evaluation of the accuracy of keypoints-based retinal image registration. In: Proc IEEE EMBS; 2017. p. 377–381.
4. Mahapatra D, Antony B, Sedai S, et al. Deformable medical image registration using generative adversarial networks. In: Proc IEEE ISBI; 2018. p. 1449–1453.
5. Maier A, Schebesch F, Syben C, et al. Precision learning: towards use of known operators in neural networks. In: Proc ICPR; 2018. p. 183–188.
6. Zhong X, Bayer S, Ravikumar N, et al. Resolve intraoperative brain shift as imitation game. In: Simulation, Image Processing, and Ultrasound Systems for Assisted Diagnosis and Navigation; 2018. p. 129–137.
7. Fu W, Breininger K, Schaffert R, et al. A Divide-and-Conquer approach towards understanding deep networks. In: MICCAI; 2019. p. 183–191.
8. Hernandez-Matas C, Zabulis X, Triantafyllou A, et al. FIRE: Fundus Image Registration Dataset. Model Opthalmol. 2017;1:16–28.
9. Fu W, Breininger K, Schaffert R, et al. Frangi-Net. In: Proc BVM; 2018. p. 341–346.

Comparison of CNN Visualization Methods to Aid Model Interpretability for Detecting Alzheimer's Disease

Martin Dyrba[1], Arjun H. Pallath[2], Eman N. Marzban[1,3,4]

[1] German Center for Neurodegenerative Diseases (DZNE), Rostock, Germany
[2] Institute of Visual & Analytic Computing, University of Rostock, Germany
[3] Clinic for Psychosomatic and Psychotherapeutic Medicine (KPM),
University Medical Center Rostock, Germany
[4] Biomedical Engineering and Systems Dept., Faculty of Engineering,
Cairo University, Giza, Egypt
martin.dyrba@dzne.de

Abstract. Advances in medical imaging and convolutional neural networks (CNNs) have made it possible to achieve excellent diagnostic accuracy from CNNs comparable to human raters. However, CNNs are still not implemented in medical trials as they appear as a black box system and their inner workings cannot be properly explained. Therefore, it is essential to assess CNN relevance maps, which highlight regions that primarily contribute to the prediction. This study focuses on the comparison of algorithms for generating heatmaps to visually explain the learned patterns of Alzheimer's disease (AD) classification. T1-weighted volumetric MRI data were entered into a 3D CNN. Heatmaps were then generated for different visualization methods using the iNNvestigate and keras-vis libraries. The model reached an area under the curve of 0.93 and 0.75 for separating AD dementia patients from controls and patients with amnestic mild cognitive impairment from controls, respectively. Visualizations for the methods deep Taylor decomposition and layer-wise relevance propagation (LRP) showed most reasonable results for individual patients matching expected brain regions. Other methods, such as Grad-CAM and guided backpropagation showed more scattered activations or random areas. For clinically research, deep Taylor decomposition and LRP showed most valuable network activation patterns.

1 Introduction

Deep convolution neural networks (CNNs) have become the state-of-the-art technique for various image classification tasks. The performance of these systems has been reported to be on par with humans. Several papers have proposed various new architectures for general-purpose image detection, which have a steady trend of improvement of model accuracy. These networks are actively being researched and developed in areas related to computer vision in many

© Springer Fachmedien Wiesbaden GmbH, ein Teil von Springer Nature 2020
T. Tolxdorff et al. (Hrsg.), *Bildverarbeitung für die Medizin 2020*,
Informatik aktuell, https://doi.org/10.1007/978-3-658-29267-6_68

fields such as self-driving cars, face recognition, object detection, and medical imaging. These systems when applied in medical imaging, could aid physicians in the early diagnosis of diseases and highlight the concerning areas in medical scans. However, there is a lack of transparency in the accuracy of results derived from these networks, as there is no direct way to identify on what basis the network performs the classification. Recently, several methods have been proposed to calculate CNN relevance maps ([1] for an extensive overview). These maps highlight regions of the input images that the network focuses on when classifying the disease. The regions identified by the network and the regions known to be affected by the disease can then be compared to check whether they match. Such plausibility checks could lead to more robust, reliable, and trustworthy CNN models; and, therefore, would also improve the clinical utility of such models.

In the literature, we only found three papers [2, 3, 4] providing CNN visualizations for 3D MRI data and disease prediction. However, a direct comparison with the most recent approaches such as layer-wise relevance propagation (LRP) and deep Taylor decomposition is still lacking.

Alzheimer's disease (AD) is the major cause of dementia in elderly people above 65 years of age. AD is characterized by the death of nerve cells (neurons) causing irreversible changes and atrophy (volume reduction) in the brain, leading to memory loss, behavioral changes, speech impairment, and difficulties in activities of daily living. AD is difficult to diagnose in its early stages due to the slow progress of the disease and due to the difficulty of discriminating accelerated atrophy in AD from normal age-related atrophy. People suffering from mild cognitive impairment (MCI), especially when involving memory, are being seen at high risk for progressing to AD dementia.

This study aims to i) detect AD or MCI using a 3D CNN for T1-weighted volumetric MRI data, and ii) compare different visualization methods with respect to the clinical utility of the derived heatmaps for indicating areas that most contribute to the classification of the scans.

2   Materials and methods

Study sample T1-weighted volumetric MRI data were obtained from the Alzheimer's Disease Neuroimaging Initiative (ADNI)[1]. In total, the sample included 662 cases consisting of 198 patients with AD dementia, 219 patients with amnestic MCI, and 254 cognitively normal controls. The subjects' demographics are shown in Tab. 1. Using common SPM8 and VBM8 software, MRI scans were segmented into grey and white matter, spatially normalized to an in-house ageing/AD-specific brain template [5] using the DARTEL algorithm, and finally modulated. Additionally, all scans were cleaned for the effects of the covariates age, gender, total intracranial volume and scanner magnetic field strength using linear regression [6]. For each voxel, models were fitted for the

---

[1] More information about the ADNI can be found on http://adni.loni.usc.edu

Table 1. Sample characteristics.

	Controls	MCI	AD	p-value
Sample size (female)	254 (130)	219 (93)	189 (80)	0.149
Age (SD)	75.4 ± 6.6	74.1 ± 8.1	75.0 ± 8.0	<0.001
Education (SD)	16.4 ± 2.7	16.2 ± 2.8	15.9 ± 2.7	0.227
MMSE (SD)	29.1 ± 1.2	27.6 ± 1.9	22.6 ± 3.2	<0.001
Delayed recall (SD)	7.6 ± 4.1	3.2 ± 3.7	0.8 ± 1.9	<0.001 .

healthy control subjects. Subsequently, these models were applied to all scans, i.e. the residualized images were taken as input for the CNN. Due to memory limitations, we defined a field-of-view including the whole brain in axial and saggital directions, but only a range of 32 coronal slices covering the temporal lobe and the hippocampus area known to be most affected by AD. The field-of-view is illustrated on the left of Fig. 1.

Validation strategy We used a ten-fold cross-validation approach, such that the sample was divided into ten test sets (10%, n=67) for determining the accuracy of the model, and nested splits into training set (80%, n=535) and validation set (10%, n=60) for model training. The test sets included approximately 17 AD dementia patients, 24 MCI patients and 26 controls. Prior to training, the training sets were augmented by adding copies of the training scans shifted by ±2 voxels in x/y/z-direction resulting in training samples of n=3745 images.

CNN model layout and paramcterization The CNN model was implemented in Keras/Tensorflow 1.15. The general 3D CNN model layout is shown in Fig. 1. Prior to training, class labels were merged for AD dementia and MCI to have a binary classification task. We specified the categorical cross-entropy as the loss function and the accuracy as the performance metric. The models were optimized by Adam running for 100 epochs with a batch size of 64 and default learning rate of 0.001. Training took approximately 55 minutes per cross-validation iteration.

Visualization methods We used the iNNvestigate library [1] implementing various visualization methods. In detail, we tested deconvnet, guided backpropagation, deep Taylor decomposition, input*gradient, and layer-wise relevance propagation (LRP) with the Z, epsilon, and alpha=1,beta=0 rules. Additionally, we used keras-vis [7] for the Grad-CAM approach. As the intensity range of the relevance maps differed greatly between approaches, it was scaled linearly to a fixed range allowing a visual comparison. In addition to the raw relevance maps overlayed on the original input data (with 50% transparency), we provide a smoothed and thresholded version containing the most prominent clusters only, i.e. the top 30 percentile of intensity values.

3   Results

For the test data, we obtained a mean accuracy of 75.2% with an area under the curve (AUC) of 0.83 for the combined dataset. When looking at the original diagnosis subsets, the CNN achieved an AUC of 0.93 for AD dementia vs. controls and 0.75 for separating MCI patients from controls.

Exemplary relevance maps for different individuals are presented in Fig. 2 for an AD dementia case, a patient with MCI, and for a healthy control.

4   Discussion

The CNN model achieved excellent diagnostic accuracy for separating AD dementia from controls, comparable to other approaches from the literature [3, 6]. For separating MCI patients from controls, accuracy was reasonable and in line with previous studies. Notably, as computational complexity is considerably higher for 3D CNN models compared to 2D CNN models used for general purpose image detection tasks, there is a high potential of model overfitting, in contrast to a very limited number of MRI scans available for training. We addressed this problem by in three ways. Firstly, we applied a sophisticated image preprocessing pipeline including segmentation, spatial normalization, and covariate cleaning as common for voxel-based statistical analyzes. Secondly, we reduced the number of layers compared to other approaches [2, 3] resulting in a more shallow network. Our CNN model included three convolutional layers with in total approximately 6,400 parameters on the cost of being less rotation/translation-invariant compared to deeper CNNs. Thirdly, we used data augmentation to multiply the data available for training and to improve the stability and robustness of the model.

The CNN relevance maps obtained from the various approaches showed diverging quality with respect to focus, smoothness and scatter (Fig. 2). This result is in line with two previous papers testing a subset of methods [2, 3]. Approximately the same image regions were highlighted across the visualization methods. As expected, the hippocampus area showed the highest relevance for the AD and MCI patients. However, the directionality of weighting (positive vs. negative) differed between the algorithms. Notably, for Grad-CAM the relevance maps substantially differed with respect to the smoothness. This is due to the approach of calculating low-resolution activations at the fully-connected layer followed by upscaling (interpolation) to the original input image resolution. The two methods deep Taylor decomposition and LRP with alpha=1,beta=0 rule showed the most promising relevance maps with strongest focus. Also, these approaches mainly showed positive relevance scores for the AD class and sup-

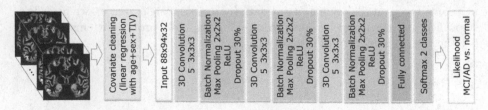

Fig. 1. Convolutional neural network model layout.

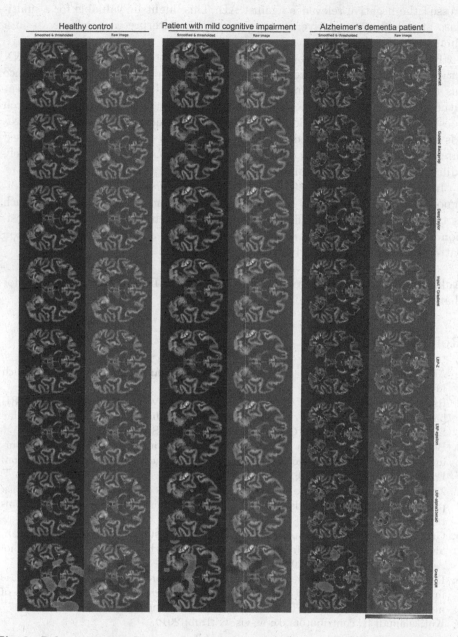

Fig. 2. Relevance maps for an individual with Alzheimer's dementia, amnestic mild cognitive impairment, and normal cognition. Raw figures in top row, smoothed and thresholded figures in bottom row. Methods by column: deconvnet, guided backpropagation, deep Taylor decomposition, input*gradient, LRP-Z, LRP-epsilon, LRP-alpha1beta0, grad-CAM. Red and blue color indicate high positive or negative activation.

pressed the negative relevance against AD. This might be valuable for a multi-class model, where negative relevance cannot be interpreted as clearly as in a binary classification task.

Two limitations have to be mentioned for the present work. Firstly, the CNN structure and parameters need to be systematically evaluated and performance has to be validated on an independent dataset, which we will do in the near future. Secondly, intensity normalization of the relevance maps is open research question. As the distribution of values differed between visualization methods and patients, we rescaled the range linearly and applied a percentile-based threshold. For clinical use, it should be considered to allow users to interactively adjust the color scale and threshold.

In conclusion, we presented a CNN structure providing both excellent diagnostic accuracy as well as relevance maps highlighting expected regions such as the hippocampus. For clinically oriented research, deep Taylor decomposition and LRP with alpha1,beta0 rule showed most valuable network activation patterns with high focus and less scatter.

Acknowledgement. We would like to thank the ADNI and contributors [2] for sharing their data.

References

1. Alber M, Lapuschkin S, Seegerer P, et al. iNNvestigate neural networks! J Mach Learn Res. 2019;20:1–8.
2. Rieke J, Eitel F, Weygandt M, et al. Visualizing vonvolutional networks for MRI-based diagnosis of Alzheimer's disease. In: Understanding and Interpreting Machine Learning in Medical Image Computing Applications. Springer; 2018. p. 24–31.
3. Böhle M, Eitel F, Weygandt M, et al. Layer-wise relevance propagation for explaining deep neural network decisions in MRI-based Alzheimer's disease classification. Front Aging Neurosci. 2019;11:194.
4. Zintgraf LM, Cohen TS, Adel T, et al. Visualizing deep neural network decisions: prediction difference analysis. In: International Conference on Learning Representations (ICLR); 2017. .
5. Grothe M, Heinsen H, Teipel S. Longitudinal measures of cholinergic forebrain atrophy in the transition from healthy aging to Alzheimer's disease. Neurobiol Aging. 2013;34(4):1210–1220.
6. Dyrba M, Barkhof F, Fellgiebel A, et al. Predicting prodromal Alzheimer's disease in subjects with mild cognitive impairment using machine learning classification of multimodal multicenter DTI and MRI data. J Neuroimaging. 2015;25(5):738–747.
7. Kotikalapudi R, contributors. keras-vis. GitHub; 2019.

---

[2] http://adni.loni.usc.edu/wp-content/uploads/how_to_apply/ ADNI_Acknowledgement_List.pdf

Abstract: Divide-And-Conquer Approach Towards Understanding Deep Networks

Weilin Fu[1,3], Katharina Breininger[1], Roman Schaffert[1], Nishant Ravikumar[1], Andreas Maier[1,2]

[1] Pattern Recognition Lab, Friedrich-Alexander University Erlangen-Nürnberg,
91058 Erlangen, Germany
[2] Erlangen Graduate School in Advanced Optical Technologies(SAOT),
91058 Erlangen, Germany
[3] International Max Planck Research School for Physics of Light (IMPRS-PL),
91052 Erlangen, Germany
weilin.fu@fau.de

Deep neural networks have achieved tremendous success in various fields including medical image segmentation. However, they have long been criticized for being a black-box, in that interpretation, understanding and correcting architectures is difficult as there is no general theory for deep neural network design. Previously, precision learning was proposed to fuse deep architectures and traditional approaches. Deep networks constructed in this way benefit from the original known operator, have fewer parameters, and improved interpretability. However, they do not yield state-of-the-art performance in all applications. In this paper, we propose to analyze deep networks using known operators, by adopting a divide-and-conquer strategy to replace network components, whilst retaining networks performance. The task of retinal vessel segmentation is investigated for this purpose. We start with a high-performance U-Net and show by step-by-step conversion that we are able to divide the network into modules of known operators. The results indicate that a combination of a trainable guided filter and a trainable version of the Frangi filter yields a performance at the level of U-Net (AUC 0.974 vs. 0.972) with a tremendous reduction in parameters (111,536 vs. 9,575). In addition, the trained layers can be mapped back into their original algorithmic interpretation and analyzed using standard tools of signal processing [1].

References

1. Fu W, Breininger K, Schaffert R, et al. A divide-and-conquer approach towards understanding deep networks. In: Proc - MICCAI 2019; 2019. p. 183–191.

© Springer Fachmedien Wiesbaden GmbH, ein Teil von Springer Nature 2020
T. Tolxdorff et al. (Hrsg.), *Bildverarbeitung für die Medizin 2020*,
Informatik aktuell, https://doi.org/10.1007/978-3-658-29267-6_69

Abstract: Fiber Optical Shape Sensing of Flexible Instruments

Sonja Jäckle[1], Tim Eixmann[2], Hinnerk Schulz-Hildebrandt[2,3,4],
Gereon Hüttmann[2,3,4], Torben Pätz[5]

[1]Fraunhofer MEVIS, Institute for Digital Medicine, Lübeck, Germany
[2]Medizinisches Laserzentrum Lübeck GmbH, Lübeck, Germany
[3]Institute of Biomedical Optics, Universität zu Lübeck, Germany
[4]German Center for Lung Research, DZL, Großhansdorf, Germany
[5]Fraunhofer MEVIS, Institute for Digital Medicine, Bremen, Germany
sonja.jaeckle@mevis.fraunhofer.de

For minimal invasive procedures like endovascular aortic repair procedures the instruments are navigated with 2D fluoroscopy imaging and digital subtraction angiography, which have several disadvantages. Optical fibers with fiber Bragg gratings (FBG), which allow to sense local strain respectively local curvature and bending angles, can be used for the guidance of medical tools to reduce the X-ray exposure and the used contrast agent. However, FBG-based shape sensing of flexible and long instruments is challenging and the computation includes many steps. In this work, we analyzed in every shape sensing step, which errors can occur, how they affect the resulting shape, and how they can be reduced or corrected [1]. The effects of different methods and parameters were analyzed with experiments done with one multicore fiber of 38 cm shape sensing length. The results of this analysis were used for an accurate shape sensing model. In an experiment different shapes were measured with the multicore fiber. Then the reconstructed 3D shapes were compared with the segmented shapes of the acquired CT scans to evaluate the accuracy of our shape sensing model. We obtained an average error of 0.35 to 1.15 mm and maximal error of 0.75 to 7.53 mm over the whole 38 cm sensing length. Furthermore, our shape sensing model was tested in a realistic endovascular setting. Therefore the fiber was inserted into a 3D printed vessel created from patient data. Here, we obtained an average and maximal error of 1.13 mm and 2.11 mm, respectively. The accuracies of our shape sensing model are promising for using fiber optical shape sensing for catheter guidance. In future work we will use electromagnetic sensors to locate the reconstructed catheter shape.

References

1. Jäckle S, Eixmann T, Schulz-Hildebrandt H, et al. Fiber optical shape sensing of flexible instruments for endovascular navigation. Int J Comput Assist Radiol Surg. 2019;.

© Springer Fachmedien Wiesbaden GmbH, ein Teil von Springer Nature 2020
T. Tolxdorff et al. (Hrsg.), *Bildverarbeitung für die Medizin 2020*,
Informatik aktuell, https://doi.org/10.1007/978-3-658-29267-6_70

Scalable HEVC for Histological Whole-Slide Image Compression

Daniel Bug[1], Felix Bartsch[1], Nadine Sarah Schaadt[2], Mathias Wien[1],
Friedrich Feuerhake[2,3], Julia Schüler[4], Eva Oswald[4], Dorit Merhof[1]

[1]Institute of Imaging and Computer Vision, RWTH Aachen University
[2]Institute for Pathology, Hannover Medical School
[3]Institute for Neuropathology, University Clinic Freiburg im Breisgau
[4]Charles River Discover Research Services Germany GmbH, Freiburg im Breisgau
daniel.bug@lfb.rwth-aachen.de

Abstract. Digital whole-slide images (WSI) are scanned representations of histological tissue at microscopic scale, enabling computer aided diagnosis and remote pathology applications. However, the data sizes may hinder a widespread use, as raw files can easily exceed 10-20GB. In this work, we explore the Scalable High Efficiency Video Coding (SHVC) as a replacement for the JPEG standard currently found in most vendor formats. Besides a comparison of the compression rates, this work comprises a user-study to estimate SHVC quantization parameters (QP) and JPEG quality level that threshold the just-noticeable distortions (JND) for a compression below the JND.

1 Introduction

Digital pathology is an emerging field in the image analysis sector. WSIs depict microscopic tissue that has been scanned patchwise and merged virtually at a very high magnification. For example, a fully digitized 2.3cm×1.7cm tissue section at 40× objective-magnification amounts to 18.4GB of raw pixel data (RGB 24bit at 91k×67k pixels). Lossless compression can achieve compression ratios up to 3:1, which is insufficient for WSI storage or transmission. A strong indication for the acceptance of lossy compression in the field is that most vendor formats, e.g. NDPI (Hamamatsu) or SVS (Leica), employ lossy compression. To handle the large image sizes in a standard compatible way, the images are processed and stored in tiles and to achieve a microscopy-like experience, e.g. zooming in and out, multiple resolutions are stored per file. Examples of the WSI data are depicted in Fig. 1.

HEVC [1] is a recent standard for video, utilizing prediction and transform coding, which can also be used for image compression. Benefits of HEVC compared to JPEG are flexible block partitioning, enhanced intra prediction, residual coding, and inloop filters to address the blocking and ringing artifacts that are otherwise common to block-based codecs. In 2015, the scalable extension

© Springer Fachmedien Wiesbaden GmbH, ein Teil von Springer Nature 2020
T. Tolxdorff et al. (Hrsg.), *Bildverarbeitung für die Medizin 2020*,
Informatik aktuell, https://doi.org/10.1007/978-3-658-29267-6_71

SHVC [2] was added to the HEVC standard, allowing spatial scaling from an image pyramid input that acts as a natural representation of a multi-resolution image.

1.1 Related Work

Liu et. al [3] present a comparison across various compression standards in medical applications, also including Hematoxylin and Eosin stained WSIs. In this study, with the WSI samples as exception, HEVC outperforms the other algorithms. This inferiority of HEVC in case of the WSIs is attributed to an unsuited rate allocation algorithm. Two works by Tuominen et. al [4, 5] research the JPEG2000 (J2k) standard for WSIs. In [4], J2k's native scaling support is evaluated and precincts are found to be an excellent solution for partitioning and random access. Herein, rate control is applied with fixed-rates between 1:25 and 1:30 which are reported to have decent quality; however, background regions are included. In [5], a method utilizing the J2k Interactive Protocol for telepathology is introduced. Furthermore, Helin et. al [6], report large gains in compression by optimizing the J2k compression settings and formulate a custom J2k-WSI protocol. Most importantly, they deploy a fore-/background subdivision and apply different compression qualities. Sanchez et al. [7] apply a lossless HEVC-intra compression to the segmented image foreground, while lossy compression is used on the background with a remaining rate budget.

Our contribution is a SHVC-based format that leverages spatial scalability and provides fast random access to regions-of-interest at arbitrary scale. Furthermore, we introduce an adaptive quantization that is well suited for WSI encoding.

2 Materials and methods

We introduce two datasets for later evaluation: 1.) For a quantitative evaluation, 12 WSIs were scanned by an Leica Aperio AT2 Scanner and saved with lossless LZW compression. This set comprises four Hematoxylin and Eosin (HE) and eight immunohistochemically stained images with Hematoxylin and Diaminobencidine (DAB). 2.) For a qualitative evaluation, four images (two HE and two DAB, Fig. 1) were extracted and compressed with different algorithms (SHVC,

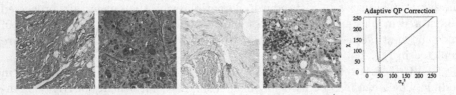

Fig. 1. Examples of WSI tiles: Hematoxylin & Eosin stain (violet/pink) and Hematoxylin & Diaminobencidine stain (blue/brown). Rightmost: corrected variance function from (2).

HEVC and JPEG) and different quality settings (five per algorithm), such that the resulting PSNRs between algorithms are comparable.

Our proposed method utilizes a scalable intra configuration for SHVC [2]. This supports arbitrary downsampling and utilizes inter layer prediction (ILP) to predict all higher resolutions above the HEVC-intra encoded base layer (BL). Thus, only the residuals of higher layers are encoded. Downsampling filters are provided to up to a ratio of 1:4 and the interpolation methods were designed for a ratio of 1:2. Note that this standard enables to decode the image pyramid only as far as needed and can stop at intermediate resolutions, which is very useful to achieve a fast random access regarding the image scale.

For the *random access* to a specific region, we expect the x, y coordinates of the largest layer $L - 1$ and the width w and height h of the region as input parameters. With this and the sizes of the largest layer W_{L-1}, H_{L-1} as side information, we can determine the Picture Order Count (position in the bitstream, Fig. 2) of the tiles in this region that need to be decoded

$$\text{POC}_{decode} = \bigcup_{i=\lfloor x/D_{L-1} \rfloor}^{\lceil (x+w)/D_{L-1} \rceil} \bigcup_{j=\lfloor y/D_{L-1} \rfloor}^{\lceil (y+h)/D_{L-1} \rceil} i + j \lceil W_{L-1}/D_{L-1} \rceil \tag{1}$$

where D_{L-1} is the tile size at the largest layer. The bitstream of HEVC and SHVC files is organized in Network Access Layer (NAL) units that have a unique prefix in the bitstream. At the start of the bitstream, NAL units containing the parameter sets (VPS, SPS, PPS) for the HEVC decoding are transmitted, which also contain layer sizes and downsampling factors. We insert a Supplemental Enhancement Information (SEI) unit right after the PPS to store the total resolution W_{L-1}, H_{L-1} of the largest layer, which is required for Eq. 1. All tiles on the BL are intra-coded as Clean Random Access (CRA) pictures. The pictures on the higher layers are CRA-P frames, which communicates that no intra-layer dependencies exist and only ILP is used. An Instantaneous Decoder Refresh (IDR) unit reinitializes the decoder at POC_0.

In term of NAL addresses, Eq. 1 does not directly reference the correct NAL unit, as the initial units produce an offset o (Fig. 2) which can easily be computed from the number of layers L and the current layer l: $o(L, l) = 3l + 1 + L$.

The biggest potential in *lossy* WSI compression is to drastically decrease the bitrate spent on brightfield background in the WSI. Following [6], our first step

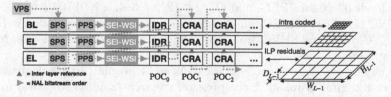

Fig. 2. Bitstream structure and order of Network Access Layer (NAL) units for the decoder. The Picture Order follows a row-wise serialization of the tiles in the image pyramid. Each tile is identified by a corresponding picture order count (POC).

is to divide the WSI into fore- and background region. For the background, a fix QP= 46 is used, while we deploy an *adaptive quantization* to control the foreground bitrate. Our goal is to remove irrelevant content via a foreground activity F in order to reduce the bitrate spent on flat-white regions. We start by calculating an auxiliary term

$$\chi = \sigma_Y^2 + e^{\alpha\left(\beta^2 2^{\mathrm{BD}\cdot 2} - \sigma_Y^2\right)} \tag{2}$$

where σ_Y^2 is the luma variance in the Y-Cr-Cb color space, BD is the encoder bit depth, and $\alpha = 0.4$, $\beta = \hat{\sigma}_Y/256$ are tuning factors, with the reference luma deviation $\hat{\sigma}_Y$ to determine the minimum of χ. This function χ, visualized in Fig. 1 for a BD = 8bit, provides a cutoff for low luma variances and a tolerance region, defined by α, β, around the empirically chosen minimum. For WSI, we found it important to include chroma (Cr and Cb) information into F and factor in the chroma range R_i in a given HEVC Coding Block (CB)

$$F = 1 + \frac{\chi}{\sqrt{\max(R_{Cb}, R_{Cr})}}, \quad \text{with } R_i = \max(\mathrm{CB}_i) - \min(\mathrm{CB}_i)$$

Furthermore, F undergoes a normalization in the encoder software[1] that can be corrupted by the white regions. Thus, we compute a weighted average, excluding low variance blocks with a threshold based on β

$$\bar{F} = \frac{\sum_k w_k \cdot F_k}{\sum_k w_k} + \epsilon, \quad \text{with } w_k = \begin{cases} 0, \text{ if } & \sigma_Y \leq \beta \cdot 2^{\mathrm{BD}} \\ 1, \text{ otherwise} \end{cases}$$

Herein, ϵ is a small constant to avoid zero division for all-white coding blocks. Finally, we compute the normalization F_n and the QP adjustment $\varDelta$QP as

$$F_n = \frac{\gamma F + \bar{F}}{\gamma \bar{F} + F}, \quad \text{with } \gamma = 2^{\frac{\varDelta\mathrm{QP}_{max}}{6}} \quad \text{and} \quad \varDelta\mathrm{QP} = \mathrm{round}[6\log_2(F_n)]$$

Herein, $\varDelta$QP$_{max}$ is the largest allowed QP adjustment.

For quantitative assessment, we evaluate the achieved Peak-to-Peak Signal to Noise Ratio (PSNR) in RGB space of the different algorithms at different bitrates. A better compression implies a high PSNR at a lower bitrate. This rate vs. PSNR is computed at varying QP $\in \{23, 26, 29, 32, 35\}$ for HEVC and SHVC, quality levels 30-90 for JPEG, and $Q_{\mathrm{step}} \in \{2, 2.7, 3, 4, 5, 7, 9\} \cdot 0.01$ for J2k. We use HEVC simulcast (HEVC-SimC) wherein each layer is intra coded individually. HEVC-SimC and SHVC are both evaluated with 1:4 and 1:2 downsampling between layers.

For qualitative assessment, we asked $N = 13$ people (3 pathologists, 5 researchers in digital histology, 2 compression researchers and 3 students) to identify the compressed image in a forced choice experiment, to identify the parameter thresholds for the just-noticeable distortion (JND), defined as the setting at

---

[1] Software and Documentation: https://hevc.hhi.fraunhofer.de

Fig. 3. Rate Distortion Curves for a large IHC and HE sample (bpp: bits per pixel). The denoted points correspond to the subjective JND thresholds.

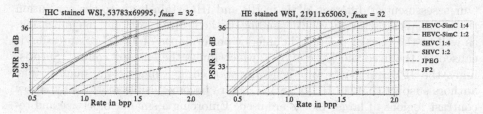

which 75% of the raters correctly recognize the compressed image [8]. As compression levels, HEVC and SHVC use the QP $\in \{23, 26, 29, 32, 35\}$ and JPEG was run with quality level $Q_l \in \{85, 70, 50, 30, 10\}$. Note that this setup already requests 60 forced choices per user and that in all cases, a higher compression level corresponds to stronger distortions.

3   Results

Fig. 3 shows representative examples of rate distortion curves (RDC) for the qualitative evaluation. We observe that HEVC-based algorithms perform much better than the JPEG compression. However, HEVC-SimC requires extra bits for the increased layer count in 1:2 versus 1:4 downsampling. SHVC shows a slight difference in the RDCs, but has superior performance for most images in the dataset in both settings. As average rate saving across all WSI, we measured 54% (SHVC compared to JPEG) and 12% (SHVC compared to J2k).

In Fig. 4, the votes of the subjective experiment are shown along with the decision times of the participants. For HEVC and JPEG, the lowest compression level (highest quality parameter) is already the limit – in case of HEVC, just barely touching the 75% threshold. The proposed SHVC with adaptive quantization tolerates the next compression level as well, but is very close to the limit. Particularly, it appears that HEVC artifacts can be spotted at higher qualities, as nearly all participants were able to spot the distortions above level two. Interestingly, JPEG had outliers, indicated by the blue background of the curve in the min/max plot, where participants did not spot errors at level three (JPEG quality 50%), which we had expected to result in severe artifacts.

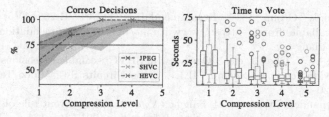

Fig. 4. Subjective JND experiment. Left: min/max graph of participant votes versus compression level, right: decision times.

4   Discussion

Our assessment of different WSIs in HE and IHC stain leads to the conclusion that rate savings strongly vary depending on the utilized stain and magnification, as well as the type of tissue. The inferior performance of JPEG compression is caused by the fixed blocksize of 8×8, which limits the entropy coding. Surprisingly, the JPEG artifacts were generally spotted at a much lower quality. The authors suspect that, in HEVC/SHVC, blurs become visible more easily in low contrast regions, if larger blocks are used. Enforcing a smaller blocksize and reducing blur is possible, but leads to decreased rate distortion performance. From this experiment, we identify the following settings: QP < 23 (HEVC), QP = 26 (SHVC), and $Q_l = 85\%$, which are highlighted as reference points in the RDCs in Fig. 3. Observing the decision times in Fig. 4, the settings of compression level two could be justified for JPEG and HEVC as well, as the raters need much more time to spot the distortions compared to the more obvious cases at higher levels.

5   Conclusion

We present an SHVC-based format for WSI compression that achieves excellent compression performance with average savings of 54% compared to JPEG and 12% compared to J2k. The method incorporates the spatial scalability inherent to WSIs, utilizes adaptive quantization, and allows for an efficient random access to image regions. In terms of the PSNR metric, SHVC-based encoding has proven to be very efficient, but there are indications that HEVC-based encodings introduce blurring artifacts, which are easier to spot than the typical JPEG blocking. We successfully counteracted this phenomenon by an adaptive quantization tailored for WSI. However, our study with 13 participants and four test images has to be taken as preliminary estimate.

Acknowledgement.   We thank the German Federal Ministry of Education and Research (BMBF) for funding this work (FKZ: 031B0006C and 01ZX1308A).

References

1. ITU-T Study Group 16.   Recommendation ITU-T H.265 (V5).   ITU-T; 2018.   Available from: https://www.itu.int/ITU-T/recommendations/rec.aspx?rec=13433&lang=en.
2. Boyce JM, Ye Y, Chen J, et al. Overview of SHVC: scalable extensions of the high efficiency video coding standard. IEEE Trans Circuits Syst Video Technol. 2016 Jan;26(1):20–34.
3. Liu F, Hernandez-Cabronero M, Sanchez V, et al. The current role of image compression standards in medical imaging. Information. 2017;8(4):131.
4. Tuominen VJ, Isola J. The application of JPEG2000 in virtual microscopy. J Digit Imaging. 2009;22(3):250–258.

5. Tuominen VJ, Isola J. Linking whole-slide microscope images with DICOM by using JPEG2000 interactive protocol. J Digit Imaging. 2010;23(4):454–462.
6. Helin H, Tolonen T, Ylinen O, et al. Optimized JPEG 2000 compression for efficient storage of histopathological whole-Slide images. J Pathol Inform. 2018;9.
7. Sanchez V, Hernández-Cabronero M. Graph-based rate control in pathology imaging with lossless region of interest coding. IEEE Trans Med Imaging. 2018;37(10):2211–2223.
8. ITU-R. Studies towards the unification of picture assessment methodology. Recommendation BT.1082-1. ITU-R; 1990. Available from: https://www.itu.int/pub/R-REP-BT.1082-1-1990.

Image Quilting for Histological Image Synthesis

Daniel Bug[1], Gregor Nickel[1], Anne Grote[2], Friedrich Feuerhake[2,3],
Eva Oswald[4], Julia Schüler[4], Dorit Merhof[1]

[1]Institute of Imaging and Computer Vision, RWTH Aachen University
[2]Institute for Pathology, Hannover Medical School
[3]Institute for Neuropathology, University Clinic Freiburg im Breisgau
[4]Charles River Discover Research Services Germany GmbH, Freiburg im Breisgau
daniel.bug@lfb.rwth-aachen.de

Abstract. Applications in digital histopathology often require costly expert labels to train modern machine learning algorithms. We introduce an adaptation of the Image Quilting algorithm for texture synthesis that is utilized to virtually multiply the tissues and labels. Potential applications are augmentation in neural network training and quality control in intra-rater experiments. We evaluate this method in a subjective expert trial and a quantitative augmented learning scenario.

1 Introduction

Digital whole-slide images (WSI) play a major role in histopathology as a tool for diagnosis and research. In both human and machine learning scenarios, quality control is essential and requires labeled data in suitable quantities. From a machine learning perspective, histological images are different from many large scale datasets, as their classes are not represented by objects, but rather textures that, in turn, sometimes incorporate certain object types such as cell nuclei. Synthesis of histological textures is used in [1] with region-synthesis methods and the goal to create realistic large-scale tumor models. In [2, 3], similar methods are developed aiming at nuclei segmentation tasks. The synthesis methods extend classical texture synthesis [2] or apply modern generative adversarial techniques [3].

In this work, we adapt the concept of texture formation through Image Quilting [4], a technique that recombines patches by computing minimum cost boundaries (MCB) in overlapping border regions, with potential applications in semantic tissue classification. As the textures are synthesized from existing image material, we can recombine corresponding label maps with the same boundaries. Thus, Image Quilting allows us to present image patches in reoccurring new contexts.

1.1 Contribution

The original method was designed to generate large realistic textures from a small selection of primary texture images. As this would not capture the diversity

© Springer Fachmedien Wiesbaden GmbH, ein Teil von Springer Nature 2020
T. Tolxdorff et al. (Hrsg.), *Bildverarbeitung für die Medizin 2020*,
Informatik aktuell, https://doi.org/10.1007/978-3-658-29267-6_72

occurring in histological images, the method is adapted for the histological field by a faster search for matching texture candidates, an improved cost function to compute the MCB and improvements to blend in image patches along the MCB.

2   Materials and methods

For a human observer study, we create three sets of 1000×1000px WSI extracts at high resolution (0.5mpp): stained 1.) strongly by immunohistochemistry (IHC) with saturated colors, 2.) by Hematoxylin and Eosin (HE), and 3.) weakly by IHC with faint colors. Each set contains ten images: four original images, three synthesized images with patch size 200×200px at an overlap of 50px, and another three images synthesized at 100×100px and a 30px overlap.

For a more quantitative evaluation, we deploy a dataset of 40 image extracts from eight HE stained WSIs. Each image has corresponding expert annotations for the tissue classes: Tumor, Stroma, Necrosis and Other.

2.1   Image quilting for histological textures

The core idea of Image Quilting is to recombine existing image patches by determining a minimum cost boundary (MCB) in an overlap area. Image construction starts from an initial patch and is then continued iteratively by finding matching patches with a high similarity in the overlapping area. The patches are blended over along the path with the MCB in terms of the sum of squared difference of the RGB pixels (Fig. 1, left).

The first challenge is to identify matches of the overlap regions in the dataset. If images from multiple sources are combined, stain normalization [5] is a crucial preprocessing step. However, a generation from a single large image is possible, too, and circumvents normalization challenges. As histological images are typically very large, the search is restricted to a random subset. The search algorithm has to keep track of the patches already extracted and their respective neighborhoods to prevent cyclic reuse of patches. Without this bookkeeping, the best matches would always be found at the border to the original neighbors of the current patch. We follow the strategy in [4] to randomly draw from a set of well-matching regions, rather than taking the best match. These randomizations

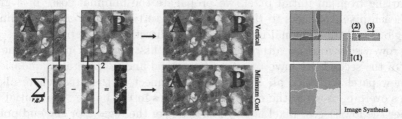

Fig. 1. Left: Minimum Cost Boundary computation, right: iterative image synthesis process with a new patch in green.

ensure that the initial patch does not fully determine the synthetic image, but leaves room for different outcomes of synthesized textures. As a final speedup of this search step, we consider only downsampled grayscale information for the search. While this seems quite restrictive, the algorithm does not depend on a ideal matches of candidates, as the MCB computation can compensate many inaccuracies.

Mathematically, we deploy the Frobenius norm as similarity measure, applied in a sliding window across the image

$$F_C(u,v) = \sum_{i,j \in \mathcal{R}} (a_{ij} - b_{u+i,v+j})^2$$

where $\mathcal{R}$ is the overlap region, A, B denote the current patch and the reference texture, and a_{ij}, b_{ij} index the pixels of A and B.

The iterative synthesis implies different overlap constellations: horizontal, vertical and a combination of both in the corner case (Fig. 1, right). As F_C is a summation, the corner matching simply adds shifted versions of the horizontal and vertical window, without further computations. After a matching candidate has been selected, it is blended into the final image along a MCB.

2.2   Minimum cost boundary (MCB)

The MCB is computed in dynamic programming fashion, utilizing the Dijkstra algorithm [6]. As cost function C_{ij}, we use the sum-squared-error of the RGB channels $C_{ij} = \sum_{r,g,b} (a_{ij} - b_{ij})^2$, with r, g, b referring to the color channels and a_{ij}, b_{ij} as the overlapping patch regions.

As we observed several cases in which this cost function leads to visible straight paths at the border of the overlapping regions, we add a term to create a cost-sink in the center of the overlap region

$$C'_{ij} = C_{ij} + \lambda \left(\frac{2i}{N} - 1 \right)^6 \quad \text{and} \quad C'_{ij} = C_{ij} + \lambda \left(\frac{2j}{M} - 1 \right)^6$$

depending on a horizontal (left) or vertical (right) border, where N and M are the width and height of a region and λ is a cost factor corresponding to the values in the images.

Starting from an initial pixel, we propagate the minimal costs in a graph, where each pixel connects to the horizontal or vertical neighbor (depending on the region) and the diagonal neighbors in the direction of the path.

In row-wise synthesis, after completing the first row and inserting the first patch of the second, we have to compute vertical and horizontal boundaries for each new patch. Ideally, all MCBs should connect in the area where all four patches overlap, to avoid the risk of visible edges in the image. The initial pixel is either the lowest cost pixel at the short edge of the region, or the end point of a previously computed MCB. For the example in Fig. 1 (right), we: 1.) compute the vertical boundary, 2.) continue from the end point of the previous horizontal boundary and compute the current horizontal boundary left/backwards (connecting the point to the previously computed boundaries), and 3.) to the right/forward, which fully blends in the current patch into the image.

Along the MCB, we linearly blend over from one patch to the other as follows: on the MCB itself, the RGB values are mixed at a ratio of 1 : 1 from A and B, while the neighboring pixels use the ratios 3 : 1 and 1 : 3, respectively. In Fig. 2, we show examples of the final result of such a quilted histological texture, boundaries and the according labels.

2.3 Evualuation

First, we perform an expert assessment of synthesized images by a group of five experts: three pathologists and two computer scientists working in digital histology. Each rater votes, whether he would rate the presented image as an original or synthesized. This vote is complemented by a confidence rating on a scale from one (uncertain) to five (convinced). It was known to the experts that the set contained a mixture of original and synthesized images, but not at what ratio. The images were presented in random order.

Second, as a quantitative evaluation, we deploy the HE dataset in an eight-fold cross-validation setting across patients (=WSI), utilizing Image Quilting as augmentation. Each time, we train a vanilla Unet architecture [7] and assess the performance in terms of the average class confusions.

3 Results

Fig. 3 shows the ratings of the experts for each presented image. Overall, most original images were recognized correctly, with a few exceptions in the faint IHC stain. Regarding the confidence, the misclassified originals were rated with *uncertain (one)*.

In the set of HE samples, only occasionally one of the experts voted falsely and these votes are mostly at the lowest confidence score. However, the confidence ratings for all synthetic images are overall slightly lower than for the originals. The exception is image nine with 3/5 expert votes for original, one even with a high confidence score of four.

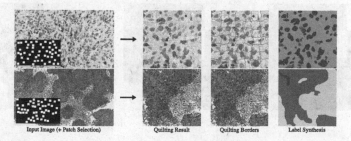

Input Image (+ Patch Selection)   Quilting Result   Quilting Borders   Label Synthesis

Fig. 2. Examples for the synthesis of IHC (upper) and HE (lower) patches. A single input image is used in both cases.

Fig. 3. Results of the expert trial. Each bar reflects a vote and a confidence score.

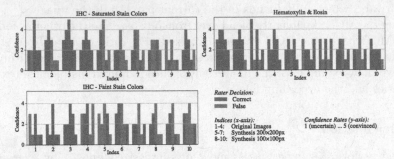

For the IHC stained images, we observe a much higher ratio of votes at higher confidences, where synthetic images are accepted as originals. Regarding the influence of the patch size during synthesis (indices 5-7 vs. 8-10 in Fig. 3), there are no notable differences.

The results of the quantitative evaluation in an augmentation scenario are presented in Fig. 4. Minor influences can be observed in the Stroma and Necrosis class. Most prevalent is the reduced misprediction of necrosis as tumor that drops from 0.36 to 0.26. The recalls of the classes after augmenting the data by a factor of five (Fig. 4, right) increase by 13% (Stroma), 8% (Necrosis), and 4% (Other), with large parts of this increase already at twice the data amount (Fig. 4, middle).

4   Discussion

Image Quilting can be adapted to synthesize realistically looking histological textures. Comparing the common stains HE and IHC, we found that the artifacts introduced by the synthesis can more easily be spotted in HE than in IHC. This summarizes the feedback that was communicated by the experts: while the images can still be considered realistic, there are some subtle and local artifacts that reveal the origin by synthesis. In most cases, these artifacts consist of visible

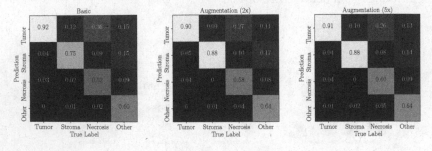

Fig. 4. Results of the augmentation for texture classification. On average in an eight-fold cross-validation the augmentation slightly increases the performance between the classes, with important gains in stroma and necrosis classification.

boundaries resulting from constellations, where no good candidate is found and even the best correlating patches are bound to introduce visible transitions from one patch to the next. An insufficient normalization is one of the main sources for this. Particularly, if the background of the tissue has a different white tone, the error effects an area along the border and is easily perceptible.

The introduced method is meant for the synthesis of large tissue patches. Global tissue structures, such as typical formations found in tumors (e.g. stroma surrounding tumor tissue with a necrotic center) are currently not represented in this method. However, first experiments of pre-selecting patches based on the annotations are promising.

This method aimed at an offline augmentation for the training of neural networks. Our quantitative evaluation confirms that the new context of patches provides an additional value to the training and creates a clearly measuable – yet not large – benefit. We conlude that the approach holds promise for the intended application and the results support investment in larger validation data sets to explore its full potential.

Another application for this method could potentially be intra-rater trials, in which an expert labels the same image multiple times, usually with long interval breaks in between, to evaluate the consistency of the annotation. Our proposed method allows the recombination of annotated images to obscure the fact that the same data that has already been labeled before. Thus, intra-rater evaluations can be included more easily into the annotation routine.

Acknowledgement. We thank the German Federal Ministry of Education and Research (BMBF) for funding this work (FKZ: 031B0006C and 01ZX1308A).

References

1. Apou G, Feuerhake F, Forestier G, et al. Synthesizing whole slide images. In: 2015 9th International Symposium on Image and Signal Processing and Analysis (ISPA). IEEE; 2015. p. 154–159.
2. Glotsos D, Kostopoulos S, Ravazoula P, et al. Image quilting and wavelet fusion for creation of synthetic microscopy nuclei images. Comput Methods Programs Biomed. 2018;162:177–186.
3. Hou L, Agarwal A, Samaras D, et al. Robust histopathology image analysis: to label or to synthesize? In: Proc IEEE CCVPR; 2019. p. 8533–8542.
4. Efros AA, Freeman WT. Image quilting for texture synthesis and transfer. In: Proc of the 28th annual conference on CGIT. ACM; 2001. p. 341–346.
5. Magee D, Treanor D, Crellin D, et al. Colour normalisation in digital histopathology images. In: Proc Optical Tissue Image analysis in Microscopy, Histopathology and Endoscopy (MICCAI Workshop). vol. 100. Citeseer; 2009. .
6. Dijkstra EW. A note on two problems in connexion with graphs. Numerische Mathematik. 1959;1(1):269–271.
7. Ronneberger O, Fischer P, Brox T. U-net: convolutional networks for biomedical image segmentation. In: PROC MICCAI. Springer; 2015. p. 234–241.

An Open-Source Tool for Automated Planning of Overlapping Ablation Zones

For Percutaneous Renal Tumor Treatment

A. M. Franz[1], B. J. Mittmann[1], J. Röser[2], B. Schmidberger[2], M. Meinke[3], P. L. Pereira[4], H. U. Kauczor[3], G. M. Richter[5], C. M. Sommer[3,5]

[1]Institute for Computer Science, Ulm University of Applied Sciences, Ulm, Germany
[2]Institute for Medical Engineering and Mechatronics, University of Applied Sciences, Ulm, Germany
[3]Clinic of Diagnostic and Interventional Radiology, University Hospital Heidelberg, Heidelberg, Germany
[4]Clinic of Radiology, Minimally-invasive Therapies and Nuclear Medicine, SLK Kliniken Heilbronn GmbH, Heilbronn, Germany
[5]Clinic of Diagnostic and Interventional Radiology, Stuttgart Clinics, Katharinenhospital, Stuttgart, Germany
alfred.franz@thu.de

Abstract. Percutaneous thermal ablation is a minimally-invasive treatment option for renal cancer. To treat larger tumours, multiple overlapping ablations zones are required. Arrangements with a low number of ablation zones but coverage of the whole tumour volume are challenging to find for physicians. In this work, an open-source software tool with a new planning approach based on the automatic selection from a large number of randomized geometrical arrangements is presented. Two uncertainty parameters are introduced to account for tissue shrinking and tolerance of non-ablated tumour volume. For seven clinical renal T1a, T1b and T2a tumours, ablation plans were proposed by the software. All proposals are comparable to manual plans of an experienced physician with regard to the number of required ablation zones.

1 Introduction

More than 14.000 patients are diagnosed with renal cancer per year in Germany. Besides surgical treatment, percutaneous ablation was established as a minimally-invasive alternative. Therefore, a needle-shaped ablation probe is inserted into the affected tissue, commonly under computed-tomography (CT) or magnetic resonance imaging (MRI) guidance. The tumour is then destroyed thermally, e.g., by using radiofrequency or microwaves. The whole tumour must be ablated for a successful treatment. Researchers proposed methods to estimate the treated area of ablations [1, 2, 3]. For example, vessel information from preoperative data can be used to compute cooling effects [4], but segmenting a vessel tree often is too cumbersome in clinical routine. Instead, physicians

© Springer Fachmedien Wiesbaden GmbH, ein Teil von Springer Nature 2020
T. Tolxdorff et al. (Hrsg.), *Bildverarbeitung für die Medizin 2020*,
Informatik aktuell, https://doi.org/10.1007/978-3-658-29267-6_73

commonly estimate a spherical or elliptical shape of a single ablation, referred to as ablation zone. These shapes are given by manufacturers for their probes depending on the ablation duration and the applied power. Usually, a security margin around the tumour is ablated to account - among other things - for uncertainties in the estimation of ablation zones. If a small tumour can be completely covered by a single ablation, the probe is inserted to the center. For larger tumours, e.g. with a maximum diameter of 4 cm (T1a for renal tumours) or 7 cm (T1b), multiple overlapping ablations zones (MOAZs) are required. Manually finding a geometric distribution that covers the whole volume in 3D with a small number of ablation zones is challenging. Algorithms for planning MOAZs can use ideal geometric combinations of spheres to fully cover a volume [5, 6]. However, this leads to relatively high numbers of ablations for larger tumours. Planning MOAZs can also be treated as an optimization problem, as proposed by Ren et al., who used a branch and bound algorithm to solve planning tasks for tumours with diameters of 2.5 cm and 3.5 cm simulated in a porcine model [7].

In this work we present an open-source software tool for a planning approach based on the automatic selection from a large number of randomized geometrical arrangements under consideration of uncertainty parameters that can be adjusted to get plans with an acceptable number of ablations. It was evaluated on renal tumours in comparison to manual plans of a physician.

2 Materials and methods

For automated planning of MOAZs, the following workflow steps are proposed: (I) segmentation of the tumour in preoperative images, (II) definition of safety margin, (III) definition of diameter for spherical ablation zones, (IV) definition of uncertainty parameters for ablation zone placement, (V) definition of a model for geometrical distribution and (VI) computation of MOAZs.

Segmentation of the tumour in step I was performed manually using the Medical Imaging Interaction Toolkit (MITK) [8]. In the following, the uncertainty parameters for step IV are described and a model based on the automatic selection from a large number of randomized geometrical arrangements for step V is presented. Finally, the open-source implementation and experiments including example parameters for step II and III are explained.

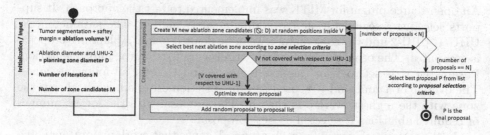

Fig. 1. Approach for automated proposal of overlapping ablation zones.

2.1 Definition of uncertainty parameters

Estimating the ablated tissue volume during a thermal ablation is usually subject to uncertainties such as tissue shrinkage after ablations [9] or other effects. Due to their experience, physicians account for these uncertainties by adapting their manual ablation plans during conventional treatment. This includes adaptation of the ablation diameter because reference values are given for the state after tissue shrinking and also tolerance of small areas of tumour tissue which is not directly treated. To account for this during automated planning, two Ulm-Heidelberg-Uncertainty-parameters (UHUs) are proposed:

- UHU-1: Tolerance of non-ablated tumour volume [% of tumour volume]
- UHU-2: Tissue shrinkage after ablation [% of ablated volume]

2.2 Approach for planning overlapping ablation zones

The proposed approach is shown in Fig. 1. For initialization, a safety margin (in mm) is added to the tumour segmentation which increases the area to be ablated to volume V. The ablation zone diameter represents the maximum reachable diameter of a single ablation. It is increased by the factor given from UHU-2 resulting in the planning zone diameter D. Further, the number of iterations, N, and the number of zone candidates, M, are defined.

A single random proposal is created by adding new zones as long as V is not covered with respect to UHU-1. A new zone is selected from M candidates according to zone selection criteria which can include coverage of new tumour volume and percentage of overlap with other zones or non-tumour tissue. If enough zones are found, the proposal is optimized by moving zones that overlap to non-tumour tissue too much towards the center of the tumour, removing zones that overlap too much with other zones and/or decreasing the diameter of single ablations if possible without loosing coverage of V.

After iteratively adding N proposals to a list, the best proposal P is selected according to the proposal selection criteria. The most important criterion typically is a low number of required ablation zones.

2.3 Open-source implementation

An open-source plugin for MITK was implemented to test the approach. It supports selecting a segmentation and adding a safety margin. The parameters N, UHU-1, UHU-2 and the zone diameter can be defined before a planning proposal is computed. The other parameters and criteria are fixed in the implementation: Parameter M is set to 1 for the starting zone and to 5 for all following zones. The overlap of a zone and V is used as zone selection criterion, while always the zone with the highest overlap is chosen. The proposal with the lowest number of required ablations is selected as best proposal.

In the optimization step for each proposal, zones that overlap more than 30% into tissue outside V are moved towards the center of the tumour until less than

Fig. 2. Computed planning proposal for a tumour (red) segmented in a MRI image with added safety margin (blue) and ablation zones (white circles).

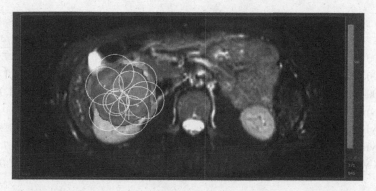

30% are outside. Afterwards, ablation zones are reduced in diameter and/or ablation zones are removed if possible without loosing coverage of V.

For the final proposal P, ablation spheres are visualized and statistical data is reported, including the number of ablation zones, the tumour volume with and without safety margin and the ablated volume. Fig. 2 shows a screenshot of the plugin and a computed planning proposal.

2.4 Experiments

For the two experiments, CT data of renal tumours from four publicly available datasets (C3N-00312, C3N-00305, C3N-00491 and TCGA-KM-8442 from collections CPTAC-CCRCC and TCGA-KICH[1]) and three anonymized clinical cases from the University Hospital Heidelberg and Stuttgart were used. A zone diameter of 3 cm was chosen which is a typical maximum diameter of spherical ablation zones, e.g. of the Emprint Ablation System (Medtronic plc., Dublin, Ireland) for renal ablations (75 watts / 5:30 minutes duration). 50 iterations were chosen because this leads to acceptable computational time of less than 5 minutes for T1a an T1b tumours and reproducible results concerning the number of required zones. All tumours were manually segmented using existing MITK plugins [8] and a safety margin of 5 mm was added.

In experiment 1, a 50 mm T1b tumour (C3N-00305) was used to test the influence of UHU-1 and UHU-2 to the planning proposals. The parameters were chosen as follows: UHU-1: 0/3/6/10/20%; UHU-2: 0/10/20/30%. For each parameter configuration, three ablation plans were automatically proposed by the software prototype. The plans were evaluated regarding the number of ablation zones and also manually examined concerning a meaningful zone distribution.

In experiment 2, all seven datasets were used to compare the automated planning proposals with manual plans of an experienced physician. For each tumour, three automated planning proposals were computed with UHU-1 of

---

[1] http://www.cancerimagingarchive.net

Table 1. Number of ablation zones (Ø:30 mm) of a manual plan of an experienced physician and three automatic proposals (UHU-1: 3%; UHU-2: 20%).

Data set	Tumour Ø[mm]	Manual plan	Automatic Proposals			
			1	2	3	$\mu \pm \sigma$
C3N-00312	40 (T1a)	5	6	5	6	5.7 ± 0.5
C3N-00305	50 (T1b)	8	5	4	5	4.7 ± 0.5
C3N-00491	45 (T1b)	10	13	13	13	13.0 ± 0.0
Anonym.1	40 (T1a)	5	7	7	7	7.0 ± 0.0
Anonym.2	60 (T1b)	14	13	14	13	13.3 ± 0.5
Anonym.3	40 (T1a)	7	7	7	6	6.7 ± 0.5
TCGA-KM-8442	>70 (T2a)	18	20	22	21	21.0 ± 0.8

3% and UHU-2 of 20%. The number of required ablations is reported for each automated planning proposal as well as for the independent manual plan.

3 Results

An installer of the software prototype will be provided in the Open Science Framework (page https://osf.io/r7f5d/) together with segmentations of the four publicly available data sets upon publication of this work. For the T1a and T1b tumours, automatic planning required up to 5 minutes (PC: core i7, 24 GB Ram). The T2b tumour required around 60 minutes.

For data set C3N-00305 with varying UHU-1 and UHU-2, the number of required MOAZs ranged from 2 ± 0 ($\mu \pm \sigma$, n=3, UHU-1:20%, UHU-2:30%) to 11 ± 0 (n=3, UHU-1:0%, UHU-2:0%). Manually examining the ablation plans, we found that too high uncertainty lead to plans that don't cover the whole tumour while low or no uncertainty leads to a too large number of ablations. Parameters of UHU-1:3% and UHU-2:20% lead to 5 ± 0 (n=3) MOAZs, which a physician confirmed to be a good trade-off for a realistic ablation plan.

The amount of required MOAZs for different tumours are shown in Tab. 2. Manual plans of an experienced physician required 5/5/7 (T1a tumours), 8/10/14 (T1b) and 18 (T2a) zones, while the automatic planning with UHU-1: 3% and UHU-2: 20% lead to 5.7/7.0/6.7 (T1a), 4.7,13.0,13.7 (T1b) and 21.0 (T2a) zones on average (n=3).

4 Discussion

The experiments confirmed, that planning MOAZs based on an automatic selection from a large number of randomized geometrical arrangements and uncertainty parameters is feasible in acceptable time for T1a and T1b tumours (less than 5 minutes). Testing the software prototype with seven clinical data sets lead to results comparable to manual plans of a physician (Tab. 2). The software was able to propose a plan for a T2a tumour, while computational time raised to around 60 minutes. Such large tumours are usually not treated with ablation therapy because it would require too much time to perform 20 or more ablations. However, ongoing studies show that even this is feasible [10].

In a first try, we implemented a model based on an ideal grid of overlapping spheres, similar to Yang et al. (Fig. 6 in [6]). Looking at the results, we found a too large number of required MOAZs in all cases (e.g., over 20 for C3N-00491).

Our approach incorporates uncertainty parameters that are subject to ongoing clinical research [9]. It needs to be shown, that a certain parameter set, such as 20% of tissue shrinking and 3% tolerance of non-ablated tumour volume as proposed in this work, leads to clinical acceptable outcome. Further, only spherical MOAZs are supported so far. While this might be sufficient for some ablation probes, future work includes an extension to elliptical ablation zones.

To improve computational time, it is planned to parallelize the implementation of the approach shown in Fig. 1 which is expected to be straight-forward, because the creation of N proposals can be done in parallel. It remains to be discussed if an algorithm highly based on random components would be acceptable in clinics, which leads to general ethical questions that also raise up for other more advanced methods, such as machine learning.

References

1. Voglreiter P, Mariappan P, Pollari M, et al. RFA guardian: comprehensive simulation of radiofrequency ablation treatment of liver tumors. Nat Sci Rep. 2018;8(1):787.
2. Pena K, Ishahak M, Arechavala S, et al. Comparison of temperature change and resulting ablation size induced by a 902-928 MHz and a 2450 MHz microwave ablation system in in-vivo porcine kidneys. Int J Hyperthermia. 2019;36(1):313–321.
3. Kath N, Handels H, Mastmeyer A. Robust GPU-based virtual reality simulation of radio-frequency ablations for various needle geometries and locations. Int J Comput Assist Radiol Surg. 2019;14(11):1825–1835.
4. Huang HW. Influence of blood vessel on the thermal lesion formation during radiofrequency ablation for liver tumors. Med Phys. 2013;40(7):073303.
5. Dodd GD, Frank MS, Aribandi M, et al. Radiofrequency thermal ablation: computer analysis of the size of the thermal injury created by overlapping ablations. AJR Am J Roentgenol. 2001 Oct;177(4):777–782.
6. Yang L, Wen R, Qin J, et al. A robotic system for overlapping radiofrequency ablation in large tumor treatment. IEEE ASME Trans Mechatron. 2010;15(6):887–897.
7. Ren H, Campos-Nanez E, Yaniv Z, et al. Treatment planning and image guidance for radiofrequency ablation of large tumors. IEEE J Biomed Health Inform. 2014;18(3):920–928.
8. Nolden M, Zelzer S, Seitel A, et al. The medical imaging interaction toolkit: challenges and advances : 10 years of open-source development. Int J Comput Assist Radiol Surg. 2013;8(4):607–620.
9. Farina L, Nissenbaum Y, Cavagnaro M, et al. Tissue shrinkage in microwave thermal ablation: comparison of three commercial devices. Int J Hyperthermia. 2018 06;34(4):382–391.

10. Schullian P, Johnston EW, Putzer D, et al. Stereotactic radiofrequency ablation of subcardiac hepatocellular carcinoma: a case-control study. Int J Hyperthermia. 2019;36(1):876–885.

Combining 2-D and 3-D Weight-Bearing X-Ray Images

Application to Preoperative Implant Planning in the Knee

Christoph Luckner[1,2], Magdalena Herbst[2], Michael Fuhrmann[2],
Ludwig Ritschl[2], Steffen Kappler[2], Andreas Maier[1]

[1]Pattern Recognition Lab, Friedrich-Alexander University Erlangen-Nürnberg,
Martensstr. 3, 91058 Erlangen, Germany
[2]X-ray Products, Siemens Healthcare GmbH,
Siemensstr. 3, 91301 Forchheim, Germany
christoph.luckner@fau.de

Abstract. Osteoarthritis is a joint disease that commonly affects the hands, feet, spine, as well as the large weight-bearing joints, i.e., the hip, and knees. Worldwide, about 3.6 % of the population suffer from osteoarthritis of the knee. If the symptoms are too severe to be treated with medication, the solution is often a total replacement. The precise preoperative planning of implants is a crucial task to achieve a good patient outcome. For planning, usually hybrid 2-D/3-D approaches are used. The main drawback of theses hybrid methods is the different patient positions during the acquisition, namely lying for the 3-D scan and standing for the 2-D scan. We proposed a method that allows acquiring both images in standing positions under natural weight-bearing without having to reposition the patient. To show the feasibility, we provide images from an anthropomorphic leg phantom. A preliminary study with medical experts has shown that the results are promising.

1 Introduction

Osteoarthritis is the degeneration of cartilage in a joint and the underlying bone. Common symptoms are joint pain, stiffness, and tenderness, which progress slowly over the years. It is believed that the primary cause of osteoarthritis is damage from mechanical stress with insufficient self-repair by joints. Moreover, also age, obesity, and changes in sex hormone levels can play a role in the development of osteoarthritis. Commonly affected are the hands, feet, spine, as well as the large weight-bearing joints, i.e., the hip, and knees. Worldwide, about 3.6 % of the population suffer from osteoarthritis of the knee, hip osteoarthritis, on the other hand, affects about 0.85 % of the population. Due to demographic changes, this rate is expected to increase in the future. As of now, knee and hip osteoarthritis rank 11th among 291 disease conditions assessed for disability [1]. If the symptoms are too severe to be treated with medication, the solution is

© Springer Fachmedien Wiesbaden GmbH, ein Teil von Springer Nature 2020
T. Tolxdorff et al. (Hrsg.), *Bildverarbeitung für die Medizin 2020*,
Informatik aktuell, https://doi.org/10.1007/978-3-658-29267-6_74

often a total replacement. According to the Agency for Healthcare Research and Quality, approximately 300.000 total hip replacements and about 600.000 total knee replacements are performed annually just in the United States. Again, with increasing prevalence, this value is also expected to grow in the future.

The precise preoperative planning of implants is a crucial task to achieve a good patient outcome. Good predictions due to precise measurements help to decrease the operation time, and thereby the risk of infections. Traditionally, the dimensioning of implants is done in simple 2-D radiographs. Recently, an incremental change from 2-D to 3-D planning is happening. The latter has the advantage that it provides more spatial information and accurate 1-to-1 mapping of the structures without magnification. Moreover, more complex musculoskeletal (MSK) measures or severe deformations can be assessed and incorporated into the planning [2]. The main drawbacks of planning in 3-D are the more complicated navigation and the higher radiation exposure compared to simple 2-D images.

Some methods combine both approaches. A typical workflow is illustrated in the top row of Fig. 1 [2]. However, 3-D CT acquisitions are usually carried out in a lying position, whereas the 2-D images are acquired in a standing position under weight-bearing. Due to the change of positioning the dynamics in the knee change. This can lead to problems during the registration of both images. Moreover, conventional 2-D radiographs suffer from inevitable magnification and distortion due to the imaging geometry. All this might cause an inaccurate dimensioning of the implants.

In this feasibility study, we focus on total knee replacements. Hence, we aim to combine a true-to-scale 2-D X-ray image of the entire leg with a 3-D scan of the knee, both of which are acquired under natural weight-bearing conditions without having to reposition the patient. The proposed workflow is depicted in the bottom row of Fig. 1.

2   Methods and materials

In this preliminary study, we use a twin robotic X-ray prototype based on the cone-beam CT (CBCT) system Multitom Rax (Siemens Healthcare GmbH, Forchheim, Germany) to acquire X-ray images. It is equipped with two independent, ceiling-mounted, fully motorized robotic arms and can perform scans along defined trajectories.

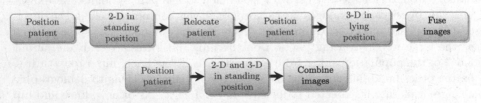

Fig. 1. Overview of the current (top) and the proposed (bottom) workflow.

The general concept of the proposed method is illustrated in Fig. 2. Before the acquisition, the knee of the patient has to be positioned in the isocenter and should be restraint to preclude or at least limit patient motion. As can be seen from the image, the acquisition process itself is split into two parts.

2.1   2-D acquisition

At first, a 2-D radiography-like image of the entire leg is acquired using an ultra--small-angle tomosynthesis-based slot scan. Therefore, a parallel-shift trajectory where source and detector move simultaneously in planes parallel to the patient is used. The acquired data forms the basis for a tomosynthesis reconstruction [3]. It builds on the famous FDK algorithm and has been highly adapted to the requirements of a slot scan reconstruction, e. g. incorporating a voxel specific weighting scheme in exchange for the redundancy weights. It has already been shown that the reconstructed radiography-like images provide a true-to-scale mapping [4]. Moreover, we need a considerably lower dose than conventional 2-D images without compromising on image quality in terms of photon noise at a resolution of up to 18 lp/cm, which is sufficient for the assessment of MSK measures [5].

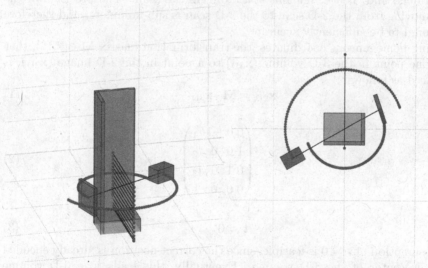

(a) 3-D view of the trajectories.   (b) Bird's-eye view (xy-plane).

Fig. 2. A schematic drawing of the acquisition process can be seen in 3-D as well as in a bird's-eye view. The 2-D acquisition is carried out first, immediately followed by the 3-D CBCT scan. The trajectories of tube and detector are indicated in red and blue, respectively. The patient support is depicted as a gray, L-shaped stand. The patient stands straight inside the patient support. The knee will be positioned at the intersection of the 2-D and 3-D scan. To mitigate artifacts due to patient motion, they will be restrained.

2.2 3-D acquisition

In the second step, the system moves on a circular trajectory around the patient while acquiring projection data, which is then used to reconstruct a 3-D volume using an algorithm proposed by Herbst et. al. [6]. It uses ánd FDK-based reconstruction with an iterative scheme for motion compensation. Both methods have the advantage of inherently being able to deal with slight inter-scan motion. For severe motion, also other motion-compensation approaches, e. g., marker-based [7] or marker-free [8, 9], could be incorporated into the algorithm. However, as the patient is positioned on a patient support and will be restrained during the scan, intra-scan motion is unlikely.

2.3 Fusion

The entire procedure is carried out without having to move or reposition the patient as the system automatically moves to the second scan. As the correspondences between both acquisitions are known precisely, it is possible to combine both images into one volume without the necessity of non-rigid registration. We geometrically align both reconstructions based on their isocenter, similarly to a method proposed by Li et. al. [10]. To this end, we assume that the patient is restrained and, hence, remains static during the scan. The precision of the robot moving from the 2-D scan to the 3-D scan is sub-millimeter and therefore considered to be sufficiently accurate.

Using homogeneous coordinates, the transformation matrix $\mathbf{M} \in \mathbb{R}^{4 \times 4}$, that maps one point in the 3-D volume ($\mathbf{x}_{3D}$) to a point in the 2-D image ($\mathbf{x}_{2D}$), is computed as follows

$$\mathbf{x}_{2D} = \mathbf{M} \cdot \mathbf{x}_{3D} \tag{1}$$

with

$$\mathbf{M} = \begin{pmatrix} 0 & 0 & -1 & t_1 \\ 1 & 0 & 0 & t_2 \\ 0 & 1 & 0 & t_3 \\ 0 & 0 & 0 & 1 \end{pmatrix} \tag{2}$$

and

$$\mathbf{t} = \mathbf{0} \tag{3}$$

The assumption of $\mathbf{t} = \mathbf{0}$ is feasible, since the correct position is already encoded in the isocenter of the 3-D volume. Eventually, this leads to a 3-D volume containing a 2-D radiograph from hip to ankle and additional 3-D information of the knee.

2.4 Evaluation

For an initial evaluation of the proposed method, the legs of an anthropomorphic full-body phantom (PBU-50, Kyoto Kagaku Ltd., Kyoto, Japan) were used for image acquisition. For an additional evaluation of the exact match of the correspondences, we also used a lead ruler in the X-ray beam path.

3   Results

In Fig. 3, the leg phantom, as well as three slices of the reconstructed volume, are depicted. It can be seen that the 2-D image of the entire leg remains static, whereas the information in the knee area changes from slice to slice. This provides a profound overview of the leg as well as a detailed and 3-D view of the knee.

4   Discussion

We have shown that it is feasible to combine a low-dose 2-D X-ray image with additional 3-D information into one volume. This fuses the better of two worlds, offering an exact 1-to-1 mapping in the 2-D as well as the 3-D image, low dose, and additional 3-D information in the knee, all of which can be utilized for implant planning. Providing both images under weight-bearing might also allow for a better assessment of the patient's conditions, and consequently, lead to a better surgery outcome. The entire procedure takes less than 30 seconds. A preliminary qualitative assessment with experts in the fields of orthopedics and medical imaging has shown that the results of the proposed method are promising. A more detailed clinical study with orthopedists and radiologists is advisable to evaluate the benefits of the proposed method - for clinicians as well as for patients.

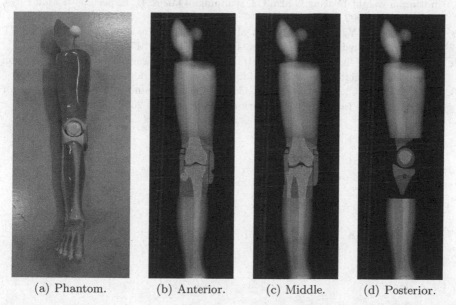

(a) Phantom.	(b) Anterior.	(c) Middle.	(d) Posterior.

Fig. 3. A picture of the leg phantom and three exemplary slices of the reconstructed CBCT volume are depicted. It can be seen, that the 2-D image remains static, whereas the displayed information in the knee area changes from slice to slice.

Disclaimer

The presented method is not commercially available. Due to regulatory reasons, its future availability cannot be guaranteed. The Siemens Multitom Rax is not available in all countries; its future availability cannot be guaranteed.

References

1. Cross M, Smith E, Hoy D, et al. The global burden of hip and knee osteoarthritis: estimates from the global burden of disease 2010 study. Ann Rheum Dis. 2014;73(7):1323–1330.
2. Sesselmann S, Tiefenböck S, Reinmuth M, et al.. Reliabilität der axialen Komponenten-Ausrichtung in der 3D-Planung von Knie-Totalendoprothesen. German Medical Science GMS Publishing House; 2017.
3. Luckner C, Sesselmann S, Mertelmeier T, et al. Parallel-shift tomosynthesis for orthopedic applications. Proc SPIE;. .
4. Luckner C, Herbst M, Ritschl L, et al. Assessment of measurement deviations: length-extended X-ray imaging for orthopedic applications. In: Proc SPIE;. .
5. Luckner C, Herbst M, Weber T, et al. High-speed slot-scanning radiography using small-angle tomosynthesis: investigation of spatial resolution. Med Phys. 2019;.
6. Herbst M, Luckner C, Wicklein J, et al. Misalignment compensation for ultra-high-resolution and fast CBCT acquisitions. In: Proc SPIE;. .
7. Choi JH, Maier A, Keil A, et al. Fiducial marker-based correction for involuntary motion in weight-bearing C-arm CT scanning of knees. II. Experiment. Med Phys. 2014;41(6):061902.
8. Berger M, Xia Y, Aichinger W, et al. Motion compensation for Cone-beam CT using fourier consistency conditions. Phys Med Biol. 2017;62(17):7181–7215.
9. Bier B, Aichert A, Felsner L, et al. Epipolar consistency conditions for motion correction in weight-bearing imaging. In: Proc BVM. Berlin; 2017. p. 209–214.
10. Li Q, Luckner C, Hertel M, et al. Combining ultrasound and X-ray imaging for mammography. In: Proc BVM. Springer; 2019. p. 245–250.

Abstract: Generative Adversarial Networks for Stereoscopic Hyperrealism in Surgical Training

Sandy Engelhardt[1,4], Lalith Sharan[1], Matthias Karck[3], Raffaele De Simone[3], Ivo Wolf[2]

[1] Working Group Artificial Intelligence in Cardiovascular Medicine, University Hospital Heidelberg, Heidelberg, Germany
[2] Faculty of Computer Science, Mannheim University of Applied Sciences, Germany
[3] Department of Cardiac Surgery, Heidelberg University Hospital, Germany
[4] Research Campus STIMULATE, Magdeburg University, Magdeburg, Germany
sandy.engelhardt@med.uni-heidelberg.de

Phantoms for surgical training are able to mimic cutting and suturing properties and patient-individual shape of organs, but lack a realistic visual appearance that captures the heterogeneity of surgical scenes. In order to overcome this in endoscopic approaches, hyperrealistic concepts have been proposed to be used in an augmented reality-setting, which are based on deep image-to-image transformation methods. Such concepts are able to generate realistic representations of phantoms learned from real intraoperative endoscopic sequences. Conditioned on frames from the surgical training process, the learned models are able to generate impressive results by transforming unrealistic parts of the image (e.g. the uniform phantom texture is replaced by the more heterogeneous texture of the tissue). Image-to-image synthesis usually learns a mapping $G : X \rightarrow Y$ such that the distribution of images from $G(X)$ is indistinguishable from the distribution Y. However, it does not necessarily force the generated images to be consistent and without artifacts. In the endoscopic image domain this can affect depth cues and stereo consistency of a stereo image pair, which ultimately impairs surgical vision. We propose a cross-domain conditional generative adversarial network approach (GAN) that aims to generate more consistent stereo pairs. The results show substantial improvements in depth perception and realism evaluated by 3 domain experts and 3 medical students on a 3D monitor over the baseline method. In 84 of 90 instances our proposed method was preferred or rated equal to the baseline. The work was presented at MICCAI 2019 [1].

References

1. Engelhardt S, Sharan L, Karck M, et al. Cross-Domain conditional generative adversarial networks for stereoscopic hyperrealism in surgical training. In: Proc MICCAI 2019;. p. 155–163.

© Springer Fachmedien Wiesbaden GmbH, ein Teil von Springer Nature 2020
T. Tolxdorff et al. (Hrsg.), *Bildverarbeitung für die Medizin 2020*,
Informatik aktuell, https://doi.org/10.1007/978-3-658-29267-6_75

Haptic Rendering of Soft-Tissue for Training Surgical Procedures at the Larynx

Thomas Eixelberger[1*], Jonas Parchent[1*], Rolf Janka[2], Marc Stamminger[4], Michael Döllinger[3], Thomas Wittenberg[1,4]

[1]Fraunhofer Institute for Integrated Circuits IIS, Erlangen
[2]Chair of Diagnostic Radiology, Department of Diagnostic Radiology, University Hospital Erlangen
[3]Division of Phoniatrics and Pediatric Audiology, Department of Otorhinolaryngology-Head and Neck Surgery, University Hospital Erlangen
[4]Chair for Computer Graphics, FAU Erlangen-Nürnberg
*These authors are joint first authors.
thomas.eixelberger@iis.fraunhofer.de

Abstract. Assistant physicians typically learn surgical techniques by observation and supervised practice on the patient or using bio-phantoms. Alternatively, surgical simulators with the possibility of new training possibilities can be used. A number of simulators is already commercially available and might in the future become as important for surgical training as flight simulators. Since so far no simulator is concerned with the training of tracheotomies, a soft-tissue model for simulating tracheotomy was developed. This soft-tissue model is integrated into our ENT surgical simulator for tracheotomy. To model the soft-tissues of the neck (skin and fat), a computed tomography (CT) scan was interactively segmented. For the interaction simulation of a scalpel with the soft-tissue, position based dynamics (PBD) was used, originally developed for the gaming industries. Initial results imply that the proposed approach is able to model soft tissues for virtual surgical training.

1 Introduction

Teaching and education in surgery is traditionally based on the concept of "see one, do one, teach one", meaning that assistant surgeons are expected to perform interventional procedures after various observations. Due to the demographic changes, the rising number of older patients along with the increasing trend to reduce expensive operation time results in less time to practice and putting patient safety at risk [1]. This circumstance can be changed by training on animal-phantoms or 3D-printed models. Nevertheless, due to rising ethical considerations and organisational limitations animal phantoms are hard to obtain, while the limit of 3D-printed models are their expense and they are used

© Springer Fachmedien Wiesbaden GmbH, ein Teil von Springer Nature 2020
T. Tolxdorff et al. (Hrsg.), *Bildverarbeitung für die Medizin 2020*,
Informatik aktuell, https://doi.org/10.1007/978-3-658-29267-6_76

only once. Thus, virtual surgery simulators are considered as alternatives for future surgical training.

In the past several virtual simulators for surgical training have been developed. Within haptic feedback they provide a high sense of realism, while minimizing expenses for animal phantoms or non-reusable material. They also provide objective feedback on the quality of the procedure and track the user's progress. A study by Iverson et al. [2] compared the success of cricothyroidotomy training on animal cadavers with the training on virtual simulators. They found no significant difference between the two groups and so simulators provide a feasible alternative to training on cadavers. Several simulators with haptic feedback are already commercially available for applications such as laparoscopy in gastroenterology or angioplasty [3]. So far no virtual simulator for tracheotomy training has been proposed.

Tracheotomy (cutting the anterior of the neck and opening the airway through an incision in the trachea) is typically performed as an open surgical procedure to ensure sufficient respiration and is applied to cases of acute swelling of the respiratory tract, to cure various facial and cervical injuries, to remove tumors of the upper respiratory tract or to operate bilateral vocal chord paresis [4]. Performing a tracheotomy is a challenging task due to possible complications such as lethal haemorrhage or loss of airway. So assistant surgeons should practice and train this procedure to avoid such complications.

Based on our previous work with respect to the immersive simulation of petrosal bone milling using haptic feedback and stereo visualization [5, 6], the goal of this work is to extend our haptic training system so it can deal with soft-tissue interventions such as tracheotomy. To its end *(a)* a soft-tissue-model of the neck (skin, epidermis and fat) was built based on interactively segmented computed tomography (CT) data, and *(b)* using so-called position based dynamics (PBD) for the interaction simulation of a scalpel with the soft-tissue model. These extensions will be described and evaluated with respect to the application example tracheotomy.

2   Materials and methods

2.1   Image data and segmentation

The anonymized CT datasets (obtained from Department of Diagnostic Radiology) of head and neck have a spatial dimension of $31.2 \times 31.2 \times 39.45$ cm and a voxel spacing of $0.609 \times 0.609 \times 0.75$ mm. For interactive segmentation of the CT data 3D Slicer was used. Specifically the skin, the underlying layer of fat, the trachea and the thyroid gland were segmented. To segment the thyroid level tracing is used. Fat and the tracheal cartilages are segmented manually. Segmenting the skin and the trachea is more complicated. For this, volume-growing based on seed points was performed, followed by morphological post-processing to clean-up the segmentation. Boney structures were not segmented, as the training system already provides iso-surface rendering of volumetric data in

the bone window. After smoothing the segmentation, the structures are visually more pleasing. Segmenting all structures separately allows setting different
material properties.

2.2   Scalpel model

A 3D scalpel model based on the shape of a no. 3 scalpel handle and a no.
10 scalpel blade by Swann-Morton Ltd. (Sheffield, UK) was used. The related
scalpel model was created using Blender. Blade and handle were modeled separately and were then united. To insure performance the model is kept simple
with 300 faces and 998 triangles. Fig. 1 shows the rendered neck and the scalpel.

2.3   Force-Feedback haptics

In order to provide realistic haptic force-feedback to the user, a Virtuose 6D
Desktop by Haption (Soulgé-sur-Ouette, France) was used. While manually
moving a replica of a real scalpel mounted at the end of the haptic arm, in the
virtual space (data space) the scalpel model (Sec. 2.2) is moved in the same
coordinate space as the head and neck image data. If in data space the tip
of the scalpel collides with the skin of the virtual patient, the deformation of
skin (and fat) and the incision of the scalpel into the skin are modeled using
position based dynamics, see next Section 2.4. Furthermore, the computed (and
changing) forces between the skin tissue and scalpel blade during the incision
are sent back to the haptic arm and are provided as force-feedback to the user.
Thus, the user obtains a realistic haptic feeling of the incision.

2.4   Position based dynamics

Position based dynamics (PBD) lacks a concrete physical basis, but the achieved
results are quite realistic and accurate enough for an application within a surgical
simulator. Previously, PBD has already been used to model cuts in a liver
model [7] and electrocautery cutting [8, 9]. PBD works directly with positions of
objects and thus allows better controllability. Furthermore, it is unconditionally

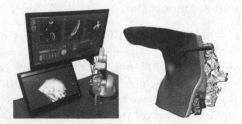

Fig. 1. Left side: setup of the surgical simulator including a haptic arm, an auto-
stereoscopic monitor and a touch screen. Right side: Screenshot of the segmented
neck-data depicting soft-tissues and bones as well as the scalpel. To allow easier visual
distinction, false colors are used for the trachea, tracheal cartilages and thyroid gland.

stable as it prevents overshooting problems, common in approaches using explicit integration. The advantage over classical methods such as finite element methods (FEM) is the gain in computational performance, and can hence be used in real-time applications. A comparison between PBD and FEM is e.g. provided by Bender et al. [10]. By using different constraints, PBD is also able to model liquids, gases and cloth, which makes it interesting for virtual surgery simulators. For implementation purposes, the Nvidia Flex library can be used.

2.5   Soft tissue simulation using Nvidia flex

Nvidia Flex is a C++ library by Nvidia (Santa Clara, CA, USA) providing a GPU accelerated implementation of PBD. With its unified solver it allows two-way interaction of rigid and soft bodies, fluids, gases, and cloths. Hence, this library fits the requirements of a virtual surgery simulator with a large number of particles. Following we will provide details about the soft tissue simulation.

After loading the pre-segmented volumes (Section 2.1) a soft tissue model is internally created. The spacing parameter P_{space} of the particles can manually be adjusted via the GUI during runtime. To achieve an accurate representation, P_{Space} is set to a value lower than 5 mm. Surface particles are created using random sampling and their number is controlled by the parameter $P_{surface} \in [0.5, ..., 10]$, whose value is internally scaled by the factor 50,000. The number of samples of the mesh's interior works in the same way and is controlled by the parameter $N_{samples} \in [0, ..., 10]$. If $N_{samples}$ is set to zero, the interior of the volume will not be sampled at all. The parameter $D \geq 1$ defines the distance between clusters of corresponding particles (shape matching clusters), and should be set to at least to 1. We use the range $D \in [1.5, ..., 6]$. In order to define the size of each particle cluster, the parameter $r_{cluster}$ is used, which is set relative to the particle spacing P_{space} and controls how much the clusters may overlap. Good values for the radius have been found to be $r_{cluster} \in [1.6, ..., 8mm]$. The stiffness S can only be set for all clusters in an object and is controlled by the parameter $S_{cluster} \in [0, ..., 1]$. It is possible to set up a cluster that consists of all particles of an object with a specified stiffness, which is created if $S_{global} > 0$. The framework also allows to set up spring-like distance constraints between particles using $r_{spring} \geq P_{space}$. Their stiffness is controlled globally using S_{spring}.

2.6   Haptic rendering of tool-tissue interaction

Through the library interface no information about a possible collision between the soft tissue and the scalpel is provided. As a continuous checking of such a collision would be computationally too expensive, and obtain an update rate of approximately 1 kHz, the scalpel object is reduced to an one-dimensional representation, as suggested by [8]. For the computation of the forces (between soft tissue and scalpel) an adapted finger-proxy algorithm [11] was applied: $F_{flex} = \frac{1}{n} \sum_{i=1}^{n} \frac{p_{i,proj} - p_i}{||p_{i,proj} - p_i||_2} ||p_i - p_{i,init}||_2$ where p_i describes the vector of the particle, $p_{i,proj}$ the projected point, $p_{i,init}$ the initial position and n the number of collisions. Hence the force is independent of the number of collisions. The simulation runs on a lower frequency than the update frequency demanded by the haptic arm necessary for realistic force feedback. Thus, the forces are extrapolated according to the approach by Picinbono & Lombardo [12]. As the forces computed by the Flex library are too large for the haptic arm, a linear scaling function is applied which clamps the force at a defined magnitude.

3   Results

For our experiments, three CT data sets of head and neck from different individuals were available. Fig. 1 depicts one state of the incision simulation where scalpel is placed in front of the skin. Using the above described Nvidia Flex library for position based dynamics (PBD), we were able to define a concept allowing a real-time interaction between a soft-tissue and a force-feedback model of a scalpel-blade including a 3D-visual feedback. Additionally, we were able to define, implement and test all necessary interfaces between the main components to enhance and extend the available surgical simulator for hard tissue towards the simulation of an incision into soft-tissue. Fig. 2 shows the implemented communication between all components for PBD (using Flex), the interface to the haptic arm (based on CHAI3D) and 3D-visualization (using OpenGL). The positions and deformations of the mesh objects are synchronised between CHAI3D and Flex. The position of the haptic arm's handle is read by CHAI3D to update the visualization and is passed on to Flex. In case of a collision between the virtual scalpel and the particles in Flex, the resulting feedback force is computed and sent to the haptic arm via CHAI3D. The visualization is handled by CHAI3D, which internally passes it on to OpenGL.

4   Discussion

A soft-tissue model for virtual surgery training with haptic feedback based on Nvidia Flex was developed and integrated into our surgical simulator. While we not find a feasible set of soft body parameters, all required components of the

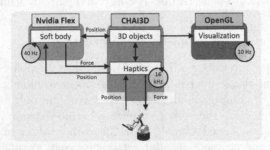

Fig. 2. Integration structure of the soft tissue model into the haptic trainer. The speed of each thread is depicted inside the circles.

simulation have been integrated including the communication of the simulation in Flex with the haptic library CHAI3D and the visualization, as well as the computation of the haptic feedback force. In many configurations of the parameters the particles move away upon collision with the scalpel even if the particles are connected to fixated points.

Position based dynamics and its implementation in Flex have several drawbacks. A soft body's stiffness depends on the number of solver iterations, which makes it difficult to set individual material properties for each tissue type. The method extended PBD [13] solves this problem but could not be integrated since Flex is closed-source.

Further work will test more parameter sets to achieve a stable simulation. Due to PBD's versatility, it will be possible to extend the simulator to model other components required in a complete surgery simulator, such as fluids and gases.

Acknowledgement. This work was supported by the German Federal Ministry of Education and Research under the grant number 16SV7559.

References

1. Kotsis S, Chung K. Application of see one, do one, teach one concept in surgical training. Plast Reconstr Surg. 2013;131(5):1194–1201.
2. Iverson K, Riojas R, Sharon D, et al. Objective comparison of animal training versus artificial simulation for initial cricothyroidotomy training. Am Surg. 2015;81(5):515–518.
3. Misra S, Ramesh K, Okamura A. Modeling of tool-tissue interactions for computer-based surgical simulation: a literature review. Presence. 2008;17(5):463–491.
4. Klemm E, Nowak AK. Tracheotomy-related deaths: a systematic review. Dt Ärzteblatt Int. 2017;114(16):273.
5. Franz D, Katzky U, Neuman S, et al. Haptisches Lernen für Cochlea Implantationen – Konzept. Proc's CURAC. 2016; p. 21–26.
6. Eixelberger T, Wittenberg T, Perret J, et al. A haptic model for virtual petrosal bone milling. Proc's CURAC. 2018; p. 214–219.
7. Pan J, Bai J, Zhao X, et al. Real-time haptic manipulation and cutting of hybrid soft tissue models by extended position-based dynamics. Comp Anim & Virt Worlds. 2015;26(3-4):321–335.
8. Berndt I, Torchelsen R, Maciel A. Efficient surgical cutting with position-based dynamics. IEEE Comput Graph Appl. 2017;37(3):24–31.
9. Lu Z, et al. Towards physics-based interactive simulation of electrocautery procedures using PhysX. IEEE Haptics Symposium. 2010; p. 515–518.
10. Bender J, Koschier D, Charrier P, et al. Position-based simulation of continuous materials. Comp & Graphics. 2014;44:1–10.
11. Zilles C, Salisbury J. A constraint-based god-object method for haptic display. Rep U S. 1995;3:146–151.
12. Picinbono G, Lombardo JC; Citeseer. Extrapolation: a solution for force feedback Int Sci Workshop on Virt Real & Prototyping. 1999; p. 117–125.
13. Macklin M, Müller M, Chentanez N. XPBD: position-based simulation of compli- constrained dynamics. Proc ICMG. 2016; p. 49–54.

Autorenverzeichnis

nger Fachmedien Wiesbaden GmbH, ein Teil von Springer Nature 2020
dorff et al. (Hrsg.), *Bildverarbeitung für die Medizin 2020*,
k aktuell, https://doi.org/10.1007/978-3-658-29267-6

Printed in the United States
By Bookmasters